CW00519612

"The Self-Care Guide to Holistic Medicine, *written by colleagues I've known for many years, is a treasure trove of practical information that can help readers address their symptoms effectively while healing on all levels: physical, emotional, and spiritual. I highly recommend this guide to tomorrow's medicine today!"*
—Christiane Northrup, M.D., author of *Women's Bodies, Women's Wisdom*

"Many books are being published today dealing with alternative and complimentary medicine. This book, however, deals with holistic medicine. It is comprehensive, easy to use, and accurately presents holistic health care. The Self-Care Guide to Holistic Medicine *effectively brings together the care and balance of body, mind, and spirit. Robert Ivker understands holistic medicine and uses it for himself, his family, and his patients. This book should be in every home."*
—Gladys Taylor McGarey, M.D., M.D. (H)
Scottsdale Holistic Medical Group, P.A.

"For almost a quarter-century, the principles of holism have been gaining momentum. Now more than ever, the one great benefit of managed care is to encourage patients to take responsibility for themselves, since managed care so often fails. The Self-Care Guide to Holistic Medicine *is a great adjunct for those ready to take this giant step forward in personal responsibility for their health."*
—C. Norman Shealy, M.D., Ph.D.
Founder, Shealy Institute for Comprehensive Health Care;
Founding President, American Holistic Medical Association; and
Chair, Energy Medicine Program, Greenwich University

"This useful book offers a clear and comprehensive overview of the basic principles of holistic medicine and applies them to a large number of acute and chronic ailments. This is important reading for anyone interested in natural healing."
—Leo Galland, M.D., FACP, FACN

"For those of you who choose to be responsible for your own health, healing, and well-being, this unique guidebook provides all the essential ingredients for taking charge of your life."
—Leonard Laskow, M.D., author of *Healing with Love*

"This is a strong, readable, eminently practical book. The authors have managed to bring the embracing spirit of holism to the details of daily treatment. I applaud them."
—James S. Gordon, M.D.
Director, Center for Mind-Body Medicine, Washington, D.C.,
and author of *Manifesto for a New Medicine*

"Robert Ivker has again made a substantial contribution with his Self-Care Guide to Holistic Medicine. *Beginning with the foundations of building and preserving health and following with the detailed integrative treatment of our most common ailments, he empowers us with critical information and confidence. His clear and friendly writing distills the complexity of health and healing into simple terms and definitive recommendations. His model of holistic health will undoubtedly transform the way we care for ourselves and the way doctors practice medicine."*
—Ralph Golan, M.D., author of *Optimal Wellness: Where Mainstream and Alternative Medicine Meet*

ALSO BY ROBERT S. IVKER, D.O.
Sinus Survival
Thriving

ALSO BY ROBERT A. ANDERSON, M.D.
Wellness Medicine
Stress Power!

ALSO BY LARRY TRIVIERI, JR.
Alternative Medicine: The Definitive Guide (editor)

The
Self-Care Guide to
Holistic Medicine

Creating Optimal Health

ROBERT S. IVKER, D.O.

ROBERT A. ANDERSON, M.D.

LARRY TRIVIERI, JR.

WITH STEVE MORRIS, N.D.,

AND TODD NELSON, N.D.

JEREMY P. TARCHER/PUTNAM
a member of
PENGUIN PUTNAM INC.
New York

Most Tarcher/Putnam books are available at special quantity discounts for bulk purchases for sales promotions, premiums, fund-raising, and educational needs. Special books or book excerpts also can be created to fit specific needs. For details, write Putnam Special Markets, 375 Hudson Street, New York, NY 10014.

Jeremy P. Tarcher/Putnam
a member of
Penguin Putnam Inc.
375 Hudson Street
New York, NY 10014
www.penguinputnam.com

First Trade Paperback Edition 2000

Library of Congress Cataloging-in-Publication Data

Ivker, Robert S., date.
    Self-care guide to holistic medicine : creating optimal health / Robert S. Ivker,
Robert A. Anderson, Larry Trivieri, Jr. ; with Steve Morris and Todd Nelson.
        p.   cm.
    Hardback ed. pub. 1999 under the title: The complete self-care guide to holistic
medicine (ISBN 0-87477-986-3)
    Includes bibliographical references.
    ISBN 1-58542-056-5 (paperback edition)
    1. Holistic medicine.   2. Self-care, Health.   I. Title: Self-care guide to holistic
medicine.   II. Anderson, Robert A. (Robert Arthur), date.   III. Trivieri, Larry, date.
    IV. Ivker, Robert S. Complete self-care guide to holistic medicine.   V. Title.
R733.I94   2000   00-056366
615.5—dc21

Printed in the United States of America
10   9   8   7   6   5   4   3   2   1

This book is printed on acid-free paper. ∞

Illustrations by Maud Kernan
Book design by Mauna Eichner

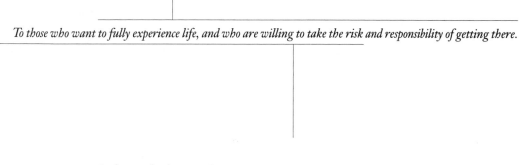

To those who want to fully experience life, and who are willing to take the risk and responsibility of getting there.

Acknowledgments

This book marks another stage in my evolution as a physician and healer. I've had the privilege of learning from a number of wonderful mentors and teachers, all of whom are gifted healers. They have taught me not only about the practice of medicine, but what optimal health looks and feels like, and what it means to "heal your life." They are: my father Morris, Carl Flaxer, Bob Anderson, Myron McClellan, Apisai Lailai, Sylvia Flesner, Gabriel Cousens, Jaison Kayn, Taulere Appel, Meredith Vaughn, Jeff Durland, Todd Nelson, Steve Morris, Mark Hofgard, Doug Shapiro, Alan Gaby, Bill Manahan, Evarts Loomis, Norm Shealy, Brugh Joy, Bernie Siegel, Chris Northrup, Andy Weil, and Deepak Chopra. My greatest teachers, however, have been the women in my life—my wife Harriet, my daughters Julie and Carin, and my mother Thelma. Thank you so much for the intensive course in unconditional love!

I would also like to thank my agent Gail Ross for helping to coordinate this project, to Joel Fotinos for asking me to write this book and for his vision as a publisher of transformational and paradigm-shifing books, to Mitch Horowitz for his incisive and masterful job of editing the manuscript, and to Steve Morris and especially Todd Nelson for their invaluable contributions to Part II. And finally, I am most grateful to my co-authors, with whom it has truly been a pleasure to work on this project. Thank you Bob and Larry for a job well done!

Rob Ivker

I express my gratitude to my fellow authors, to the thousands of patients who taught me much over the last four decades, and to my family for graciously ceding me the time to make my contributions to this book.

Bob Anderson

I wish to thank my parents, for their many gifts and blessings; and my brothers and sisters, and nieces and nephews, for the joy and community they provide. Grateful thanks, as well, to my friends, especially Paul Witte, Richard Stark, Karen Defuria, Bob Cohen, Ted Allen, Lynne Sable, Lucille Kall, Don Elefante, Jim Hagan, Marc Smith, Marc Wilson, Peter Wild, Marc Rohrer, Janet Roberts, Rich Stone, and Cary Sullivan, for their much-valued love and support. Thanks, too, to friend and healer Eyhraune Jau Saune, for first pointing out this path so many years ago. And special thanks to Rob and Bob, for their friendship, mentorship, and living embodiment of the principles of Holistic Medicine.

Larry Trivieri, Jr.

Contents

Introduction
How to Use This Book

THE BASIS OF medicine in the twenty-first century will be self-care. With that in mind, this book was written to show you how you can immediately begin applying the principles of *holistic medicine*, medicine's newest specialty. It is the only field of medicine that addresses the whole person—body, mind, and spirit—to create a greater experience of *optimal health* in all areas of your life. In the pages that follow you will learn how to practice the various therapies that comprise holistic medicine, both complementary and conventional, so that you can treat the most common acute and chronic illnesses at home, as part of your overall self-care regimen.

We recognize that many of our readers purchased this book in order to learn how to relieve a specific disease condition. If you fall into that category, you will most likely want to begin your healing journey by locating your condition in part II, "A Self-Care Guide for Treating Disease Conditions Holistically." There you will discover proven self-care approaches for treating over 60 conditions, ranging from alcoholism and addiction to sciatica and sinusitis. Each condition is addressed from the perspective of body, mind, and spirit, ensuring that you understand the multiple factors that may be contributing to your condition, as well as a variety of treatment options to either improve it, cure it, or prevent it from recurring. You will be able to use many of these treatment options on your own, without the need of a physician. Yet when professional assistance is required, you will also find which therapies, both conventional and complementary, are scientifically verified as being your most appropriate professional-care choices.

This book is far more than a self-care guide for treating disease, however. Throughout the book you will encounter a definition of health that goes far beyond the mere absence of discomfort or illness. The goal of holistic medicine is to lead each of us into a dynamic and daily experience of improved health at all levels—physically, environmentally, emotionally, mentally, spiritually, and socially—

while connecting us to life's most powerful medicine, unconditional love. To learn how to achieve this, you will need to read all the chapters in Part I, "A Holistic Blueprint for Optimal Health." Here you will begin the process of discovering your own unique path to loving and nurturing your body, mind, and spirit. The information outlined in Part I goes to the heart of what holistic medicine is all about—maintaining and enhancing optimal wellness in each of these areas, and understanding the difference between *healing* and *curing*, and *disease* and *dis-ease*. In chapter 1, you will find an overview of what holistic health means, and a questionnaire that you can use to gauge how well you are thriving in all three areas of your life—*body, mind, and spirit*. In chapter 2, you will learn how to establish a solid foundation for achieving physical and environmental well-being through the proper use of diet, nutritional supplements, herbs, physical exercise and activity, and environmental medicine. In chapter 3, you will discover powerful tools to heal your mind and emotions, while chapter 4 outlines proven principles to improve your spiritual health, including your social relationships. Finally, in chapter 5, you will be taught a series of action steps that you can take in each of these areas to immediately begin healing your body, mind and spirit.

The material in Part I serves as a comprehensive foundation on which the recommendations shared in Part II can most effectively be built. At times, however, you may need professional treatment for your health care needs. To help you choose which therapeutic approaches may be best suited for you, in the appendix you'll find descriptions of various types of practice, lists of resource organizations, an online database and medical library, and recommended books to enable you to become a much better informed holistic health care consumer.

The information provided in these pages has worked for countless people throughout the United States and around the world, giving them the opportunity to experience a quality of life they never knew was possible. Now the same information can work for you as well. All that is necessary is your commitment to your own health, and a willingness to apply in your daily life the principles that we share with you.

ROBERT S. IVKER, D.O.
ROBERT A. ANDERSON, M.D.
LARRY TRIVIERI, JR.

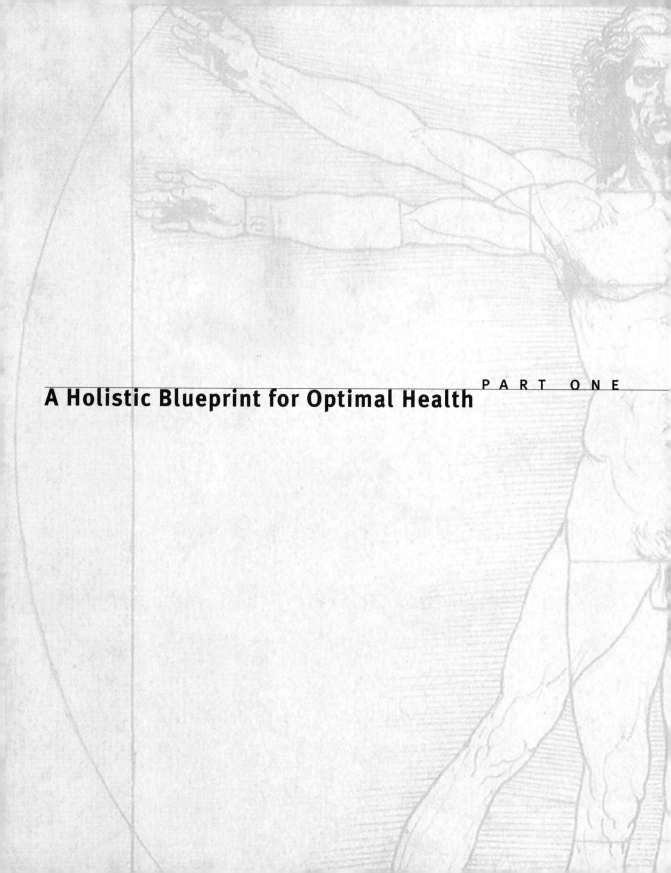

PART ONE

A Holistic Blueprint for Optimal Health

1

How Healthy Are You?
The Wellness Self-Test

The only thing I know that truly heals people is unconditional love.
ELISABETH KÜBLER-ROSS, M.D.

ARE YOU HEALTHY?

Your answer to this question is most likely based on whether you suffer from symptoms of disease or have a chronic ailment or nagging condition that never quite goes away. If you don't, then you may automatically assume you are healthy, since the conditioning that the majority of us have grown up with has taught us to define health as the absence of illness. Yet the words *health*, *heal*, and *holy* are all derived from the same Anglo-Saxon word *haelen*, which means to make whole. Viewed from this perspective, two questions that more directly and accurately address the issue of health are: "Do you love your life?" and "Are you happy to be alive?" For health is far more than simply a matter of not feeling ill. It is the daily experience of *wholeness and balance—a state of being fully alive in body, mind, and spirit*. Such a condition could also be called optimal, or *holistic*, health. Helping you to achieve this state of total well-being is the primary objective of this book.

THE HALLMARKS OF OPTIMAL HEALTH

Optimal health results from harmony and balance in the physical, environmental, mental, emotional, spiritual, and social aspects of our lives. When this harmonious balance is present, we experience the *unlimited and unimpeded free flow of life force energy throughout our body, mind, and spirit*. Around the world, this energy is known by many names. The Chinese call it *qi* ("chee"), the Japanese refer to it as *ki*, in India it is known as *prana*, and in Hebrew it is *chai*. But in the Western world, the phrase that comes closest to capturing the feeling generated by this energy is *unconditional love*, regarded by holistic physicians as *our most powerful medicine*.

Though each of us has the capacity to nurture and to heal ourselves, most of us have yet to tap into this infinite wellspring of loving life energy. Yet there is no one who can better administer this life-enhancing elixir to you than yourself.

By committing to caring for yourself in the manner recommended in the following pages, you will in essence be learning how to better *give and receive love*—to yourself and others. As a result, you will be enhancing the flow of life force energy throughout every aspect of your life. This holistic healing process will also provide you with the opportunity to safely and effectively treat any physical, mental, or spiritual conditions that may be restricting the flow of healing energy.

Living a holistically healthy lifestyle can facilitate the realization of your ideal life vision in accordance with both your personal and professional goals. But since the majority of us are only aware of health as a condition of not being sick, a mental image of what living holistically means is usually needed in order to achieve it. Briefly, let's examine this state of optimal well-being to give you a glimpse of what it looks and feels like.

A list of the six components of health follows; the first italicized item in each category encompasses the essence of that component. For example, physical health can be simply described as a condition of *high energy and vitality*, while mental health is a state of *peace of mind and contentment*. The italicized items can also serve as a health gauge you can use to measure your progress in each area.

Physical Health

High energy and vitality

Freedom from, or high adaptability to, pain, dysfunction, and disability

A strong immune system

A body that feels light, balanced, strong, flexible, and has good aerobic capacity

Ability to meet physical challenges

Full capacity of all five senses and a healthy libido

Environmental Health

Harmony with your environment (neither harming nor being harmed)

Awareness of your connectedness with nature

Feeling grounded

Respect and appreciation for your home, the Earth and all of her inhabitants

Contact with the earth; breathing healthy air; drinking pure water; eating uncontaminated food; exposure to the sun, fire, or candlelight; immersion in warm water (all on a daily basis).

Mental Health

Peace of mind and contentment

A job that you love doing

Optimism

A sense of humor

Financial well-being

Living your life vision.

Emotional Health

Self-acceptance and high self-esteem

Capacity to identify, express, experience, and accept all of your feelings, both painful and joyful

Awareness of the intimate connection between your physical and emotional bodies

Confronting your greatest fears

Fulfilling your capacity to play

Peak experiences on a regular basis

Spiritual Health

Experience of unconditional love/absence of fear

Soul awareness and a personal relationship with God or Spirit

Trust in your intuition and willingness to change

Gratitude

Creating a sacred space on a regular basis through prayer, meditation, walking in nature, observing a Sabbath day, or other rituals

Sense of purpose

Being present in every moment

Social Health

Intimacy with a spouse or partner, relative, or close friend

Forgiveness

Sense of belonging to a support group or community

Touch and/or physical intimacy on a daily basis

Selflessness and altruism

THE WELLNESS SELF-TEST

Now that you understand the six categories that comprise optimal health, it's time to measure how close you are to *thriving* in each area. The following questionnaire is designed to provide you with a much clearer idea of the status of your health in all six areas. You can use the results of the test to guide you through this book, and it can become a blueprint for restructuring your life. You can also measure your progress by taking the test again every two or three months.

Answer the questions in each section and total your score. Each response will be a number from zero to five. Please refer to the frequency described within the parentheses (e.g., "2 to 3x/week") when answering questions about an *activity*, for example, "Do you maintain a healthy diet?" However, when the question refers to an *attitude* or an *emotion* (most of the mind and spirit questions), for example, "Do you have a sense of humor?" the response is more subjective, less exact, and refers to the terms describing frequency, such as "often" or "daily," but not to the numbered frequences in parentheses.

0 = Never or almost never (once a year or less)

1 = Seldom (2 to 12x/year)

2 = Occasionally (2 to 4x/month)

3 = Often (2 to 3x/week)

4 = Regularly (4 to 6x/week)

5 = Daily

BODY: Physical and Environmental Health

_____ 1. Do you maintain a healthy diet (low fat, low sugar, fresh fruits, grains and vegetables)?

_____ 2. Is your water intake adequate (at least one-half ounce per pound of body weight; 160 pounds = 80 ounces)?

_____ 3. Are you within 20 percent of your ideal body weight?

_____ 4. Do you feel physically attractive?

_____ 5. Do you fall asleep easily and sleep soundly?

_____ 6. Do you awaken in the morning feeling well rested?

_____ 7. Do you have more than enough energy to meet your daily responsibilities?

_____ 8. Are your five senses acute?

_____ 9. Do you take time to experience sensual pleasure?

___ 10. Do you schedule regular massage or deep-tissue body work?

___ 11. Does your sexual relationship feel gratifying?

___ 12. Do you engage in regular physical workouts (lasting at least 20 minutes)?

___ 13. Do you have good endurance or aerobic capacity?

___ 14. Do you breathe abdominally for at least a few minutes?

___ 15. Do you maintain physically challenging goals?

___ 16. Are you physically strong?

___ 17. Do you do some stretching exercises?

___ 18. Are you free of chronic aches, pains, ailments, and diseases?

___ 19. Do you have regular effortless bowel movements?

___ 20. Do you understand the causes of your chronic physical problems?

___ 21. Are you free of any drug (including caffeine and nicotine) or alcohol dependency?

___ 22. Do you live and work in a healthy environment with respect to clean air, water, and indoor pollution?

___ 23. Do you feel energized or empowered by nature?

___ 24. Do you feel a strong connection with and appreciation for your body, your home, and your environment?

___ 25. Do you have an awareness of life force energy or *qi?*

Total BODY Score: ___

MIND: Mental and Emotional Health

___ 1. Do you have specific goals in your personal and professional life?

___ 2. Do you have the ability to concentrate for extended periods of time?

___ 3. Do you use visualization or mental imagery to help you attain your goals or enhance your performance?

___ 4. Do you believe it is possible to change?

___ 5. Can you meet your financial needs and desires?

___ 6. Is your outlook basically optimistic?

___ 7. Do you give yourself more supportive messages than critical messages?

___ 8. Does your job utilize all of your greatest talents?

___ 9. Is your job enjoyable and fulfilling?

___ 10. Are you willing to take risks or make mistakes in order to succeed?

___ 11. Are you able to adjust beliefs and attitudes as a result of learning from painful experiences?

____ 12. Do you have a sense of humor?

____ 13. Do you maintain peace of mind and tranquillity?

____ 14. Are you free from a strong need for control or the need to be right?

____ 15. Are you able to fully experience (feel) your painful feelings such as fear, anger, sadness, and hopelessness?

____ 16. Are you aware of and able to safely express fear?

____ 17. Are you aware of and able to safely express anger?

____ 18. Are you aware of and able to safely express sadness or cry?

____ 19. Are you accepting of all your feelings?

____ 20. Do you engage in meditation, contemplation, or psychotherapy to better understand your feelings?

____ 21. Is your sleep free from disturbing dreams?

____ 22. Do you explore the symbolism and emotional content of your dreams?

____ 23. Do you take the time to let down and relax, or make time for activities that constitute the abandon or absorption of play?

____ 24. Do you experience feelings of exhilaration?

____ 25. Do you enjoy high self-esteem?

Total MIND Score: ____

SPIRIT: Spiritual and Social Health

____ 1. Do you actively commit time to your spiritual life?

____ 2. Do you take time for prayer, meditation, or reflection?

____ 3. Do you listen to and act on your intuition?

____ 4. Are creative activities a part of your work or leisure time?

____ 5. Do you take risks or exceed previous limits?

____ 6. Do you have faith in a God, spirit guides, or angels?

____ 7. Are you free from anger toward God?

____ 8. Are you grateful for the blessings in your life?

____ 9. Do you take walks, garden, or have contact with nature?

____ 10. Are you able to let go of your attachment to specific outcomes and embrace uncertainty?

____ 11. Do you observe a day of rest completely away from work, dedicated to nurturing yourself and your family?

____ 12. Can you let go of self-interest in deciding the best course of action for a given situation?

___ 13. Do you feel a sense of purpose?

___ 14. Do you make time to connect with young children, either your own or someone else's?

___ 15. Are playfulness and humor important to you in your daily life?

___ 16. Do you have the ability to forgive yourself and others?

___ 17. Have you demonstrated the willingness to commit to a marriage or comparable long-term relationship?

___ 18. Do you experience intimacy, besides sex, in your committed relationships?

___ 19. Do you confide in or speak openly with one or more close friends?

___ 20. Do you or did you feel close to your parents?

___ 21. If you have experienced the loss of a loved one, have you fully grieved that loss?

___ 22. Has your experience of pain enabled you to grow spiritually?

___ 23. Do you go out of your way or give your time to help others?

___ 24. Do you feel a sense of belonging to a group or community?

___ 25. Do you experience unconditional love?

Total SPIRIT Score: ___

Total BODY, MIND, SPIRIT Score: ___

Health Scale:

325–375	Optimal Health: THRIVING
275–324	Excellent Health
225–274	Good Health
175–224	Fair Health
125–174	Below Average Health
75–124	Poor Health
Less than 75	Extremely Unhealthy: SURVIVING

Once you have completed this questionnaire, pay attention to which categories you need to make the most improvements in, and start to implement the tools and suggestions that are outlined in chapters 2, 3, and 4. Chapter 2 gives you a blueprint for improving your physical and environmental health; chapter 3 outlines similar approaches for mental and emotional health; chapter 4 will help you enhance your spiritual and social health. Begin where you are most comfortable and take your time. You are committing to a life-changing process, one that requires patience and dedication, so proceed at your own pace. Remember, too, that everyone is unique and no two of us will follow the exact same healing path. While the science of holistic medicine provides a universal foundation and structure, its *art* lies in the writing of your own personal prescription for optimal health, so feel free to adapt the techniques in the pages ahead to tailor-make the holistic self-care program that is most ideally suited for you. Your heart will be your primary guide on this odyssey of realizing your full potential as a human being.

2

Healing the Body

Health is the proper relationship between the microcosm, which is man, and the macrocosm, which is the universe.
YESHE DONDEN,
Physician to the Dalai Lama

COMPONENTS OF OPTIMAL PHYSICAL HEALTH

high energy and vitality

Freedom from, or high adaptability to, pain, dysfunction, and disability

A strong immune system

A body that feels light, balanced, strong, flexible, and has good aerobic capacity

Ability to meet physical challenges

Full capacity of all five senses and a healthy libido

IN CHAPTER 1 you learned that optimal health depends on achieving a state of wholeness in body, mind, and spirit. This requires you to address the underlying dis-eases or imbalances that may be present in each of these aspects of your life. Realistically, however, it is usually difficult for most of us to improve our mental and spiritual health before we first *focus on the physical*. If you are in constant physical pain, have no energy, or are suffering from a nagging or chronic health problem, your thoughts and attitudes can easily become negative, resulting in painful emotions, such as fear or hopelessness, that can leave you feeling isolated from loved ones and God.

Unfortunately, in our society there is a tendency to wait until our physical condition becomes practically unbearable before we seek help to correct it. Far too many of us settle for merely surviving in our bodies, instead of *thriving* in them. This unhealthy behavior (it takes much longer to cure a disease than to prevent it), combined with our increasingly stress-filled, sedentary lifestyles, goes a long way toward explaining why the United States, the world's wealthiest nation, is entering the twenty-first century with its population beset with record levels of chronic illness. Despite decades of research and untold billions of dollars spent on drug-based treatments and conventional surgical procedures, the incidence of both cancer and cardiovascular disease remain our country's top medical concerns; obesity levels have reached all-time highs; diabetes and arthritis are commonplace; and over one hundred million American adults now suffer from a chronic health ailment.

While these facts are cause for serious concern, the picture they paint isn't hopeless. As practitioners of holistic medicine well know, there are many methods available to all of us that can successfully reverse these trends. This chapter examines key areas in which you can immediately begin achieving and maintaining op-timal physical health—*high energy and vitality*—and environmental health, *har-mony with your surroundings*. These holistic approaches not only will enable you to improve your physical health, they will also help you develop a deeper awareness of your body. Over time, you'll learn to "listen" to the messages your body com-municates to you on a daily basis, as it instructs you on the best ways to nurture it, and in this way you will become more energetic and more resistant to illness. You will also find yourself moving away from physical limitations you once regarded as normal and toward a fuller experience of increased physical activity and perfor-mance. In short, you'll be experiencing greater love for your body, and greater joy in being alive.

SELF-CARE KEYS FOR IMPROVED PHYSICAL WELL-BEING

One of the ironies surrounding America's proliferation of chronic illness is how often we neglect various lifestyle factors that can go a long way toward reversing disease and enhancing our physical well-being. These safe and simple measures are available to us all, are inexpensive and easy to implement, and for the most part can be undertaken without professional supervision. Yet all too often they re-main ignored. In order to experience optimal health, you must make a commit-ment to include them in your daily routine.

These measures, which fall into three categories—nutritional medicine, exer-cise and physical activity, and environmental medicine—are essential components in the practice of holistic medicine.

Nutritional medicine includes your diet, the water you drink, nutritional sup-plements, fasting and detoxification, and hidden food allergies that may be drain-ing your energy. Exercise and physical activity encompass proper breathing, aerobic exercise, strength conditioning, stretching and limbering, yoga, and t'ai chi; and environmental medicine deals with ways of ensuring that both your home and work environments avoid toxic and allergenic challenges.

As you become more familiar with these categories and begin to master the recommendations and activities suggested for each of them, you will gain power-ful self-help tools that will enable you and your family to dramatically improve and maintain physical health.

NUTRITIONAL MEDICINE

Proper assessment of an individual's complete nutritional requirements is best performed by a holistic physician. A variety of tests, such as blood testing, urinal-ysis, and liver function testing, are available from many holistic practitioners, and

No illness which can be treated by diet should be treated by any other means.

MAIMONIDES
(1135–1204)

can help you tailor-make an overall nutritional program that is best suited to your unique biochemical individuality. These practitioners can also help determine if you are suffering from food sensitivities or allergies and can provide professional guidance in any detoxification measures that might be advisable. But even without a physician's supervision, there is much that you can undertake right now in the area of nutritional medicine that can set you on the road to lifelong wellness. Nowhere is this more true than in the areas of the foods we eat, the air we breathe, and the water we drink.

SUPPLEMENTATION AND BIOCHEMICAL INDIVIDUALITY

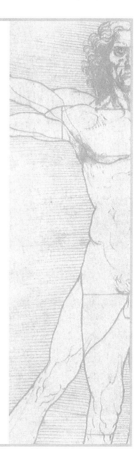

While the recommendations given for diet and nutritional supplementation in this chapter will create positive results for most people, certain individuals may require professional guidance from a holistic practitioner in creating their dietary and supplement programs before they notice dramatic improvements in their health. The reason for this has to do with each person's *biochemical individuality,* a term introduced by the late Roger Williams, Ph.D., in the 1930s. Through his research and clinical observations, Dr. Williams found that the amount of nutrients required for health can vary by as much as 700 percent from person to person. This variance is primarily due to the fact that each person's genetic makeup is unique. In addition, whether or not we need to use nutritional supplements, and in what dosages, is determined by the quality of the foods we eat, as well as our age, the environment we live in, and any stressors—physical, emotional, or chemical—we may be facing. Food allergies and our ability to properly digest and assimilate the nutrients we consume are also important factors to be considered.

Recognizing each person's unique biochemical individuality is one of the hallmarks of holistic medicine. If you follow the nutritional recommendations in this chapter and do not begin to notice an increase in your overall well-being within a few weeks, consulting with a holistic physician is likely to be beneficial. He or she can provide a variety of advanced diagnostic tests to determine your nutritional profile and eliminate any nutritional imbalances you may have, while tailor-making a dietary and supplement plan that is most appropriate for your specific needs.

Diet

There is no one universal diet that ideally suits every individual. Certain lab tests (including blood type), a comprehensive nutritional history, and personal experimentation (trial and error), along with the guidance of a holistic physician, can assist you in determining the diet best suited to your unique requirements. The following guidelines, however, are self-care approaches to diet from which most people will be able to derive benefit.

The importance of a healthy diet in relation to health has been emphasized for centuries in both the East and West. While proper diet alone may not be enough to entirely reverse certain types of disease, most chronic medical conditions can be significantly improved by a diet of nutrient-rich foods and adequate intake of purified water. Unfortunately, our society, with its overreliance on fast foods and snacks, affords great temptation to stray from healthy eating habits. And even when we do resolve to change our diet for the better, many of us wind up confused about what foods to actually eat and how they should be prepared, due in great part to the steady introduction of bestselling books touting the "latest and greatest" cure-all diet. While such books may be well intentioned, not all of them contain scientifically supported recommendations, and those that do often contradict equally well-researched information that made the bestseller list the year before. As a result, a number of polls now indicate that growing numbers of Americans are literally "fed up" with the amount of dietary and nutritional information that is becoming increasingly prevalent in our society.

A good dose of "common sense" can go a long way toward alleviating this confusion. There is a great deal of truth to the old adage "You are what you eat." The foods you consume become the fuel your body uses to carry out its countless functions. Therefore, it makes good sense to eat those foods that are the best "fuel sources." This means foods that are rich in vitamins, minerals, enzymes, essential fatty and amino acids, and other necessary nutrients and are free of preservatives, pesticides, and other substances that deplete the body's energy and can damage your vital organs.

In January 1992, the U.S. Department of Agriculture (USDA) unveiled its recommended dietary pyramid as a guideline for meeting these nutritional needs. At the base of this pyramid are whole grains, such as brown rice, bulgur, wheat (breads and pasta), oats, barley, millet, and cereals, with a recommended six to eleven servings from this food group per day. The next section of the pyramid is divided into the categories of fruits and vegetables, with a recommended two to four servings of the former and three to five servings of the latter. Moving upward, we find a recommended two to three servings each of dairy products (milk, yogurt, and cheese) and the meats, poultry, fish, eggs, dry beans, and nut group; with fats, oils and sweets at the top and used sparingly.

While the USDA food pyramid is a good place to start, a number of recent studies now indicate that our daily need for carbohydrates from whole grains may not be as vital as our need for fresh fruits and vegetables. A good deal of this research has been popularized by Barry Sears, Ph.D., in his books about the "Zone diet." The harmful effects of excessive intake of carbohydrates that he and other researchers have found include the following:

- Overstimulation of insulin production, which can lead to excess storage of fat in the body, hypoglycemia, and diabetes
- Diminished physical and mental capacity
- Fluctuating energy levels and mood swings
- Predisposition to other chronic diseases, including arthritis, heart disease and skin disorders

As a result, practitioners of holistic medicine now emphasize the fruits and vegetable groups, recommending more servings of these two food groups than of whole grains, breads, pasta, and cereal. In addition, it is recommended that milk—other than 1 percent or skim—be eliminated, and that your daily intake of butter, margarine, and cheese be reduced.

You should also reduce your intake of red meat, and when you do eat it, choose only the leanest cuts. In its place, have two to three servings per day of either poultry, fish, beans, or nuts. Also avoid all cooking fats and oils derived from animal products and those from vegetable sources that are hydrogenated and found in most margarines, many brands of peanut butter, and hydrogenated cooking fats. Instead, use vegetable oils, such as olive, safflower, and canola. Flaxseed oil, a particularly rich source of vital omega-3 essential fatty acids, can also be used. The best fats are from whole vegetables, grains, nuts, and seeds that are unprocessed, polyunsaturated, and nonoxidized.

Also pay attention to the various food additives that are commonly found in the typical American diet. These include all chemical preservatives, such as BHA, BHT, sodium nitrate, and sulfites; artificial coloring agents; and artificial sweeteners, such as saccharin, aspartame (NutraSweet), and cyclamates. These additives pose potentially enormous health risks. To avoid their use, stay away from processed or canned foods and get in the habit of reading labels whenever you go shopping.

Finally, if you aren't already in the habit of doing so, consider selecting fruits and vegetables that are grown organically, and meats and poultry derived from free-range animals. In the former case, you will be eating foods that are richer in nutrients and free of pesticides, artificial fertilizers, preservatives, and other additives. Free-range meats and poultry are the end products of animals that are not subject to the injections of growth hormones, antibiotics, and irradiation commonly found in commercially raised meats and poultry.

A list follows of a variety of nutritious foods that can be added to your diet for their rich nutrient value.

Fruits and Vegetables. Fresh fruits and vegetables should be a staple of your daily diet. Not only are they rich in nutrients, they also possess vital cleansing properties and high fiber content, which helps rid the body of waste and toxins, creating greater levels of energy. Be sure to eat at least part of your daily servings of fruits and vegetables raw, since in this form you will be receiving the highest nutrient content. Lightly steaming vegetables is another healthy way to prepare them. Boiling or overcooking vegetables, on the other hand, can destroy their abundant vitamins, minerals, and enzymes.

Among the fruits and vegetables with the greatest nutritional value (especially vitamin C and carotenes) are: oranges, cantaloupe, strawberries, apples, guavas, red chili peppers, red and green sweet peppers, kale, parsley, greens (mustard, collard, and turnip), broccoli, cauliflower, brussels sprouts, carrots, yams, spinach, mangoes, winter squash, romaine lettuce, asparagus, tomatoes, onions, garlic, mushrooms, peaches, papayas, bananas, cherries, grapefruit, watermelon, grapes, plums, blueberries, and sprouts. *NOTE: Although they are extremely rich sources of vitamins, minerals, and fiber, fruits impede the digestion of other foods and are therefore best not eaten at meal times.*

Whole Grains and Complex Carboydrates. Whenever possible, whole grains, beans, and legumes should be your primary source of carbohydrates, as they, too, provide many essential vitamins and minerals. Most grains also contain about 10 percent of excellent quality protein. Recommended whole grains include: amaranth, bulgur, millet, brown rice, basmati rice, quinoa, barley, oats, wheat, and couscous.

Other sources of complex carbodyrates are starchy vegetables and legumes. Complex carbohydrates provide sustained boosts of energy and are digested slowly, releasing their sugars into the bloodstream gradually. This gradual release of sugars helps to maintain insulin balance and contributes to the production of *adenosine triphosphate* (ATP) in the cells, thereby strengthening the immune system. Good sources of starchy vegetables include: potatoes, sweet potatoes, yams, acorn and butternut squash, and pumpkins. For legumes, choose black beans, garbanzo beans (chick peas), lima beans, aduki beans, navy beans, kidney beans, lentils, black-eyed peas, or split peas.

Proteins. Proteins are the nutrients your body uses to build cells, repair tissue, and produce the basic building blocks of DNA and RNA. Bones, hair, nails, muscle fibers, collagen, and other connective tissues are all composed of protein, and protein itself is second only to water in terms of the body's overall composition.

The main sources of protein for a healthy diet are: fish, chicken, and turkey (choose cuts that are free-range and free of hormones and antibiotics), soy products (soy milk, tofu, miso, and tempeh), sunflower seeds, almonds, cashews, peanuts, pine nuts, pecans, walnuts, and sesame seeds. Red meats and dairy products are not on this list due to their higher concentration of unhealthy fats, which can contribute to a host of disease conditions, especially heart disease and hardening of the arteries.

Fats and Oils. Contrary to popular belief, all of us need a certain amount of fat in our diet. Fats supply energy reserves that the body draws on when not enough fat is present in the foods we eat. Fats also serve as a primary form of insulation and help to maintain normal body temperature. In addition, fats help to transport oxygen; absorb fat soluble vitamins (A, D, E, and K); nourish the skin, mucous membranes, and nerves; and serve as an anti-inflammatory. Healthy fat is utilized by the body in the form of essential fatty acids (EFAs).

Excessive fat intake, however, can contribute to a variety of illnesses, especially obesity and heart disease. Fat intake that is too low can also pose health risks. One of the keys to optimal health, then, is to make sure that you are getting an adequate supply of fats in your diet and that they are "good" fats, not fats that are harmful. These good fats, in the form of oils, are those that remain liquid at room temperature.

The best food sources of healthy fats are the whole foods from which the oils are derived. These include foods such as nuts and seeds, soybeans, olives, avocados, and wheat germ. Healthy fats in the form of oils include: olive, canola, safflower, flaxseed (do not use for cooking), wheat germ, sesame, and sunflower oils. Essential fatty acids are found in two groups, the omega-3s and the omega-6s. Good sources of omega-3 EFAs include cold water fish (salmon, sardines, tuna), wild game, flaxseeds and flaxseed oil, canola oil, walnuts, pumpkin seeds, soybeans, fresh sea vegetables, and leafy greens. Good sources of omega-6 EFAs include vegetable oils, legumes, all nuts and seeds, and most grains, breast milk, organ meats, lean meats, leafy greens, borage oil, evening primrose oil, and gooseberry and black currant oils.

Fiber. Fiber is one of the most overlooked components of a healthy diet; the average American diet supplies only one-fourth to one-third of the amount necessary for optimum health. High fiber diets are associated with less coronary heart disease, lower cholesterol and triglyceride levels, lower blood pressure, lower incidence of cancer (especially colon and rectum), better control of diabetes, and lower incidences of diverticulitis, appendicitis, gall bladder disease, ulcerative colitis, and hernias. Lack of fiber is also the major cause of constipation and hemorrhoids.

Fiber includes the nondigestible substances in the foods that we eat. Good sources of fiber include fruits; the bran portion of whole grains, such as whole wheat, rolled oats, and brown rice; and raw and cooked green, yellow, and starchy vegetables, such as spinach, romaine lettuce, squash, carrots, beans, and lentils.

"The Sickening Six." There are six substances in the American diet that should be substantially eliminated—sugar, unhealthy fats, caffeine, salt, refined carbo-hydrates, and alcohol. These "sickening six" can lead to a variety of disease con-ditions. While it is all right to enjoy these substances in moderation, keeping their intake to a minimum can pay big dividends. Here are a number of rea-sons why:

Sugar

The use of sugar in your diet can pose many harmful health risks, yet the average American consumes 150 pounds each year. This is the equivalent of over 40 tea-spoons of sugar every day. The following are only a few of sugar's health-depleting effects:

- Sugar has been shown to be a risk factor for heart disease, *and may be more harm-ful than fat.*

- Sugar weakens the immune system, increasing susceptibility to infection and al-lergy and further exacerbating all other diseases caused by diminished immune function.

- Sugar stimulates excessive insulin production, thereby causing more fat to be stored in the body; lowers levels of HDL cholesterol (the healthy cholesterol); in-creases the production of harmful triglycerides; and increases the risk of arte-riosclerosis (hardening of the arteries).

- Sugar contributes to diminished mental capacity and can cause feelings of anxiety, depression, and rage. It has also been implicated in certain cases of attention deficit disorder (ADD).

- High sugar intake is associated with certain cancers, including cancer of the gall bladder and colon. Recently, sugar has also been implicated as a causative factor in cases of breast cancer.

- Excessive sugar in the diet is a primary contributor to candidiasis (intestinal yeast overgrowth), which can lead to a host of health problems, including gastrointesti-nal disorders, asthma, bronchitis, sinusitis, allergies, and chronic fatigue.

If you still feel a need to satisfy your sweet tooth, substitute modest amounts of pure honey or maple syrup to decrease the risk of these adverse effects.

Unhealthy Fats

The regular intake of good fats is essential to our health. Unfortunately, most of us are getting too much unhealthy fat in our diets. Primary sources of these harmful fats include red meats, milk and other dairy products, and the hydrogenated trans fats found in margarine, cooking fats, and many brands of peanut butter. These fats are also found in many packaged foods, including most commercial cereals, which also tend to be loaded with sugar.

Unhealthy fats lead to arteriosclerosis and the build-up of plaque on the inner lining of the arteries, where over time they obstruct the flow of blood and the transport of oxygen and nutrients to the body's internal organs. This obstruction, in turn, can lead to heart attacks, angina, stroke, kidney failure, and pregangrene in the legs.

The excessive intake of unhealthy fats is also associated with certain cancers, including cancer of the breast, colon, rectum, prostate, ovaries, and uterus. This is particularly true of the saturated fats derived from meat products.

Obesity, which is increasing to epidemic proportions in this country, is also directly related to excessive fat (and sugar) intake. Obesity is a serious disease condition by itself, but if prolonged, it can contribute to many other forms of illness, including adult-onset diabetes.

Becoming aware of your fat intake and minimizing the amount of harmful fats you consume is an important step toward optimal health.

Caffeine

Caffeine is a drug to which more than half of all Americans are addicted. On average, we drink at least two and a half cups of coffee a day, or 425 mg of caffeine. Because caffeine acts as a stimulant, we consume it in order to have more energy. But the quick fix it provides usually only lasts for a few hours, leaving us with greater fatigue and irritability once its effects wear off. Typically, when this happens, we reach for another cup of coffee to keep us going. The result is a roller coaster of ups and downs that, over time, can result in a number of health hazards.

While caffeine in moderation (200 mg or less per day) is relatively safe, the regular consumption of greater amounts can result in elevated blood pressure; increased risk of cancer, heart disease, and osteoporosis; poor sleep patterns; anxiety and irritability; dizziness; impaired circulation; urinary frequency; and gastrointestinal disorders. Caffeine also causes loss of calcium from muscle cells and can interfere with the blood clotting process by decreasing platelet stickiness.

Taken in moderation, however, caffeine has been shown to enhance mental functioning, improve both alertness and mood, and reduce risk for gallstones; it appears that 200 mg or less of caffeine per day may be safely tolerated by most individuals.

If you consider yourself addicted to caffeine, the best way to break your habit is to reduce your intake *very gradually*, over a period of a few weeks or even months. Start by substituting noncaffeinated drinks such as herbal tea or a roasted grain beverage for one of your normal cups of coffee each day. Over time, cut back further while increasing the number of substitute beverages, and beware of possible withdrawal symptoms such as headache, nervousness, and irritability. Typically, these will pass within a day or two. Also avoid other caffeine sources, such as soft drinks (particularly colas), cocoa, chocolate, and nonherbal teas.

Salt

Salt is another ingredient that is far too prevalent in many diets, and it poses particular dangers for certain people who suffer from high blood pressure. Many of us have been conditioned since childhood to crave salt, but its overuse draws water into the bloodstream. This, in turn, increases blood volume, causing higher blood pressure levels. Too much salt also upsets the body's sodium-potassium balance, thereby interfering with the lymphatic system's ability to draw wastes away from the cells.

Although some salt can be used in cooking, a good rule of thumb is to avoid adding salt to your food once it is served.

Refined Carbohydrates

Refined, or simple, carbohydrates, such as those found in white breads and in pastas made from white flour, are another group of health-threatening agents. When eaten in excess, these types of foods overstimulate insulin production and produce the same excessive fat storage in the body that results from eating too much sugar. This can lead to the onset of diabetes and obesity. The rise in obesity among American children is due in part to a diet heavy in sugars and refined carbohydrates and lacking in nutritious alternatives, notably fruits and vegetables.

Several recent studies have shown that certain carbohydrates previously promoted as being "whole" sources of starch are very rapidly digested and absorbed. As a result, they elevate blood sugar fully as much as sugar itself, contributing to all the problems cited earlier for sugar. Most carbohydrates have been carefully analyzed and assigned a *glycemic index* rating. A high glycemic index indicates that a food acts much as sugar does in the body; food sources with a low glycemic index are assimilated much more slowly and therefore offer much better nutritional value. High glycemic index foods include corn flakes, puffed rice, instant and mashed potatoes, white bread, maltose, and, of course, sugar itself. Foods with a low glycemic index include whole grain cereals (oats, brown rice, amaranth, ka-mut, millet), legumes (beans, peas, peanuts, soybeans), pumpernickel breads, whole wheat pastas, pearled barley, bulgur wheat, sweet potatoes, apples, oranges, yogurt, and fructose.

Alcohol

Alcohol is another example of a substance that when taken in moderation may en-hance health but when consumed in excess can cause a variety of serious problems. A growing body of research now indicates that one or two beers or a glass of wine per day can be beneficial to health as a way to relieve stress and to improve diges-tion. In fact, studies have shown that complete abstainers from alcohol have a slightly shorter life expectancy than those who drink in moderate amounts. Un-fortunately, for many men especially, alcohol and moderation usually "don't mix."

Although most people drink in order to feel better, evidence indicates that al-cohol can significantly contribute to feelings of depression, loneliness, restless-ness, and boredom, according to studies conducted by the National Center for Health Statistics. In addition, very moody people are also three times more likely to be heavy drinkers (three or more drinks per day).

Aside from the social stigma surrounding excessive alcohol consumption, too much alcohol can contribute to obesity; increased blood pressure; diabetes; colon, stomach, breast, mouth, esophagus, laryngeal, and pancreatic cancers; gastroin-testinal disorders; impaired liver function; candidiasis; impaired mental function-ing; and behavioral and emotional dysfunctions. If you are having difficulty in bringing your alcohol consumption under control, seek the help of a professional counselor and follow the protocols outlined in chapter 7.

Water. Next to oxygen, water is our most essential nutrient, and drinking enough water to satisfy your body's needs may be the simplest, least expensive self-help measure you can adopt to maintain your good health.

Our adult bodies are 60 to 70 percent water (an infant's body is about 80 per-cent), and water is the medium through which every bodily function occurs. It is the basis of all body fluids, including blood, digestive juices, urine, lymph, and perspiration, which explains why we would die within a few days without water.

Water is vital to metabolism and digestion and helps prevent both constipa-tion and diarrhea. It is also critical to healthy nerve impulse conduction and brain function. Some of water's other vital functions in the body are:

- Enhancing oxygen uptake into the bloodstream (The surface of the lungs must be moistened with water to facilitate oxygen intake and the excretion of carbon diox-ide.)

- Maintaining a high urine volume, helping to prevent kidney stones and urinary tract infections
- Regulating body temperature through perspiration
- Maintaining and increasing the health of the skin
- Maintaining adequate fluid for the lubrication of the joints and enhancing muscular function, particularly during and after exercise or other strenuous activity
- Moistening the mucous membranes of the respiratory tract, which in turn increases resistance to infection and allows the sinuses to drain more easily.

Because water is so important to our health, all of us need to make a conscious effort to stay well hydrated, since most of us lose water faster than we replace it. For example, we lose one pint of water each day simply through exhalation. We also lose the same amount through perspiration, as well as three additional pints per day through urination and defecation. Exercise and heat exposure, especially in a dry climate, also increase water loss in the body. The percentage of body water content also decreases with age. All told, on average, each of us loses two and a half quarts of water (80 ounces) per day under normal conditions. Therefore, it is essential that the same amount or more be replenished daily.

Unfortunately, most Americans don't come close to consuming that much water per day. As a result, many of us are chronically dehydrated. When we think of dehydration, we may envision a lost soul in the desert dying of thirst. However, most conditions of dehydration are not that dramatic, so that dehydration all too often is unsuspected and therefore undiagnosed. Meanwhile, its insidious effects can wreak havoc on our health by chronically impacting every one of our bodily functions. The results are:

- Reduced blood volume, with less oxygen and nutrients provided to all muscles and organs
- Reduced brain size and impaired neuromuscular coordination, concentration, and thinking
- Excess body fat
- Poor muscle tone and size
- Impaired digestive function and constipation
- Increased toxicity in the body
- Joint and muscle pain
- Water retention (edema), which can result in a state of being overweight and also impede weight loss

- Hyperconcentration of blood with increased viscosity, leading to higher risk of heart attack

Even though you may not be feeling thirsty, you may nonetheless be one of the millions of Americans who are chronically dehydrated. Observation of your urine is one simple way to determine if you are. If your urine is heavy, cloudy, and deep yellow, orange or brown in tint, it's more than likely that you are dehydrated. The urine of a properly hydrated body tends to be light and nearly clear in color, similar in appearance to unsweetened lemonade. As your water intake approaches your daily need for it, you will notice the appearance of your urine changing accordingly. (Remember that B vitamins will also turn urine a dark yellow.)

Because dehydration is so deceptive—it can occur without symptoms of thirst—in general, we need to drink more water than our thirst calls for. This does not mean coffee, soft drinks, or alcohol, all of which contribute further to dehydration. Even processed fruit juices and milk are not healthy substitutes for water because of the sugar and possible pesticides in the former and the hormones and antibiotics in the latter.

The exact amount of water a person needs depends on a number of individual factors, such as body weight, diet, metabolic rate, climate, level of physical activity, and stress factors. Some health professionals recommend that we all drink 8 eight-ounce glasses of water a day. A more accurate rule of thumb is to drink half an ounce of water per pound of body weight if you are a healthy but sedentary adult, and to increase that amount to two-thirds of an ounce per pound if you are an active exerciser. This means that a healthy, sedentary adult weighing 160 pounds should drink about 10 eight-ounce glasses of water per day, while an active exerciser should drink 13 to 14 eight-ounce glasses. If your diet is particularly high in fresh fruits and vegetables, your daily water intake needs may be less, since these foods are 85–90 percent water in content and can help restore lost fluids. Herbal teas, natural fruit juices (without sugar added and diluted 50 percent with water), and soups that are sugarless and low in salt (the thinner the better) are also acceptable substitutes for drinking water.

Nearly as important as the amount of water you drink is the *quality* of your water. Simply put, if you aren't drinking filtered water, then your body is forced to become the filter. Still, it's impossible to generalize about whether you should drink tap, bottled, or filtered water. (Distilled water is not recommended for drinking because it lacks necessary minerals and can also leach them from your body.) In some communities, water purity is so high that it requires no treatment, while other water sources are contaminated with high concentrations of lead and radon, the two worst contaminants.

Another issue related to our drinking water is chlorination. Since chlorine was first introduced into America's drinking water supply in 1908, it has eliminated epidemics of cholera, dysentery, and typhoid. Multiple studies, however, now suggest an association between chlorine and increased free radical production, which can lead to a higher incidence of cancer. On the positive side, chlorine is effective in eliminating most microorganisms from drinking water. (One notable exception is the parasite *Cryptosporidium*, which is resistant to chlorine.)

Unless you live in one of the communities that supplies pure water, drinking tap water is not recommended, especially since the majority of health-related risks present in drinking water occur from contamination that is added *after* the water leaves the treatment and distribution plant. This includes pipes that run from municipal systems into your home, lead-soldered copper pipes, and fixtures that contain lead and may leach lead or other toxic metals (such as cadmium, mercury, and cobalt) into your tap water. Therefore, if you drink tap water, it would be a good idea to have the water from your tap tested, regardless of the claims from your local water utility. You can get started by calling your local health department for a referral for testing.

Because of the growing concerns regarding tap water, increasing numbers of Americans now choose bottled water for drinking and cooking purposes. This can not only prove to be expensive, but may also not be as safe as you think. Regulations mandated for the bottled-water industry are similar to those followed by the public water treatment industry and currently do not include required testing for *Cryptosporidium* and many other contaminants. Moreover, 25 percent of bottled water sold in this country comes from filtered municipal water that is then treated. For this reason, perhaps the healthiest choice regarding your drinking water is to invest in a water filter.

Since it is impossible to always know for certain whether what we drink or eat is completely safe, do the best you can. To get in the habit of drinking enough water, spread your intake throughout the day (drinking very little after dinner), and don't drink more than four eight-ounce glasses in any one-hour period. It's also best to drink between meals so as not to interfere with your body's digestive process. Make your water drinking convenient; keep a container of water at hand, in your car or at your desk, and don't wait until you feel thirsty to start drinking.

Nutritional Supplements

Following the dietary recommendations just outlined is a vital first step in creating optimal health for yourself and your loved ones. Sadly, however, a healthy diet alone, even one that is rich with pure, organically grown foods, is no longer enough to ensure total physical well-being. Due to our unhealthy environment and the stresses of daily life, most of us also need to supplement our diets in some fashion. On a daily basis we are exposed to stress in the form of chemicals, emo-

I believe that you can, by taking some simple and inexpensive measures, extend your life and your years of well-being. My most important recommendation is that you take vitamins every day to optimum amounts, to supplement the vitamins you receive in your food.

LINUS PAULING, PH.D., two-time Nobel Prize Laureate, who lived a full and productive 93 years by following his own advice.

tions, and infection. Chemical stress may come from polluted air and water, food pesticides, insecticides, heavy metals, and even radioactive wastes. More than ever before, foreign chemicals can be found in our foods and environment. Many of these are commerically synthesized, but quite a few are naturally occurring as well. In 1989, the Kellogg Report stated that one thousand newly synthesized compounds are introduced into our environment every year. That's the equivalent of three new chemicals per day. Currently, there are approximately one hundred thousand of these foreign chemicals, or *xenobiotics*, in the world. They include drugs, pesticides, industrial chemicals, food additives and preservatives, and environmental pollutants. As a result, it's very easy for toxic chemicals to find their way into our bodies via the air we breathe, the foods we eat, and the water we drink. We also ingest these chemicals whenever we use drugs (both medicinal and illicit), alcohol, or tobacco.

Compounding this problem is the fact that the soil in which our foods are grown is greatly depleted of the trace minerals needed to create and maintain health. Many of our foods are shipped, frozen, stored, and warehoused, reaching us weeks or months after being harvested. Degeneration of their nutrient value occurs at each stop. Cooking methods, such as boiling and frying, also contribute to nutrient loss once the food reaches our kitchens and restaurants. Moreover, the standard American diet has become increasingly devoid of nutrients and overburdened with empty calories and nonfood additives. Therefore, even though the body is marvelously designed to eliminate toxins, in today's environment it needs help in doing so.

Free Radicals and Antioxidants. One of the biggest threats to our health are free radicals, highly toxic molecules that play a causative role in many disease conditions, particularly degenerative disorders such as arthritis, heart disease, cancer, cataracts, macular degeneration, high blood pressure, emphysema, cirrhosis of the liver, ulcers, toxemia during pregnancy, and mental disorders. Free radicals also increase susceptibility to infection and accelerate the aging process by damaging the cells.

Since free radicals are the primary agents of most cellular damage, minimizing their harmful effects is important. Fortunately, our bodies manufacture antioxidant enzymes within the cells to neutralize and protect against free radicals. Working in tandem with antioxidant nutrients supplied by our diet, such as vitamin A, carotenes, vitamin C, vitamin E, copper, manganese, selenium, and zinc, these enzymes maintain healthy cell function in a variety of ways. As a result, so long as there is an adequate supply of oxygen, water, antioxidant nutrients, and enzymes in the body, cell damage is kept to a minimum. But when our bodies become deficient in any one of these health-enhancing agents, the cells are overrun by free radicals and the antioxidant defenses become unable to maintain their protective shield. This occurs whenever the body's production of antioxidant enzymes and our intake of antioxidant nutrients fall below what is needed to maintain good health. Poor diet, physical and emotional stress, exposure to pollutants, and lack of sleep all contribute to this decline in enzyme production. Escaping such stressors altogether is practically impossible in today's fast-paced world, but there are vitamins and other nutritional antioxidant supplements that can offer substantial help in preventing disease and maintaining proper immune function.

The following table contains recommended dosages for the most common antioxidant vitamins and minerals, all of which should be part of your daily regimen for creating and maintaining optimal health. There are a number of multivitamin formulas on the market that contain the ingredients listed here, or you can take them separately. Use the higher dosages whenever you are experiencing higher levels of stress, diminished sleep, or increased exposure to pollutants and other sources of toxicity or when you are not eating as well as you should be. Otherwise take at least the minimum dose every day, preferably with your meals.

Recommended Daily Nutritional Supplements

Vitamin C (as polyascorbate or Ester C)—1,000 to 2,000 mg, three times

Beta-carotene—25,000 I.U. one or two times

Vitamin E—400 I.U. one or two times

B-complex vitamins—50 to 100 mg of each B vitamin

Selenium—100 to 200 mcg

Zinc picolinate—15 to 40 mg

Calcium citrate or apatite—1,000 mg

Magnesium citrate or aspartate—500 mg

Chromium polynicotinate (ChromeMate®)—100 to 200 mcg

Manganese—10 to 15 mg

Copper—1 to 2 mg

Iron—10 to 18 mg

In addition, supplementing with either grape seed extract or pycnogenol (100 mg one to two times daily between meals) is also advisable. The antioxidant properties of these supplements have been found to be 20 times greater than vitamin C and 50 times greater than vitamin E.

Daily supplementation of flaxseed oil, evening primrose oil, or other sources of essential fatty acids are recommended as well.

Herbal Remedies

Herbs, from which approximately 25 percent of all prescription drugs are derived, have been used for millennia by cultures throughout the world to maintain health and treat and prevent disease. Their proper use is also one of the components of holistic medicine.

While it is not a good idea to employ herbal remedies indiscriminately and without the guidance of a trained herbalist, the following herbs can be safely used by anyone to enhance and maintain health:

Garlic. A member of the lily family, garlic is a perennial plant cultivated around the world, and has been used for thousands of years for its therapeutic properties. Garlic is effective as an antibacterial, antiviral, antifungal, antihypertensive, and anti-inflammatory agent, and, according to the National Cancer Institute, it shows promise in fighting both stomach and colon cancer. For all of its health-giving properties, however, garlic is also renowned for its distinct odor and the bad breath that it causes. Still, raw garlic, up to a clove per day, is the best way to take it. Otherwise, many brands of processed garlic are now available in pill, capsule, and liquid forms.

Cayenne (Red Pepper). As a general tonic, cayenne is useful in a variety of ways. It has beeen shown to increase blood flow and circulation, and can help stimulate digestion. According to James Braly, M.D., a specialist in the treatment of food allergies, cayenne can also serve as an anti-inflammatory agent and can prevent allergic reactions in people with food sensitivities. An excellent way to take cayenne is to use it as a seasoning with your meals. It is also available in capsule form.

Ginger. Ginger has been used medicinally in China and India as far back as the fourth century B.C., primarily to stimulate the gastrointestinal tract and to treat indigestion and flatulence. More recently, ginger has been shown to aid in the treatment of nausea, motion sickness, and coughs and asthma caused by allergy or inflammation. Ginger, along with garlic and onion, has also been found to reduce blood platelet aggregation, indicating that it may be useful in reducing the risk of cardiovascular disease. Ginger can be taken as a tea or in capsule form, and can also be eaten raw and added to meals for flavoring.

Echinacea. Native to the American Midwest, echinacea is a perennial herb renowned for its immune-enhancing properties. In addition to its ability to stimulate the immune system, it is effective as a wound healer, an antiviral and antibacterial agent, and an anti-inflammatory. It can be taken alone as a liquid tincture, or in combination with goldenseal, in a dosage of 40 drops taken three times per day. It is also available in capsule form.

According to Steve Morris, N.D., an authority in herbology, echinacea should be regarded as a natural antibiotic. It must be taken regularly in order to have a therapeutic effect, but if taken for periods longer than three weeks, a tolerance to it may occur, thereby negating its effectiveness. Dr. Morris recommends that his patients take the herb daily until their symptoms are completely gone, and then continue for another three to four days to ensure that they do not return. If you choose to use it for longer periods, stop for at least a week following each three-week period of use before resuming again.

Ginkgo Biloba. One of the world's oldest living tree species, Ginkgo biloba is believed to have survived for two hundred million years. In China the ginkgo tree is considered sacred, and in traditional Chinese medicine ginkgo biloba is commonly prescribed for respiratory ailments and to maintain and improve brain function. Ginkgo has been shown to increase circulation to the brain and is therefore helpful with dementia, Alzheimer's disease, memory loss, concentration problems, vertigo, tinnitus, and dizziness. It can also be used in cases of peripheral vascular disease, such as Raynaud's syndrome, intermittent claudication (severe pain in the calf muscle brought about by walking), numbness, and tingling. Studies have also reported ginkgo's usefulness in improving cases of head injury, macular degeneration, asthma, and impotence. The usual daily dose is 120 mg.

Food Allergy

Food allergy ranks as one of the most common conditions in the United States. Compounding this problem is the fact that millions of Americans are unaware that they are having negative reactions to the foods they eat. Ironically, the foods to which we react are the foods we crave the most. The foods that most commonly cause allergy are cow's milk and all dairy products, wheat and other grains, chocolate, corn, sugar, soy, yeast (both brewer's and baker's), oranges, tomatoes, bell peppers, white potatoes, eggs, fish, shellfish, cocoa, onions, nuts, garlic, peanuts, black pepper, red meat, coffee, black tea, and beer, wine, and champagne. Aspirin and artificial food colorings can also cause allergic reactions. But as holistic physicians know, any food can cause an unsuspected allergic reaction, even water.

Doris Rapp, M.D., past president of the American Academy of Environmental Medicine and author of *Allergies and Your Family*, recommends the following method for detecting food allergies. Take your pulse in the morning, on an empty stomach. Count your heartbeat for a full minute. Then eat the food you wish to test. Wait 15 to 30 minutes, then retake your pulse. If your heart rate has increased by 15 to 20 beats per minute, chances are that you are sensitive to the food you ate.

The symptoms of food allergy are many and usually occur within four days after eating the food in question, further contributing to food allergies being often overlooked as an underlying cause of poor health. In the case of effects on the joints, the symptoms can take seven to twelve days to manifest. Nearly every organ system of the body can be the target of food reactions, including the brain (foggy-headedness, headache), heart (rhythm disturbances), lungs (asthma), sinuses (postnasal drip), gastrointestinal tract (ulcers, colitis), veins (phlebitis), bladder (frequency, urgency, bedwetting), and joints (arthritis). If you suspect you suffer from food allergies, consult a holistic physician or practitioner of environmental medicine; they offer a more comprehensive perspective on allergies and food sensitivities than do more conventional allergy specialists. To find such a physician in your area, contact the American Academy of Environmental Medicine, 10 E. Randolph, New Hope, PA 18938; (215) 862-4544.

For more information on treating allergies, see chapter 6.

EXERCISE, PHYSICAL ACTIVITY, AND REST

No discussion of physical health would be complete without including the subject of exercise and physical activity. Regular exercise can contribute more to optimal health than any other health practice, with the possible exception of diet. Yet in spite of exercise's many proven benefits, we are becoming an increasingly sedentary nation. This is especially true of our children, who are becoming fatter (25 percent are overweight), weaker, and slower than ever before.

Numerous studies show that sedentary people, on average, don't live as long or enjoy as good health as those who get regular aerobic exercise in the form of brisk walking, running, swimming, cycling, rebounding, or similar workouts. In fact, some researchers now believe that lack of exercise might be a more significant risk factor for decreased life expectancy than the *combined* risks of cigarette smoking, high cholesterol, being overweight, and high blood pressure. Simply put, *being unfit means being unhealthy.*

The benefits of regular exercise and physical activity include dissipation of tension; *decreased* "fight or flight" response, depression, anxiety, smoking, drug use, and incidence of heart disease and cancer; *increased* self-esteem, positive attitudes, joy, spontaneity, mental acuity, mental function, aerobic capacity, and enhanced energy; *increased* muscular strength and flexibility; and *improved* quality of sleep. Regular exercise also results in an increased muscle to fat ratio and increased longevity (people who are least fit have a mortality rate three and a half times that of those who are most fit).

Some of the more pronounced benefits of regular exercise occur with older women. A seven-year study conducted by the University of Minnesota School of Public Health tracked the physical activity levels of over 40,000 women, all of whom were postmenopausal and ranged in age from 55 to 69. The results showed that women who exercised at least four times a week at high intensity had up to a 30 percent lowered risk of early death as compared to women in the same age group who were sedentary. But even infrequent exercisers among participants in the study (once per week) experienced reduced mortality rates.

In selecting an exercise program, choose a blend of activities that will increase *aerobic capacity, strength,* and *flexibility.* A regimen focused solely on strength conditioning, such as weight lifting, while providing strength, does little to increase aerobic capacity and can even diminish flexibility. Adding a stretching routine and an aerobic workout on alternate days will provide a much more effective exercise practice.

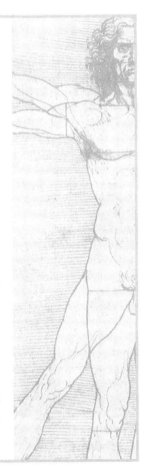

THE IMPORTANCE OF PROPER BREATHING

We can live for weeks without food and days without water, but typically if we stop breathing for more than two or three minutes, we die. Breathing is the single most important physical function we perform, yet almost all of us breathe inefficiently. For the most part, we aren't even conscious of our breath, and spend hour after hour breathing shallowly into the chest, depriving ourselves of the tremendous energy and revitalizing power that proper breathing can provide.

The primary purpose of breathing is to deliver oxygen to every cell in every tissue and organ in the body, while removing carbon dioxide. Oxygen's primary role in the body is to produce the energy required for every basic bodily function via its interaction with ATP. Since the cellular content of ATP is responsible for the body's total energy levels and its ability to perform all of its functions, adequate oxygen levels are essential for our overall health. When our oxygen intake is reduced, ATP is diminished as well.

A variety of environmental factors can also contribute to oxygen deficiency, including high carbon monoxide and smoke pollution, smog, and high altitude. (Oxygen content decreases by over 3 percent every thousand feet above sea level.) The primary cause of chronic reduced oxygen levels in the body, however, is shallow and inefficient breathing patterns. Typically, most of us habitually breathe in through the chest, failing to breathe deeply and fully. This unconscious and inefficient method of breathing significantly reduces our oxygen supply. By simply learning how to improve the way you breathe, you can considerably improve your health and ensure that your cells remain in an oxygen-rich state. Specific breathing exercises to improve your health are outlined in the action steps in chapter 5.

Aerobic Exercise

The word *aerobic* means *with oxygen.* Aerobic exercise refers to prolonged exercise that requires extra oxygen to supply energy to the muscles. In general, aerobic activities cause moderate shortness of breath, perspiring, and doubling of the resting pulse rate. A few words of conversation should be possible at the height of activity; otherwise the workout may in fact be too strenuous.

Aerobic exercise is based on maintaining your *target heart rate*, producing greater benefits to the cardiovascular system and providing more oxygen to the body than any other form of exercise. To determine what your target heart rate should be, use the following formula: 220 minus your age, multiplied by 60 to 85 percent. Keep in mind that 60 percent is considered low intensity aerobic exercise, with 70 percent being moderate, and 85 percent being high intensity. For example, a 40-year-old's target heart rate is between 108 and 153 beats per minute. To accurately determine your pulse, use your index and middle finger to feel the pulse on the thumb side of your wrist or at your neck, just below the jaw. Using a watch with a second hand, count the number of beats in 60 seconds, which will give you your heart rate in beats per minute (or count for 15 seconds and multiply by 4).

When you have attained your target heart rate (after about five to ten minutes of exercising), try to maintain it for at least twenty minutes. It is also beneficial to cool down by working out at a slower heart rate and with less intensity for an additional five to ten minutes before you end your session.

The most convenient forms of aerobic exercise involving the least amount of wear and tear on the body are brisk walking, hiking, swimming, rebounding (jumping on a mini-trampoline), and cycling. Cross-country skiing, if convenient, can also provide a very good aerobic workout. Jogging can also be effective, but due to the rising number of patients with running-related complaints, it is recommended that you stretch thoroughly before and after each run, use good running shoes and orthotics—if indicated—and supplement with vitamin C and calcium to strengthen your bones, cartilage, muscles, and tendons. Treadmills, rowing machines, stair climbers, stationary bikes, and cross-country ski machines also offer an opportunity for excellent indoor aerobics, as do low impact aerobics classes. Racquetball, handball, badminton, singles tennis, and basketball provide good aerobic workouts as well.

The keys to a successful aerobic routine are consistency and comfort. Aerobic conditioning does not have to entail a great deal of time, nor does it have to be painful. Find an activity that you can enjoy and keep it fun. Remember, too, that low to moderate aerobic exercise for 45 minutes is just as beneficial as high intensity for 20 minutes. Exercise outdoors whenever possible, as long as it is convenient and safe to do so, as the combination of fresh air and sunshine provides greater health benefits than indoor exercise.

Do not begin any aerobic activity in the heat of an emotional crisis, especially intense anger. Wait at least 15 to 20 minutes to avoid the risk of heart attack or arrhythmias that can be triggered under such circumstances. In addition, make sure your aerobic exercise precedes meals by at least half an hour, or follows them by at least two and a half hours, in order to avoid indigestion.

Strength Conditioning

Building and maintaining muscle strength is another essential component of your overall exercise program. Strength conditioning falls under the following three categories. *Strengthening without aids* includes calisthenics such as sit-ups, push-ups, jumping jacks, and swimming. *Strengthening with aids* includes chin-ups, dips, weight lifting, and training on weight machines. And *strengthening with aerobics* involves various forms of interval training that can be done running, bicycling, jumping rope, circuit training with weight machines, and working out on a heavy bag. The goal of interval training is to work intensively, reaching your maximum heart level for a short interval, then lower the level of activity to recover. Repeating this process while maintaining your heart rate in its target zone reduces recovery time, strengthens various muscle groups, and conditions the cardiovascular system.

Weight training is perhaps the most popular form of strength conditioning exercise. To design a weight program to meet your specific needs, consult with a personal trainer, who will most likely advise you to work out two or three times a week. It isn't necessary to lift a lot of weight to build and tone muscle. If muscle tone and definition is your goal, best results will be achieved using less weight and more repetitions. To build mass, increase the amount of weight you use and do fewer repetitions. Remember to breathe out as you exert effort, and for free-weight exercises it is advisable to work with a spotter. Also wear a weight belt to help keep your spine properly aligned. If you are unable to work with a personal trainer, refer to the list of recommended books for helpful guidelines in designing your strength conditioning program.

Increasing Flexibility

The final component of a good exercise program addresses flexibility. This includes stretching exercises, yoga, t'ai chi, and the Feldenkrais Method. Exercise that promotes flexibility also significantly contributes to strength and function by allowing the body's muscle groups to perform at maximum efficiency. Lack of flexibility can severely inhibit physical performance, increase the potential for injury, and compromise posture. Muscles exist in a state of static tension wherein contrasting sets of muscles exert similar force to create a state of balance. When muscles become weak or inflexible, this balance is disrupted, resulting in reduced function or postural misalignment. Additional benefits of muscle flexibility include improved circulation, enhanced suppleness of connective tissue (tendons and ligaments), decreased risk of injury, and greater body awareness.

Stretching exercises. Some form of stretching is recommended before and after both aerobic and strengthening workouts. Before you begin stretching, do five minutes of movement to warm up your muscles and body core. This will enhance your circulation and make stretching easier. Never stretch to the point of pain. Ideally, you should feel a tension in the affected muscle or muscle group that you are working. As you do, breathe into the stretch to elongate and relax the muscle group as you hold the posture for 20 to 30 seconds. Repeat each stretch at least twice. You should notice that your range increases on the second and third repetition. A few minutes of daily stretching will noticeably improve your well-being over time.

Yoga. Yoga, a Sanskrit word meaning *to yoke*, refers to a balanced practice of physical exercise, breathing, and meditation to unify body, mind, and spirit, making yoga one of the most effective and ancient forms of holistic self-care. The benefits of this five-thousand-year-old system of mind/body training to improve flexibility, strength, and concentration are well documented. There are a number of yogic systems; *hatha yoga* is most well known in the West. Hatha yoga postures, or *asanas*, affect specific muscle groups and organs to impart physical strength and flexibility, as well as emotional and mental peace of mind.

There are a variety of hatha yoga forms available, and initially it is a good idea to receive instruction for at least a few months, due to the subtleties involved in yoga practice that are not apparent without firsthand experience of its practice under the guidance of a qualified yoga instructor.

T'ai chi. Sometimes referred to as *meditation in motion*, t'ai chi, like yoga, is thousands of years old. It involves slow-motion movements integrated with focused breathing and visualization and is practiced daily by tens of millions of people in mainland China. The goal of t'ai chi is to move qi (pronounced "chee"), or *vital life force energy*, along the various meridians, or energetic pathways, of the body's various organ systems. According to traditional Chinese medicine, when the flow of qi is balanced and unobstructed, both blood and lymph flow are enhanced and the body's neurological impulses function at optimal capacity. The result is greater vitality, resistance to disease, better balance, stimulation of the "relaxation response," increased oxygenation of the blood, deeper sleep, and increased body/mind awareness. Although not as well known as yoga in this country, t'ai chi is rapidly gaining in popularity, and t'ai chi instructors can be found in most metropolitan areas. After being taught the basic movements of t'ai chi, you can practice them almost anywhere to instill a centeredness and sense of calm, and to alleviate stress.

Sleep And Relaxation

While diet, the use of supplements, and exercise can all benefit physical health and improve immune function, perhaps the most powerful and overlooked key to overall well-being is sleep. The average person requires between eight and nine hours of uninterrupted sleep, yet in the United States we average between six and eight hours, with an estimated 50 million Americans suffering from insomnia.

Lack of sleep and its resulting depression of the immune system can be a factor in many chronic health conditions, and is a common cause of colds. Additional sleep is therefore an essential component in the holistic treatment of such conditions. Besides lowered immune function, sleep deprivation can also cause a decrease in productivity, creativity, and job performance and can affect mood and mental alertness. In cases of insomnia, most incidents of sleep deprivation are due to a specific stress-producing event. While stress-induced insomnia is usually temporary, it may persist well beyond the precipitating event to become a chronic problem. Overstimulation of the nervous system (especially from caffeine, salt, or sugar) or simply the fear that you can't fall asleep are other common causes.

Researchers have identified two types of sleep: *heavy* and *light*. During heavier, or nonrapid eye movement (NREM) sleep, your body's self-repair and healing mechanisms are revitalized, enabling your body to repair itself. During lighter, rapid eye movement (REM) sleep, you dream more, releasing stress and tension. (For more on dreams, see chapter 3.)

Conventional medicine commonly prescribes sleeping pills for insomnia and other sleep disorders, but as with almost all medications, there are unpleasant side effects to contend with, as well as the risk of developing dependency. A more holistic approach to ensuring adequate sleep begins with establishing a regular bedtime every night so that you can begin to reattune yourself to nature's rhythms. According to Ayurvedic medicine (see the appendix), the circadian rhythm, caused by the earth rotating on its axis every 24 hours, has a counterpart in the human body. Modern science has confirmed that many neurological and endocrine functions follow this circadian rhythm, including the sleep-wakefulness cycle. Ayurveda teaches that the ideal bedtme for the deepest sleep and for being in sync with this natural rhythm is 10 P.M. Unfortunately, most people with insomnia dread bedtime and go to bed later, when sleep tends to be somewhat lighter and more active. Ayurveda also states that eight hours of sleep beginning at 9:30 P.M. is twice as restful as eight hours beginning at 2 A.M. It is also important in resetting your biological clock to get up early and at the same time every day, regardless of when you go to bed. Establishing an early wake-up time (6 or 7 A.M.) is essential for overcoming insomina. You'll eventually begin to feel sleepier earlier in the evening, and even if you aren't actually sleeping by 10 P.M., you'll benefit just by resting in bed at that hour.

Most importantly, don't worry about lost sleep, since, in most cases, anxiety is what caused the problem in the first place. If you can learn to relax without drugs, you will have cured your sleeping problems while giving your immune system a powerful boost. (A fuller discussion on how to holistically treat sleep problems can be found in chapter 7).

Relaxation is another essential ability that promotes physical health. Derived from the Latin *relaxare*, meaning *to loosen*, relaxation is a way to allow the mind to return to a natural state of equilibrium, creating a state of balance between the right and left brain. It is also a highly effective means of stress-reduction.

Relaxation is a skill that can be improved upon with practice; therefore, it is recommended that you take time each day to relax. This can be achieved as easily as taking a few deep breaths or simply shifting your focus away from your problems and concerns, or through any activity that engages your creative and physical faculties. Such activities include reading and writing, gardening, taking a walk, painting, singing, playing music, doing crafts, or any other hobby that you enjoy for its own sake, without the need to be concerned about your performance. Committing two to three evening hours a week to the hobby or activity of your choice will help make relaxation a natural and regular part of your daily experience. The ability to relax and shift gears away from the competitive drive that impels most of us in our society holds the key to greater health.

ENVIRONMENTAL MEDICINE

COMPONENTS OF OPTIMAL ENVIRONMENTAL HEALTH

harmony with your environment (neither harming nor being harmed)

Awareness of your connectedness with nature

Feeling grounded

Respect and appreciation for your home, the Earth and all of her inhabitants

Contact with the earth; breathing healthy air; drinking pure water; eating uncontaminated food; exposure to the sun, fire, or candlelight; immersion in warm water (all on a daily basis).

As discussed above, our environment is increasingly becoming burdened with a proliferation of toxic chemicals and pollutants. Environmental medicine deals with these environmental hazards, as well as communicable disease and the potential health risks that are becoming increasingly common in work and social settings. The modern-day roots of environmental medicine go back to the late 1940s and the work of Theron G. Randolph, M.D., one of the first physicians to notice the negative impact that chemicals in the environment could have on the body. Today, Dr. Randolph's work is primarily carried on by the American Academy of Environmental Medicine (AAEM) (see page 497), an organization that trains physicians in treating illnesses caused by environmental factors.

The range of diseases that have been linked to the environment is both extensive and growing. The body systems affected include the immune, cardiovascular, respiratory, endocrine, gastrointestinal, nervous, genitourinary, and musculoskeletal. Environmental factors also play a role in many pediatric diseases; eyes, nose, ear, and throat conditions; skin conditions; and mental illness and have also been linked to certain forms of cancer. Among the elements that can contribute to environmentally caused illness are poor nutrition and diet; stress; air- and waterborne chemical exposures; infection; heredity and genetic predisposition; dental mercury amalgam fillings; the overuse of antibiotics and other medications; glandular and hormonal imbalances; and electromagnetic radiation.

Like food allergy, environmental illness is often undiagnosed. If you suspect that environmental factors may be impacting your health, contact the AAEM for a referral to a physician in your area. Overall, professional guidance is usually required to deal with serious cases of environmental illness, but there are also a variety of self-care measures that you can use preventively and therapeutically.

Nothing is more important to our health than the air we breathe. The healthiest air is clean, moist, warm, and high in both oxygen and negative ion content. According to the Environmental Protection Agency (EPA), however, 60 percent of all Americans live in areas where poor air quality is a health risk. An additional detriment lies in the adverse effects that many newer, air-conditioned buildings and office spaces can have in the form of "sick building syndrome." Researchers in France, for instance, have found that such indoor environments are twice as likely to cause or contribute to respiratory problems among workers as compared to workers who work outdoors or in buildings without air-conditioning. Moreover, their findings indicate that such buildings are breeding grounds for airborne bacteria and fungi and contribute to a greater incidence of asthma, colds, sinus infections, runny noses, and sore throats. Compounding this problem is the fact that the majority of Americans spend 90 percent of their time indoors, where, according to the EPA, the air can be as much as one hundred times more polluted than outdoor air.

To safeguard against the harmful effects of bad air and other environmental factors, supplement with antioxidants, especially if you live in a city. Proper diet and good drinking water are also essential. Creating a setting of indoor plants where you work and at home can also be helpful. Not only do plants oxygenate the air and create more moisture, they also filter out carbon monoxide and organic chemicals, add beauty to the environment, and can enhance feelings of well-being. Also consider the use of a negative ion generator and humidifier.

Negative ions, which are air molecules containing an excess of electrons, can substantially vitalize the air we breathe. Some studies have suggested that negative ions increase the sweeping motion of the cilia on the respiratory mucosa, thereby enhancing the movement of mucus and the expulsion and filtration of inhaled pollutants. They also help reduce pain, heal burns, suppress mold and bacteria, and stimulate plant growth. Positive ions, by contrast, have an opposite effect and are largely the by-product of manmade pollutants such as auto and truck exhaust, smokestacks, and cigarette smoke. Heating and filtration systems also tend to produce air high in positive ion content, as do window air conditioners, air cleaners (including HEPA filters), television sets, and computer monitors. Airplane cabins contain an inordinate amount of positive ions as well. The use of a negative ion generator can significantly increase negative ion content in an indoor environment, minimizing positive ion effects.

Dry air, especially if it is cold, is also harmful to health and is quite common in many modern buildings. Dry air is a major contributor to sinusitis and chronic bronchitis and is also a factor in allergies. Optimum indoor air quality contains 35 to 55 percent relative humidity, which can easily be achieved by using a room humidifier. Humidifiers are particularly useful in the winter months because most heating systems dry the indoor air considerably. Of the variety of room humidifiers available, warm-mist units are most effective. These produce a mist just slightly warmer than room air, use tap water, and require no filter; some are able to kill bacteria. Be sure to clean them at least weekly with vinegar. Their only limitation is that they also tend to require more electricity than other models.

Another important strategy for minimizing indoor environmental pollution is the use of materials that emit no pollutants. Natural products such as wood, cotton, and metals are preferable to synthetic materials such as particle board, fiberboard, polyester, and plastics. Synthetic carpets are also high in potentially toxic ingredients. Beware of formaldehyde from insulation materials, unpainted particle board, and plywood as well. Substitutes of cellulose and white fiber-glass insulation are recommended. Cleaning substances can also be a source of indoor pollution, due to their chemical content. In their place, use nontoxic substances, including ordinary soap and vinegar.

Other self-care steps you can take to protect yourself from environmental pollution include:

- Avoiding secondhand tobacco smoke (If you are a smoker, see chapter 7 and seek professional help in order to quit.)
- Using highly efficient furnace filters in your home
- Reducing use of coal- or wood-burning fireplaces and stoves
- Sleeping with your bedroom window open to ensure a stream of fresh air
- Taking frequent breaks away from your computer
- Making a habit of spending regular periods of time outdoors in an unpolluted, natural setting
- Moving to a healthier neighborhood or city
- Cleaning carpets and rugs regularly with nontoxic cleaners to prevent build-up of mold and bacteria
- Ensuring that both your home and workplace benefit from good ventilation

Becoming environmentally healthy requires conscious attention and effort. Remember, environmental health is a state of respect and appreciation for your home, community, nature, and the Earth. It is a relationship of harmony with your environment so that you are enhanced and enlivened by your surroundings instead of harming or being harmed by them. The more you become involved in improving the conditions of your environment, the healthier you will be.

Summary

Committing yourself to a consistent program of physical fitness based on the recommendations in this chapter will enable you to achieve improvements in your physical well-being in as little as a few weeks. Before long, you should find that your reserves of energy are greater, and that you are physically stronger and more flexible. You will also develop a more positive self-image and feel better about how your body looks and performs. Such benefits are just the beginning of your journey to optimal wellness and will continue to become more noticeable as you continue to follow these guidelines in the months and years ahead. In the process, you will be creating the foundation necessary for healing the other aspects of holistic medicine's triumvirate—*mind and spirit.*

3

Healing the Mind

*The greatest discovery of any
generation is that human beings can
alter their lives by altering the
attitudes of their minds.*
ALBERT SCHWEITZER

ONE OF THE MOST exciting developments in the field of medicine in recent decades has been the scientific verification that our physical health is directly influenced by our thoughts and emotions. The reverse is also true; overwhelming evidence now exists showing that our physiology has a direct correlation to the ways we habitually think and feel. While Eastern systems of medicine, such as traditional Chinese medicine and Ayurveda, have for centuries recognized these facts and stressed the importance of a harmonious connection between body and mind, in the West this mind-body connection did not begin to be acknowledged until research conducted in the 1970s and 1980s conclusively revealed the ability of thoughts, emotions, and attitudes to influence our bodies' immune functions. In fact, many of the scientists exploring this relatively new field have concluded that there is *no separation between mind and body*.

In order to heal our minds and emotions it helps to know what we mean by the term *mental health*. From the perspective of holistic medicine, the essence of mental health is peace of mind and feelings of contentment. Being mentally healthy means that you recognize the ways in which your thoughts, beliefs, mental imagery, and attitudes affect your well-being and limit or expand your ability to enjoy your life. It also means knowing that you always have choices and are aware of your gifts, and are practicing your special talents, working at a job that you enjoy, and being clear about your priorities, values and goals. People who have made a commitment to their mental health live their lives with rich reserves of humor, forgiveness, gratitude, and hope. You can determine your own state of mental health by referring to the appropriate section of the wellness test at the end of chapter 1 and then use the information in this chapter to improve the areas you may need to work on.

The term *mental health* can be interpreted to include not only our thoughts and beliefs, but also our feelings. These aspects of ourselves—mental and emotional—are for the most part inextricably related and together form the "mind" aspect of holistic health. As your healing journey progresses, you will increasingly come to recognize how your own distorted or illogical thoughts are the underlying cause of feelings such as anger, depression, anxiety, fear, and unfounded guilt. Learning how to free yourself from such distorted thinking patterns is the goal of this chapter, and of behavioral medicine, the aspect of holistic medicine that deals with this interconnectedness among physical, mental, and emotional health. Behavioral medicine includes professional treatment approaches such as *psychotherapy*, *mind/body medicine*, *guided imagery and visualization*, *biofeedback therapy*, *hypnotherapy*, *neurolinguistic programming (NLP)*, *orthomolecular medicine* (the use of nutritional supplements to treat chronic mental dis-ease), *flower essences*, and body-centered therapies like *Rolfing, massage therapy*, and *Hellerwork*. (For an overview of what these therapies are and how they work, see the appendix.) The focus in this chapter, however (with the exception of psychotherapy), is on proven self-care approaches that you can begin using immediately to heal the mind. They include *beliefs, affirmations, breathwork, guided imagery, visualization, meditation, dreamwork, journaling*, and your approaches to both *work* and *play*. Each of these methods can help you become more aware of your habitual thoughts, emotions, and beliefs—both pleasurable and painful—in order to create a mindset conducive to experiencing optimal health and more effectively meeting your personal and professional goals.

THE BODY-MIND CONNECTION

Growing numbers of Western scientists and physicians now recognize that *body* and *mind* are not separate aspects of our being but interrelated expressions of the same experience. Their view is based on the findings of researchers working in the field of *psychoneuroimmunology (PNI)*, also referred to as *neuroscience*, which for the past three decades has shown that thoughts, emotions, and attitudes can directly influence immune and hormone function. In light of such research, scientists now commonly speak of the mind's ability to control the body. In large part this perspective is due to the scientific discovery of "messenger" molecules known as *neuropeptides*, chemicals that communicate our thoughts, emotions, attitudes, and beliefs to every cell in our body. In practical terms, this means that all of us are capable of both weakening or strengthening our immune system according to how we think and feel. Moreover, scientists have also proven that these messages can originate not only in the brain but in every cell in the body. As a result of such studies, scientists now conclude that the immune system actually functions as a "circulating nervous system" that is actively and acutely attuned to our every thought and emotion.

Among the discoveries which have occurred in the field of PNI are the following:

- Feelings of loss and self-rejection can diminish immune function and contribute to a number of chronic disease conditions, including heart disease.
- Feelings of exhilaration and joy produce measurable levels of a neuropeptide identical to interleukin-2, a powerful anticancer drug that costs many thousands of dollars per injection.
- Feelings of peace and calm produce a chemical very similar to Valium, a popular tranquilizer.
- Depressive states negatively impact the immune system and increase the likelihood of illness.
- Chronic grief or a sense of loss can increase the likelihood of cancer.
- Anxiety and fear can trigger high blood pressure.
- Feelings of hostility, grief, depression, hopelessness, and isolation greatly increase the risk of heart attack.
- Repressed anger is a factor in causing many chronic ailments, including sinusitis, bronchitis, headaches, and candidiasis.
- Acknowledgment and expression of feelings strengthens immune responses.
- Anger decreases immunoglobulin A (a protective antibody) in saliva, while caring, compassion, humor, and laughter increase it.
- Chronic stress has a broad suppressive effect on immunity, including the depression of natural killer cells, which attack cancer cells.

The implications of these discoveries are enormous and are producing a paradigm shift in physicians' approaches to treating chronic disease. They are also tremendously empowering for anyone committed to holistic health. Once you accept the fact that there is an ongoing, instant, and intimate communication occurring between your mind and your body via the mechanisms of neuropeptides, you can also see that the person best qualified to direct that communication in your own life is you. Learning how to do so effectively can enable you to become your own 24-hour-a-day healer by becoming more conscious of your thoughts and emotions and managing them better to improve all areas of your health. The first step in this process is acknowledging that you can no longer afford to continue feeding yourself the same limiting messages you most likely have been conditioned to accept since early childhood. Scientists now estimate that the average person has approximately 50,000 thoughts each day; yet 95 percent of them are the same as the ones he or she had the day before. Typically, such thoughts are not only unconscious but often critical and limiting. For example, "Why did I say (or do) that? I should have said (or done) it this way." Or: "I'll never be able to overcome this _____ (any chronic condition). I'm going to have to live with this for the rest of my life." *By consciously taking control of your thoughts and recognizing how they govern your behavior, you can dramatically change your life.* You will gain the freedom to think, feel, and believe as you choose, thereby flooding your body's cells with positive, life-affirming messages capable of producing optimal health. The remainder of this chapter provides a variety of approaches to help you do so.

PSYCHOTHERAPY

The field of psychotherapy, an outgrowth of the theories and discoveries of Sigmund Freud, continues to evolve more than a hundred years since its inception. In addition to the mental and emotional benefits commonly attributed to psychotherapy, a growing body of research has documented that physical benefits can also occur. For example, in a study conducted at the UCLA School of Medicine by the late Norman Cousins, a group of cancer patients receiving psychotherapy for 90 minutes a week showed dramatic improvement in their immune systems after only six weeks. During that same period, the control group of other cancer patients who received no counseling showed no change in immune function whatsoever.

Psychotherapy, by its very nature, is not a self-care protocol, but can be extremely valuable for individuals struggling with deeply rooted mental and emotional problems. The most popular forms of psychotherapy are *classical* or *Freudian psychoanalysis, Jungian psychoanalysis, family therapy, cognitive/behavioral therapy, brief/solution-focused therapy,* and *humanistic/existential therapy. Though they all share the same goal of helping patients achieve mental health, their approaches can vary widely.*

If you feel that psychotherapy might help you, you will gain the most benefit by choosing the approach best suited to your specific needs and objectives. In addition, be aware that the work of psychotherapy is increasingly being conducted by nonpsychiatrists, including psychologists, social workers, and pastoral counselors. One of the reasons for this, perhaps, lies in the fact that many of today's patients seeing psychiatrists are given a psychiatric diagnosis (manic-depressive, obsessive-compulsive, etc.) and then treated with drugs, such as the antidepressant Prozac. This trend within psychiatry, a departure away from counseling toward greater drug therapy, makes it a less desirable choice for someone interested in a holistic and self-care approach. While psychotherapeutic drugs can be effective at times, especially over the short term, each of the drugs commonly prescribed by psychiatrists has the potential to cause unpleasant side effects. Equally important, by focusing on treating psychological symptoms with drugs, many psychiatrists are depriving their patients of the opportunity to change their attitudes and behavior and to learn how to understand and grow from their emotional pain. Finally, whichever type of psychotherapist you choose, make sure that he or she is someone with whom you are comfortable. Psychotherapy can only be effective in a situation of trust, so you may wish to interview a number of therapists before making your choice.

BELIEFS AND AFFIRMATIONS

In his classic treatise *The Science Of Mind*, noted spiritual teacher Ernest Holmes wrote: "Health and sickness are largely externalizations of our dominant mental and spiritual states . . . A normal healthy mind reflects itself in a healthy body, and conversely, an abnormal mental state expresses its corresponding condition in some physical condition." At the time Holmes wrote those words, in the mid-1920s, modern science was far behind him in understanding how *our thoughts directly influence our physical health*. But today a growing body of evidence not only verifies this fact but also indicates that it is our predominant, habitual beliefs that determine the thoughts we primarily think. Socrates stated that the unexamined life was not worth living. Based on today's research in the field of behavioral medicine, we might paraphrase his statement to say: *"The unexamined belief is not worth believing in."* Yet most of us have never taken the time to actually examine the beliefs we hold and therefore remain unaware of how they may be influencing our well-being.

The importance of beliefs in the overall scheme of human functioning is confirmed by placebo studies. A placebo is a dummy medication or procedure possessing no therapeutic properties that works because of our belief in it. Detailed analysis of 13 placebo studies from 1940 to 1979, including 1,200 patients, found an 82 percent improvement resulting from the use of medications or procedures that subsequently proved to be placebos. The power beliefs have to affect health is also dramatically demonstrated by patients dealing with life-threatening illness. The vast majority of these patients who accept their physicians' prognoses die at a time very close to the end of their predicted life expectancy. By contrast, patients who challenge their physician's "death sentence" tend to survive longer, and many of them go on to achieve full recoveries.

All too often our predominant beliefs were handed down to us when we were children by our parents, teachers, and other influential adults in our lives. We

SELF-CARE TECHNIQUES FOR DEALING WITH ANGER

Unexpressed anger, or anger that is expressed inappropriately, is both harmful and extremely common in our society. Most of us were taught very early in life that anger was an unacceptable emotion. When it was expressed it often elicited fear in us, and it was usually equated with bodily harm and loss of control. ("He's really lost it." "He's out of control.") This inability to safely express anger has been shown to produce many serious health consequences. For example, Dr. Robert Ivker has found that repressed anger is the primary emotional factor triggering sinus infections. Today, many psychotherapists are combining sound and body movement techniques to help their patients deal with their anger, finding that such approaches can be far more effective than simply talking about it. The following techniques can be safely employed by anyone to release the highly charged emotional energy of anger. They are most effective when employed regularly as preventive measures, instead of allowing anger to build up into a state of chronic, health-impacting tension, much less explosive rage.

Screaming. This is the most common anger release technique due to the fact that all of us already know how to do it. In his novel *Tai Pan,* James Clavell wrote that the chieftains of ancient Scotland for centuries maintained the custom of the "screaming tree." From the time they entered adolescence, men of the clan were instructed to go into the forest and select a tree to which they could express their discontent. Then, whenever their troubles grew too great to otherwise deal with, they would go to the forest alone and scream with the tree as their witness until their emotions settled.

The value of screaming is no secret to young children, who commonly scream when they are greatly upset, only to exhibit a smiling face moments afterward. For adults, the biggest

(continued on next page)

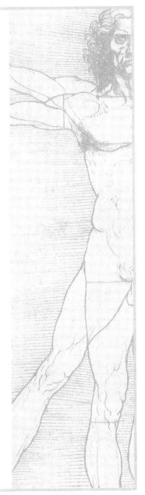

then grew up continuing to hold them in order to comply with the norms and standards defined by our society, usually never asking ourselves if we in fact agreed with them. Once you commit yourself to your own healing, however, becoming aware of your beliefs becomes vitally important. By making unconscious beliefs conscious, you gain the power to change or eliminate those that don't serve you and to replace them with more positive beliefs that do, rejuvenating your health, vitality, and behavior in the process.

A very simple yet powerful exercise that can help you become more conscious of your thoughts, beliefs, and emotions is to take 15 minutes and write out everything that you are thinking during that time. Do this when you are not likely to be disturbed, and don't edit anything out. After a few days of practicing this technique, many of your predominant beliefs will have been expressed on paper. Read them over. If they don't build confidence and self-esteem, regenerate you, or

(continued from previous page)

difficulty here is finding a place to scream in privacy. Screaming when you are home alone, in the basement or closet, in the car with the windows up, or in a secluded spot outdoors are all possibilities. To get the most benefit, take a deep abdominal breath before you scream, and then direct the scream from your diaphragm or deep within your chest cavity, as this will protect your vocal cords. As you scream, slowly move your upper body from side to side or up and down. Usually, after two or three screams in succession, you will begin to feel much better.

The angry letter (not sent). This technique is increasingly employed by therapists to help their clients release their anger. It involves writing a letter to the person with whom you are angry, listing all the reasons why you are upset with them. As you write, allow yourself to express whatever comes to mind, no matter how harsh or offensive it might seem. Once the letter is written, read it over, and if anything else occurs to you that you wish to express, write that down too before signing it. Then either burn the letter or tear it up into small pieces.

Punching. Punching a bag, pillow, or sofa is another effective method of dissipating anger. Remember to grunt or yell with each punch. A variation of this method is to take hold of a pillow and hit it against the floor, sofa, or wall. With either approach, it only takes a few moments before you will start to feel your anger transforming into satisfaction and even joy. Remember, anger in and of itself is not a negative emotion to be shunned. It's only when it remains bottled up inside of us unexpressed that it becomes unhealthy. Safely and appropriately expressing your anger in socially acceptable ways can dramatically improve the way you feel, both emotionally and physically.

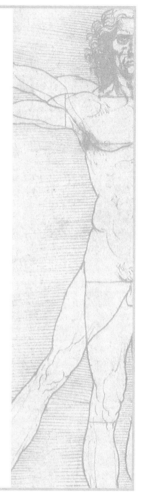

feel nurturing, clearly they are not serving you and need to be either eliminated or changed. Pay particular attention to the "shoulds," "coulds," and "nevers." Before you discard what you write, examine your statements for possible clues to aspects of your life that may require more of your attention. For instance, if one of your statements reads "I hate going to work," more than likely you may need to change your attitude about your job or leave it for one that is more fulfilling and better suited to your talents. (If the thought of leaving your job raises the thought "How will I provide for myself and my family?" realize that this in itself can be a limiting thought. Numerous options will become available to you once you liberate yourself from your old assumptions and beliefs.)

Once you have identified beliefs that are holding you back from your goals and desires, or negatively impacting your health, the next step is to begin to *reprogram* your mind with thoughts, ideas, and images more aligned to what you want. One of the most effective ways to do this is through the use of *affirmations*, or positive thoughts that you repeat to yourself either verbally or in writing in order to produce a specific outcome. Affirmations create images that directly affect the unconscious, shaping patterns of thought to direct behavior. In doing so, they act as powerful tools to unleash and stimulate the healing energy of love present in great abundance within each of us.

The purpose of affirmations is to replace habitual, limiting thought patterns and beliefs with more appropriate images of how you want your life to be. When affirmations are practiced regularly, they have the power to create optimal health by infusing the immune system with the life energy of *hope*, which triggers the activity of neuropeptides in the cells. Affirmations can be used to address virtually all aspects of your life, enhancing self-esteem, improving the quality of relationships, dealing with illness, and launching a more rewarding career.

Because of the simple nature of affirmations, the greatest challenge in using them is to suspend judgment long enough to allow them to produce the results you desire. Keep in mind that the way your life is today is the direct result of the thoughts and beliefs you have held for most, if not all, of your life. Replacing these old thought patterns can take time, although it is quite possible that you will begin to experience the results you want much sooner than you expect. In addition, it helps to *feel* your affirmations as you recite or write them, since this brings more energy to the experience. Make the process as vivid and real as possible.

There are a variety of ways to use affirmations. Some people find they get their best results by writing each affirmation 10 to 20 times a day. Others prefer to say them out loud, or to record them onto a cassette that they can then play to themselves daily. One powerful technique suggested by Louise Hay, author of *You Can Heal Your Life*, is to stare into a mirror and make eye contact with your reflection while verbally repeating each affirmation. Hay notes that this experience tends to bring up feelings of discomfort at first, and recommends that you continue the process until such feelings lessen or fade away altogether. You can experiment with these and other methods until you find the one that works best for you. Here are some other guidleines to ensure that you get the best results from your affirmation program:

- Always state your affirmation in the present tense and keep it positive. For example, if one of your goals is to be free of job-related stress, the affirmation *I accomplish my daily responsibilities with ease and satisfaction* will produce far more effective results than statements such as *My job no longer makes me stressful* or *I will meet my responsibilities with ease.* The reason affirmations work is because the unconscious accepts them as statements of fact and immediately begins to reorganize your life experience to match what you are telling it. So state *what you desire*, not what you wish to be free from, and write and say your affirmation in the present tense *as if your desire is already accomplished.*

- Keep your affirmations short and simple, and no longer than two brief sentences.

- Say or write each affirmation at least 10 to 20 times each day.

- Whenever you experience yourself thinking or hearing a habitual negative message, counteract it by focusing on your affirmation. Over time, you will find that your tendency to give yourself negative messages will diminish.

- Schedule a time each day to do your affirmations and adhere to it. Doing something regularly at the same time each day adds to the momentum of what you are trying to achieve and eventually will become a positive, effortless habit.

- Repeat your affirmations in the first, second, and third person, using your name in each variation. Using affirmations in the first person addresses the mental conditioning you have given yourself, while affirmations in the second and third person help to release the conditioning you may have been accepting from others. For example, if your name is Tom and one of your goals is to make more money, you might write: *I, Tom, am earning enough money to satisfy all my needs and desires, You, Tom, are earning enough money to satsify all your needs and desires,* and *He, Tom, is earning enough money to satisfy all his needs and desires.* In each case, write out or repeat the affirmation 10 times.

- Make a commitment to practice your affirmations for at least 60 days or until you begin experiencing the result you desire.

Perhaps the most effective method for deriving benefit from affirmations is to write, recite, and *visualize* them (see Guided Imagery and Visualization below). Using this method, you would write down your affirmation while reciting it aloud, and then close your eyes and imagine what the affirmation looks and/or feels like, engaging as many of your senses as possible.

GUIDED IMAGERY AND VISUALIZATION

Visualization is a skill all of us have and one that we use every day. Most of the time, however, we do so unconsciously, as when we daydream. The 50,000 thoughts we have each and every day are often accompanied by inner pictures, or imagery, with corresponding emotions. Since the 1970s, researchers, physicians, and other health care professionals have been examining how to harness these mental images in order to use them consciously to create improved states of well-being. Due to their continued work, thousands of individuals nationwide are learning how to use visualization and guided imagery to enhance their health. In many cases, their

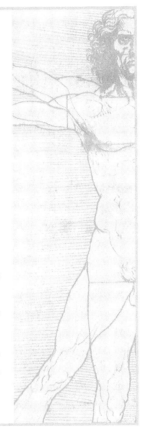

DISCOVERING YOUR GOALS

Often when people who express dissatisfaction with their lives are asked the question "If you could do what you would most enjoy, what would it be?" the answer is "I don't know." A more accurate response is usually that they haven't taken the time to find out. Not having clear goals is common and can have a significant influence on your state of well-being. In order to regularly experience a sense of thriving in your life, you need to know what you want. The following exercise can help you determine what you want and reconnect to the passion that makes life worth living.

Answer these questions: What are you good at and what do you most appreciate about yourself? What do you most enjoy? What is most meaningful to you? Where do you see yourself in five or ten years and what will you be doing? What do you wish for in each area of your life—physical, environmental, mental, emotional, spiritual, and social?

To answer the first question, make a list of your talents, gifts, qualities, and attributes. Set aside all personal judgments as you do this part of the exercise, and don't be afraid if your answers at first seem irrational. All of us have numerous gifts and abilities that make us special. Take the time to write down as many as you can think of, based on the criteria of what you are *good at* and *most appreciate about yourself.*

Now list the things you most enjoy, both activities and states of being. This part of the exercise will help you discover the activities that you most enjoy and have a talent for and are able to do with more skill and less effort than other people.

(continued on next page)

results have been astounding. Since 1971, radiation oncologist O. Carl Simonton, M.D., for instance, has been a pioneer in developing imagery as a self-care tool for cancer patients to use to bolster their response rate to traditional cancer treatments, with remarkable success. The first patient to whom he taught his techniques was a 61-year-old man who had been diagnosed with a "hopeless" case of throat cancer. In conjunction with his radiation treatments, the man spent 5 to 15 minutes three times a day imagining himself healthy. Within two months, he was completely cancer free.

A similarly remarkable case is that of Garrett Porter, a patient of Patricia Norris, Ph.D., another leader in the field of guided imagery. Garrett, who was nine, had been diagnosed with an inoperable brain tumor. Using biofeedback techniques in conjunction with imagery based on his favorite TV show, *Star Trek* (he pictured missles striking and destroying his tumor), Garrett was able to completely reverse his condition within a year, with brain scans confirming his tumor's disappearance. Numerous studies also confirm the health benefits of imagery and visualization. For example, college volunteers who practiced imagery twice daily

(continued from previous page)

After you have identified your talents and what you enjoy, list the things that have the most meaning for you. This is important, because if your goal doesn't meaningfully encompass more than one area of your life, or have benefit to others in some way, more than likely it is incomplete, and you will lack the passion necessary to commit to it. As you list the meaningful things in your life, you will more easily recognize the talents and activities you enjoy that are most worth your while.

Now visualize yourself five or ten years in the future. Make the image as detailed as you can. Based on what you have discovered about yourself and your goals, your vision will showcase for you a new belief system that reflects the type of life you are best suited for—one in which you can contribute the most benefit to yourself, your loved ones, and your community.

The final step of this exercise, your wish list, will help you sort out which goals are most important to you. Write down all that you wish for in each of the six categories of health described above. When you finish, identify the items in each list that most appeal to you and are your more immediate needs and desires (rather than those that you see for yourself ten years from now). You will probably discover that they are also the ones for which your unique special gifts are best suited. Moreover, you now have a map of *where you want to go* and *how you want to get there,* based on what you've discovered about yourself. This will make it much easier for you to make life-changing decisions and to commit to doing whatever is necessary to make your dreams become a reality.

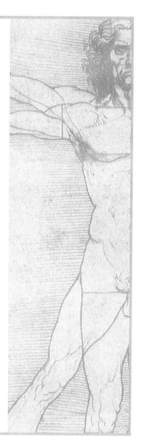

for six weeks experienced a marked increase in salivary immunoglobulin A as compared to a control group who did not practice imagery. In another study, the well-known drop in helper T-immune cells in students facing the stress of final examinations was greatly reduced in a group utilizing relaxation and imagery each day for a month before exams. And patients scheduled for gall bladder surgery who listened to imagery tapes before and after their operations had less wound inflammation, lower cortisone levels, and less anxiety, compared to controls who were treated with comparable periods of quiet only.

Like most of the other therapies outlined in this chapter, one of the most exciting things about guided imagery and visualization is that both techniques are powerful self-healing tools that can be used to create positive change in almost any area of your life. Besides health issues, imagery can help you feel more peaceful and relaxed, assist you in further developing your creative talents, create more fulfillment in your relationships, improve your ability to achieve career goals, and dissolve negative habit patterns. All that is necessary is a commitment to practice the techniques on a regular basis.

Guided imagery and visualization work to improve and maintain health because of their ability to directly affect our bodies at a cellular level, particularly
with regard to neuropeptides. In addition, the use of imagery can often provide
greater insight about causes and treatment for chronic conditions, guiding us
toward the most personalized and effective solutions for our particular health
problem. This occurs because our mental images are so deeply connected to our
emotions, which, as we have discussed, are usually interconnected with the events
in our lives. By using imagery, you can become better aware of what emotional issues may lie beneath the surface of your life and begin the process of healing
them.

There are two types of guided imagery and visualization: preconceived or
preselected images employed by you or your health care professional in order to
address a specific problem and achieve a specific outcome, and imagery that occurs spontaneously as you sit comfortably, eyes closed and breathing freely. Both
forms have value, so try them both and see which works best for you. What follows are two techniques you can use to make imagery a part of your self-care
holistic health routine. The first is a form of guided imagery, while the latter is
conducive for allowing spontaneous imagery to occur on its own.

The Remembrance Technique. This exercise can be adapted to improve issues or
conditions in any area of your life. It's called the Remembrance Technique because in our core selves we are already whole. In many respects, healing is simply
a remembrance of that state in order to reconnect with it. Begin this exercise by
sitting comfortably in a chair or lying down in bed. Select a time and place when
you will not be disturbed. Close your eyes and focus on your breathing. Take a few
deep, unforced breaths to help yourself relax. With each inhalation, imagine that
soothing, relaxing energy is flowing through all areas of your body. As you exhale,
visualize the cares and concerns of the day gradually disappearing. Do this for two
or three minutes, allowing your breath to carry you to a place of calm relaxation.

Now choose the issue you want to focus on for the rest of the exercise, and recall a time when the outcome you desire was something you already experienced.
For example, if you have a cold, remember a time when you felt healthy and could
breathe freely. Allow yourself to reexperience that time, using all of your senses to
make what you are imagining as vivid as possible. Once you have reconnected to
the experience, bring it into the present *as if it were actually happening now.* Stay
with the experience for at least five more minutes, mentally affirming that you *are*
experiencing the state you desire here in the present.

Spontaneous imagery. In this exercise, instead of preselecting a specific outcome, you are going to allow your own unconscious to communicate with you
through imagery about whatever situation in your life you choose to focus on. As
in the preceding exercise, sit or lie down comfortably in a quiet place, close your

eyes, and focus on your breath until you feel yourself settling into a deeper state of relaxation. Now focus on the area in your life into which you desire to gain greater insight, allowing thoughts and images to freely and spontaneously emerge. You may be surprised by what you experience, but don't judge it. Trust that your unconscious knows what you most need to understand, and allow your imagery to lead you to that answer. Continue this exercise for five to ten minutes, and when you complete it, write down what you experienced so that you can contemplate it for possible further insight. As a variation of this exercise, you can first ask a question of yourself and then see what image appears. From there, you may find yourself engaged in a dialogue between yourself and your unconscious that results in answers and solutions you did not know were possible.

When you first begin to practice mental imagery techniques, don't be discouraged if at first "nothing seems to be happening." Like any new skill, achieving results in imagery takes time. Remember that the language of your unconscious, like the symbolism of your dreams, is usually not literal or rational. It may take some time before you are able to grasp the messages of the images you perceive. Keeping a written log of your experience can make learning this new "language" easier.

BREATHWORK AND MEDITATION

The benefits of learning to breathe properly and consciously go far beyond the physical. Proper breathing can also improve your mood, make you mentally more alert, and help you to become more aware of deeply held and often painful feelings. Most importantly, by working with the breath, you can begin to heal the wounded, rejected, unacknowledged, and disowned parts of yourself and bring them into wholeness.

The primary reason so many of us breathe unconsciously and inefficiently lies in the fact that our breathing process began traumatically at birth. We were forcibly expelled from the security of the womb and compelled to take our first breath on our own when we encountered the outside world. Often that first breath came as a harsh and unexpected shock, accompanied by pain and confusion. In order to suppress such pain, newborns typically follow their first inhalation by pausing and holding their breath for a moment as they struggle to make sense of their new environment. Today, a number of researchers in the field of mental health speculate that this first pause in our breath not only sets the stage for a lifetime of shallow, inefficient breathing, but also conditions us to suppress our painful emotions, instead of learning how to accept and relax into them. You can observe this pattern in yourself the next time you find yourself feeling shock, fear, pain, or worry. If you take a moment to observe yourself in the initial experience of such emotions, more than likely you will find that you are also holding your breath or breathing very shallowly.

Breathwork, also known as *breath therapy*, is a means of learning how to breathe consciously and fully in order to deal with emotional pain more effectively and healthfully. There are many approaches to breathwork, ranging from ancient breathing techniques found in the traditions of *yoga*, *t'ai chi*, and *qigong*, to modern-day methods such as *rebirthing* (also known as *conscious connected breathing*), developed by Leonard Orr, and *holotropic breathwork*, developed by Stanislav Grof. All of them have in common a focus on the breath and the ability to move energy through the body and connect you with suppressed emotions and limiting beliefs in order to heal them.

Most breathwork therapies use the technique of connected breathing, first pioneered by Leonard Orr. In connected breathing, each inhalation immediately follows the exhalation of the preceding breath without pause. (Typically, we breathe unconsciously, pausing between inhalation and exhalation.) The pattern of respiration can vary according to the technique. Sometimes it is rapid; sometimes it is deep, slow, and full. In addition, some approaches recommend breathing in and out through the mouth, instead of the nose, and both abdominal and chest breathing can be used. In rebirthing, sometimes the therapy is performed in a tub or under water with the use of a snorkel, although this usually does not occur until after the client has had a number of "dry" connected breathing sessions and has become comfortable with the movement of energy and the integration of emotions that commonly occur during the rebirthing process. Because of the emotional release that can result from breathwork, it is advisable to learn the techniques under the direction of a skilled breath therapist. Once you gain proficiency, however, you will have at your disposal a powerful self-healing technique that you can practice daily on your own.

Meditation. There are numerous meditation techniques, but all of them can be accurately described as conscious breathing methods. Meditation's many physiological benefits include improved immune function; reduced stress, including decreased levels of adrenaline, cortisone, and free radicals; increased oxygen intake; relief from chronic pain and headache; lower blood pressure and heart rate; and a reduction of core body temperature, which has been linked to increased longevity. Among the psychological benefits of meditation are greater relaxation, improved focus on the present instead of regrets and worries about the past and future, enhanced creativity and cognitive functioning, heightened spiritual awareness (including insights leading to the healing of past emotional trauma), improved awareness and management of beliefs and emotions, and a greater compassion and recognition of others and oneself as parts of a greater whole.

The following is a simple meditation technique that utilizes breathing to promote mental calm. Select a quiet place and sit in a chair, with your back straight and your feet on the floor. Close your eyes and begin abdominal breathing, inhaling and exhaling through your nose at a rate of three to four full breaths (inhale and exhale) per minute. The object of this exercise is to stay focused on your breath, allowing whatever thoughts you have to come and go without being absorbed by them. Should you find your attention wandering, bring it back to your breath. You can also enhance the process by silently repeating a short affirmation, or a positive phrase, such as *God, love,* or *peace,* on both the inhale and the exhale. At first try to do this exercise for five minutes once or twice a day, gradually working up to 20 minutes twice daily. Don't be discouraged if at first you find this exercise difficult to practice. For most Americans, sitting and breathing without thinking or external stimulation is not easy. With time and continued practice, especially in the morning and before you go to bed, you will begin to notice the benefits meditation affords. (For more on meditation, see chapter 8.)

DREAMWORK AND JOURNALING

Dreams can play an important role in our healing journey. Serving as symbolic expressions of our inner emotional life, our dreams often provide the clues we need to better understand our mental and emotional states, as well as the guidance we may need to heal personal life situations. Dreams can also sometimes reveal how to heal physical disease conditions. This was illustrated in a dream of Alexander the Great recounted in Pliny's *Natural History.* One of Alexander's friends, Ptolemaus, was dying of a poisoned wound. Alexander dreamt of a dragon holding a plant in its mouth; the dragon said that the plant was the key to curing Ptolemaus. Upon awakening, Alexander dispatched soldiers to the place he had seen in his dream. They returned with the plant and, as the dream had predicted, Ptolemaus, as well as many others of Alexander's troops suffering from similar wounds, was cured.

In American society, dreams are often overlooked or ignored, although researchers like Stephen LaBarge, Ph.D., have in recent decades done much to scientifically demonstrate their importance. The two biggest obstacles that prevent us from getting the most benefit from our dreams are that we either do not remember or quickly forget them, or we do not know how to interpret the symbolism and imagery that dreams contain. Dream recall is a skill that anyone can develop with time and practice, however. One of the keys to dreamwork is to commit to focusing attention on your dreams. A deceptively simple way to do this is to tell yourself each night before you fall asleep that when you wake up you will remember what you dreamt during the night. At first you might not experience much success, but regular affirmation of this technique will instruct your unconscious to eventually make your dreams recallable.

As you start to remember your dreams, keep a pad and pencil or a tape recorder by your bed so that you can either write down or verbally record them immediately after you awaken. All of us dream an average of three or four times each night. With practice, many people who make the commitment to record and study their dreams are able to train themselves to spontaneously awaken after each dream cycle to record the gist of their dreams before settling back to sleep until after their next dream stage. Recording your dreams *immediately* after you awaken provides the best results, since dreams are quickly forgotten once you get out of bed and begin your day. At first, all you may recall are fragments of your dream experience. Don't be discouraged if this is the case. Over time, the regular recording of your dreams will begin to yield more details. In addition, after you have recorded your dreams for a few weeks or months, as you read over your dream diary, you will start to notice how certain symbols and events tend to recur. Pay attention to such common themes; usually they contain the most important messages that your dreams have for you.

Learning how to interpret the symbolism of your dreams takes time and practice. Certain psychotherapists, especially those with a background in Jungian theory, are skilled in dream interpretation and can help you, and a number of books on the subject can also guide you. Bear in mind, however, that your dreams are highly personal, and though many dream symbols do seem to be common to what Jung called the collective unconscious, there is no such thing as a standard for dream interpretation that will work for everyone. As the dreamer of your own life, you are ultimately the person best suited to appreciate your dreams and discern their deepest meanings. By taking the time to do so, you can improve your mental and emotional health immeasurably.

Journaling is another simple but very effective way to become more conscious of your mental and emotional life and to help you better express your feelings. Studies have also shown that it can strengthen your immune system in addition to improving physical symptoms. The practice of journaling entails keeping a written record of your thoughts, emotions, and any other daily experiences that you would like to better understand. Instead of recording your dreams, you will be keeping a journal of your waking activities. When journaling is done on a regular basis it usually results in increased self-knowledge, often with insights that are both enlightening and enlivening. In a very real sense, journaling can help you become your own therapist or best friend. Your journal becomes your own emotional diary.

Many people who begin the practice of journaling are amazed to discover how the simple act of writing out one's daily experiences can lead to sudden or deeper insights into what they are feeling. Journaling can also help you become better aware of your beliefs, providing you with the opportunity to recognize and change those that may be limiting you. As you use your journal, you will also start to take more control over what you are thinking and feeling, becoming less reactive to your life experiences and more creative in your approaches to dealing with them. Journaling also makes communicating with yourself easier and allows greater clarity, since you are free from judgment or criticism from others. Your journal is for you alone and isn't meant to be shared. Nor do you have to worry about spelling or grammar.

A number of researchers, including James W. Pennebaker, Ph.D., author of the book *Opening Up*, have documented the benefits that journaling can provide by writing about upsetting or traumatic experiences. For people who have difficulty in expressing their emotions, particularly those that are judged to be negative, such as anger, journaling can be especially valuable as a tool for self-healing. The results of a recent study measuring the effects of writing about stressful experiences on symptom reduction in patients with asthma and arthritis were published in the *Journal of the American Medical Association* in April, 1999. The subjects in the study were asked to write about the most stressful event of their lives for 20 minutes daily for 3 consecutive days. Four months later, researchers found a significant improvement in lung function in the asthmatics and a reduction in the severity of disease in the arthritics.

For best results with journaling, try to write in your journal at the same time each day. This will help you make journaling a healthy habit. Just before you go to bed can be an ideal time for journaling. You can express the emotions that you've been containing all day and can achieve resolution of the day's events prior to going to sleep. Journaling and dreamwork not only will help you to heal mentally and emotionally but can also open up new vistas of adventure that can last you a lifetime.

WORK AND PLAY

Do you enjoy your job? Does your work utilize your greatest talents? Is your job fulfilling and challenging? Sadly, for the majority of Americans the answer to these questions is no. Recent studies reveal that an alarmingly high proportion of our society—nearly 70 percent of us—do not experience satisfaction from our jobs. Unfortunately, there is a significant price to be paid, both physiologically and psychologically, for not loving your work. For example, in a study conducted by the Massachussetts Department of Health in the late 1980s, it was found that the two greatest risk factors for heart disease lie in one's self-happiness rating and one's level of job satisfaction. Low scores in these two areas were shown to be better indicators of the likelihood for developing heart disease than high cholesterol, high blood pressure, excess weight, and a sedentary lifestyle. No wonder, then, that in the United States more heart attacks occur on Monday morning around nine o'clock than at any other time of the week.

Your job is a vital aspect of your mental health. If you find yourself working at a job that you do not enjoy, chances are that you continue to do so due to one or more of the following limiting beliefs: *I don't have a choice; I need the money. I'll never be able to make enough money doing what I love. I have no idea what I'd enjoy doing or what my greatest talents are.* By using the techniques outlined in this chapter, especially in the sections "Beliefs and Affirmations" and "Discovering Your Goals," you can begin to liberate yourself from these unhealthy beliefs. You'll dis-

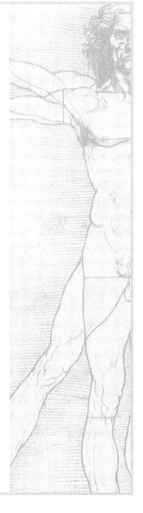

OPTIMISM AND HUMOR

In the Bible it is written, "A cheerful heart is good medicine, but a downcast spirit dries up the bones" (Proverbs 17:22). Science is now beginning to verify this ancient truth, revealing that optimism and humor are integral factors in one's overall health, providing both physical and mental benefits. One of the most famous anecdotes illustrating this point concerns Norman Cousins, who in his book *Anatomy of an Illness,* attributed his recovery from ankylosing-spondylitis (a potentially crippling arthritic condition) to the many hours he spent watching Marx Brothers movies and reruns of *Candid Camera* while taking megadoses of vitamin C. The more he laughed, the more his pain diminished, until eventually his illness completely disappeared, never to return. Based on his experience with humor, Cousins went on to explore mind/body medicine at UCLA. Today a number of institutions are studying the healing potential of humor, such as the appropriately named Gesundheit Institute in Arlington, Virginia, founded and directed by Patch Adams, M.D.

Some of the most in-depth research in this area has been conducted by Robert Ornstein, Ph.D., and David Sobel, M.D., who presented their findings in their book *Healthy Pleasures.* They discovered that the people who are optimally healthy also tend to be optimistic and happy and to possess the belief that things will work out no matter what their difficulties may be. Such people maintain a vital sense of humor about life and enjoy a good laugh, often at their own expense. According to Ornstein and Sobel, they also expect good things of life, including being liked and respected by others, and experience pleasure in most of what they do.

Optimistic people also tend to laugh a lot, something that most likely plays an important role in their health. Studies have shown that laughter can strengthen the immune system. One study, for instance, found that test subjects who watched videotapes of the comedian

(continued on next page)

cover that you are not bound to your job for life, and you do have the ability to find a job for which you are better suited and which is more fulfilling. Every one of us is blessed with at least one God-given talent, and there is at least one activity that we enjoy doing that we do quite well. *That* is where you need to begin to investigate what your gifts are. Write down your talents as outlined in the goal-setting section on page 50, followed by a list of activities you truly enjoy. Then brainstorm all the possible ways you can think of in which you could earn a living combining your talents with each of the activities you wrote down. List every idea that occurs to you, regardless of how ridiculous it might seem. As you continue to practice this exercise, you will have a much clearer idea of new job options. At the same time, acknowledge that you are seeking a greater level of fulfillment, are willing to change and take a risk, and are committed to begin the exploration that

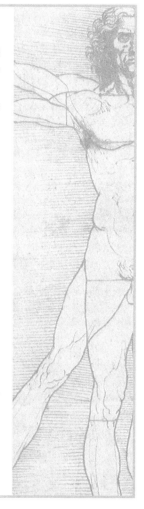

(continued from previous page)

Richard Pryor produced increased levels of antibodies in their saliva. Furthermore, subjects in the study who said they frequently used humor to cope with life stress had consistently higher baseline levels of those antibodies that help to combat infections such as colds.

Hearty laughter is actually a form of gentle exercise, or "inner jogging." Describing the physiological effects of laughter, Ornstein and Sobel write:

A robust laugh gives the muscles of your face, shoulders, diaphragm, and abdomen a good workout. With convulsive or side-splitting laughter, even your arm and leg muscles come into play. Your heart rate and blood pressure temporarily rise, breathing becomes faster and deeper, and oxygen surges through your bloodstream. A vigorous laugh can burn up as many calories per hour as brisk walking or cycling. . . . The afterglow of a hearty laugh is positively relaxing. Blood pressure may temporarily fall, your muscles go limp, and you bask in a mild euphoria. Some researchers speculate that laughter triggers the release of endorphins, the brain's own opiates; this may account for the pain relief and euphoria that accompany laughter.

In short, laughter's benefits are many and profound.

Both optimism and a sense of humor are directly related to our beliefs. If you wish to become more optimistic and experience more humor and fun in your life, practice the exercises outlined in this chapter. It may take time before you achieve the results you desire, but your commitment will prove well worth it. Nothing quite epitomizes the free flow of life force energy as laughter, and all of us can stand to laugh even more than we do. Be advised, however. There is one side effect to this powerful form of self-healing—more pleasure.

will lead you to work that you love doing. In the process, you may discover that your capabilities are limitless.

Even if you are fortunate to have a job you do enjoy, you may still be prey to another modern-day dis-ease, *workaholism*. According to the Economic Policy Institite in Washington, D.C., the majority of Americans are working longer and harder than they used to. Our yearly workload has increased by 158 hours, compared to that of 20 years ago, including longer commuting times and a reduction of paid holidays and vacation time. That's the equivalent of an extra month's work per year. To counter this tendency, it is essential that you regularly engage in the counterbalance to work—*play*.

Many of us have unfortunately relegated play to childhood, yet play is a crucial aspect of mental health and is unrivaled as a means of expressing joy, passion, exhilaration, even ecstasy. The word *play* comes from the Dutch *pleien*, which means *to dance, leap for joy, and rejoice*, all activities that suggest a vibrantly healthy mental state. Play has also been defined as any activity in which you lose track of time. Believing that play is not appropriate adult behavior is both limiting and unhealthy.

If your work involves your greatest talents and is something you truly enjoy doing, work and play for you can seem virtually indistinguishable. Even so, to optimize mental health, find at least one other activity to participate in, besides your work, that you can thoroughly enjoy. Such activities include sports, games, dance, and active creative pursuits such as playing a musical instrument, acting, singing, painting, crafts, or gardening. Although many people derive great pleasure from playing cards, chess, and other board games, or stamp or coin collecting, all of these are mental pursuits. To create a healthier balance, select activities that utilize your body, allow you to better express your feelings and creativity, and perhaps even bring you to a greater level of spiritual attunement. Ideally, the activity should be something so consuming and absorbing that it requires your total attention, providing a pleasurable escape from your normal tension, stress, and habitual thought patterns. Choose something that instinctively appeals to you and do it on a regular basis, for at least an hour three times a week. Be prepared to make mistakes and look silly. That's part of the risk, and the excitement, of doing something new. The more you commit to and practice whatever activity you choose, the better you'll become at it and the more you'll enjoy the benefits it provides.

We live in a society where work has become the greatest addiction, and the majority of us gauge our self-worth according to our achievements and financial income. For this reason alone the importance of play cannot be overemphasized. All of us, for a short time, at least, need to regularly let go of that responsible, mature, working adult part of ourselves to reconnect with our woefully neglected playful "inner child."

SUMMARY

The biggest obstacles each of us must overcome in order to achieve optimal mental health are our largely unconscious denial and repression of emotional pain and our limiting thoughts, beliefs, and attitudes, which combine to create our unhealthy behaviors. The tools in this chapter will enable you to heighten your awareness, allowing you to consciously transform your life in harmony with your greatest needs and desires. The more you practice the methods outlined here, the more profound the impact you will have on your mental health, as well as your physical health. *You will become more conscious of your behavior and gain the freedom to choose how you wish to think, feel, and behave.* By letting go of your fear of experiencing life more fully, you can embrace and be more accepting of all your thoughts, beliefs, and emotions. This will allow you the joy of realizing your life's goals and the exhilaration of the unimpeded free flow of life force energy. Remember, only through fully experiencing *both pain and joy* can you truly use your unique gifts and talents to thrive and fulfill your life purpose.

4

Healing the Spirit

*What profit does a man receive
if he gains the whole world only
to lose his soul?*
MATTHEW 16:26

**COMPONENTS OF OPTIMAL
SPIRITUAL HEALTH**

*Experience of unconditional
love/absence of fear*

Soul awareness and a
personal relationship
with God or Spirit

Trust in your intuition and
willingness to change

Gratitude

Creating a sacred space
on a regular basis through
prayer, meditation,
walking in nature,
observing a Sabbath day,
or other rituals

Sense of purpose

Being present in
every moment

THE ULTIMATE OUTCOME of healing ourselves holistically is the recognition that we are truly spiritual beings, and the heightened awareness of the transcendent power known as God or Spirit. By making the commitment to become spiritually healthy, we open ourselves to the underlying life force energy to which all religions refer, known in holistic medicine as *unconditional love.* Learning to love yourself in body, mind, and spirit is also the simplest and most effective way to learn to love God. (Most religions teach that all human beings have been created in the image of God.) To heal yourself spiritually means developing a relationship with Spirit in your own life and attuning yourself to its guidance in all aspects of your daily existence. By doing so, you will begin to experience a profound reduction in your feelings of fear and a greater capacity for loving yourself and others unconditionally. You will also become better able to identify your special talents and gifts and use them to fulfill your life's purpose, *while fully experiencing the power of the present moment.*

In the deepest sense, all *dis-ease* can be seen as a disconnection between ourselves and Spirit. From that perspective, spiritual health encompasses not only a conscious awareness of the Divine but also an intimate connection to ourselves and our families, friends, and communities. Just as mental health encompasses emotional health, spiritual health embraces social health. You cannot have one without the other. This truth is illustrated in the lives of the world's great spiritual teachers, including Moses, Jesus, Mohammed, Krishna, and Buddha, all of whom remained closely connected to their communities throughout the course of their ministry. Despite the apparent differences in their instructions to us, at their core, their messages are actually the same: *Place God first in all that you do, and love your neighbors as you love yourself.* As you reclaim your spiritual health, you fulfill their intention.

ACCESSING SPIRIT

Every advance in knowledge brings us face to face with the mystery of our own being.

MAX PLANCK,
father of quantum physics

You may believe that you are incapable of experiencing Spirit in your life, but that is not the case. *Spirit is present in any moment when we feel profoundly alive.* During these special moments, our predominant emotions are exhilaration and joy. The Jesuit priest and scientist Teilhard de Chardin described *joy* as "the most infallible sign of the presence of God." Usually, these fleeting moments surprise us: our perception of reality is suddenly free of our normal judgments and concerns. Time seems to slow as we lose ourselves in *pure awareness*. Examples of these moments include experiencing the birth of your child, time spent with your beloved, being present at the death of someone you love, witnessing a sunset, entering "the zone" while playing sports, and being in the presence of inspirational works of art. Such peak experiences can also occur unexpectedly and spontaneously during the course of your normal routine, sparked by something as innocuous as hearing your favorite song on the radio. For most of us, these moments may seem to be accidental occurrences.

The purpose of this chapter is to help make your encounters with Spirit a more frequent and conscious part of your life. As you learn to master the techniques that follow, recognize that Spirit operates in much the same fashion as sub-atomic particles—both can be identified without being directly observed. Most often, and especially at the beginning of your spiritual journey, Spirit will be identified by the traces it leaves behind as it flows through you. With time and attention, each of us can deepen our perception of Spirit in our lives. Among the ways of doing so are *prayer, meditation, gratitude, spiritual practices, reconnecting with nature*, and *working with spiritual counselors*.

Prayer

The most common form of spiritual exercise engaged in by most Americans is prayer. Nearly 90 percent of us pray, and 70 percent of us believe that prayer can lead to physical, emotional, or spiritual healing. Most people who pray have a greater sense of well-being than those who don't, and, when polled, the majority of people who pray say that through prayer they experience a sense of peace, receive answers to life issues, and have even felt divinely inspired or "led by God" to perform some specific action. Interestingly, people who experience a "sense of the Divine" during prayer also score the highest on ratings of general well-being and satisfaction with their lives.

In recent years, a great deal of scientific study has focused on the beneficial effects of prayer. Among the studies is one by the National Institute of Mental Health (NIMH) in 1994, which examined nearly three thousand North Carolini-

ARE WE SPIRITUAL BEINGS? THE NEAR DEATH EXPERIENCE

Most of us spend our lives deluded by the belief that our traits, habits, and actions are the sum total of who we are. In actuality, these characteristic behaviors only comprise our conscious personality, or the sense of self that psychology refers to as the ego. Our ego is the source of our thoughts, judgments, and comparisons, which usually are based on past experience or future concerns. Largely fear-based, the ego diverts our attention from appreciating the reality that exists in the present moment. We live most of our waking hours in this ego state, yet our true nature extends well beyond the limits of comprehension of the human intellect.

Letting go of the ego entails a surrender of mind and body that most of us equate with death. The thought of our death can be overpoweringly frightful. Yet it is also one of the surest methods for reconnecting with our true spiritual natures. Every experience we have of transcendence and Spirit is also one in which we feel exhilarated and access a dimension of being beyond body and mind. If death is the freeing of our deeper self from the physical plane, isn't it possible that it, too, can be an exhilarating experience? Certainly that is the report given by the vast majority of people who have had near death experiences. These episodes, also known as NDEs, involve people who were considered clinically dead in emergency or operating rooms, or at the scenes of accidents, and were subsequently resuscitated. In almost every case, these people report experiencing profound feelings of peace and unconditional love, as well as a reluctance to leave the spiritual dimension to return to their bodies.

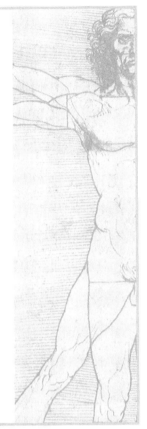

(continued on next page)

ans and found that those who attended church weekly had 29 percent less risk of alcoholism than those who attended less frequently. In the same study, the risk of alcoholism decreased by 42 percent among those who prayed and read the Bible regularly. Another NIMH study conducted in the same year found that frequent churchgoers also had lower rates of depression and other mental problems.

A survey of 212 medical studies examining the relationship between religious beliefs and health by Dale Matthews, M.D., associate professor of medicine at Georgetown University, found that 75 percent of the studies showed health benefits for those patients with "religious commitments." Among patients with hypertension, regular prayer reduced blood pressure in 50 percent of all cases.

Among the pioneers in the study of the physiological effects of prayer and meditation is Herbert Benson, M.D., a Harvard cardiologist. In 1968, Benson began studying people who regularly practiced transcendental meditation (TM). The subjects meditated by focusing on a mantra, such as *Om*, that had no apparent meaning to its user. Benson discovered that repetition of the mantra resulted

(continued from previous page)

The consistency of the reports of NDEs confirms the observation of many physicians and researchers who have scientifically studied the phenomena of death and dying that the soul (the individualized expression of Spirit) remains intact beyond the death of the body. One of the leaders in this field, known as thanatology, is Elisabeth Kübler-Ross, M.D., who pioneered this investigation for most of her professional career. After nearly thirty years of scientific research, she has concluded, "Death does not exist . . . all that dies is a physical shell housing an immortal spirit." She also describes the time that we spend on earth as but a brief part of our total existence, and that *to live well while we are here means to learn to love*— which is an active recognition, engagement, and appreciation of Spirit in ourselves and others. In one of her studies of over two hundred people who had experienced a near death experience, almost all reported that they went before God and were asked the question: "How have you expanded your ability to give and receive love while you were down there?"

Whether or not you choose to believe the data being gathered in the fields of thanatology and NDEs, there is mounting evidence strongly suggesting the existence of Spirit beyond the realms of mind and body. Choosing to believe this theory can heighten your creativity, enhance your healing capacity, free you to realize your life's purpose, diminish the level of fear in your life, and release the self-imposed limitations of past traumas. By becoming aware of that part of yourself that does not die, you will be better able to take risks and pursue the dreams of your life.

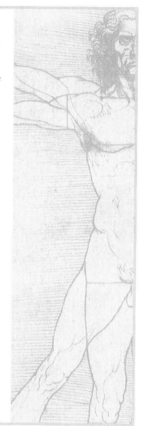

in a lower metabolic rate, slower heart rate, lower blood pressure, and slower breathing. He dubbed this physiological effect the *relaxation response*. Benson then turned his attention to Christians and Jews who prayed instead of meditating, instructing them to repeat religious phrases such as the first line of the Lord's Prayer, "Hail Mary, full of grace," "The Lord is my shepherd," or "Shalom." He found that the phrases all produced the same relaxation response that is triggered by meditation, and that the degree of physiological benefit is determined by the degree of faith on the part of the person praying.

Since 1988, Benson and psychologist Jared Klass have been conducting a series of programs at the Mind/Body Medical Institute at New England Deaconess Hospital, inviting priests, rabbis, and ministers to investigate the spiritual and health implications of prayer. In their studies, a psychological scale developed by Benson and Klass for measuring spirituality is employed. People scoring high in spirituality—defined by Benson as a feeling that "there is more than just you" and as not necessarily religious—score higher in psychological health. They also:

- Were less likely to get sick, and were better able to cope if they did
- Had fewer stress-related symptoms
- Gained the most from meditation training
- Showed the greatest rise on a life-purpose index
- Exhibited the sharpest drop in pain

To begin the practice of prayer, start with any prayer you are comfortable with or recall from your religious training as a child. You can also use a favorite psalm or passage from the Bible or prayer book you find especially meaningful. In addition, you can engage in personal prayer, talking to God as if you were speaking to your best friend. State your need or concern and ask for God's help. (It is more effective to pray for the peace that would result from having what you desire, than for the specific things themselves.) Whichever form of prayer you choose, try to establish a regular routine and repeat your prayer morning and night.

Meditation

In the West, meditation has primarily been studied for its mental, emotional, and physiological benefits, while in the East it has primarily been used for thousands of years to still the mind in order to contact Spirit. During meditation, practitioners enter into a neutral emotional state, becoming a witness to their passing thoughts and feelings as they move into a state of heightened attention that can ultimately result in pure awareness.

As with prayer, there are many ways to meditate. Meditation can be performed while sitting or in a supine position, or while on the move—walking, jogging, and even during sports. What all forms of meditation have in common is a focusing on the breath and an emptying of the mind of thought. With regular practice, meditators typically report increased feelings of calm and peace, improved mental functioning and enhanced powers of concentration, and a deeper connection to Spirit, which is often perceived as a quiet, inner voice guiding them in their actions. Other reported benefits include increased equanimity toward, and detachment from, life events; increased energy and joy; feelings of bliss and ecstasy; and increased dream recall.

Ideally, it is best to learn meditation under the guidance of a qualified instructor, but a variety of books and audiotapes are also available on the subject. The simplest method of meditation is to sit in a quiet place, resting comfortably in a chair, with your spine erect and your feet flat on the floor. Close your eyes and begin focusing on your breathing, keeping your awareness on each inhalation and exhalation. To improve your concentration, you may wish to silently repeat the word *in* as you inhale, and *out* as you exhale. Or you can repeat a word or mantra, such as *love, peace, God, Om,* or *Hu* (the latter two are names for the Divine). Allow your thoughts to come and go, without lingering on them, as if your awareness is a running stream and your thoughts are simply leaves floating by. At first, it may seem as if you are deluged with thoughts. Each time you find yourself distracted, simply bring your attention back to your breathing. Eventually, you may notice longer periods of silence between each thought. It may take months to quiet your mind to this extent, but with consistent practice your meditation *will* become deeper and easier. Try to sit for at least ten minutes once or twice a day, gradually working up to two half-hour sessions per day. It's important to keep your practice regular and consistent, but don't force things. If you find yourself too distracted or pressed for time, end your session until the next time, instead of sitting rest-lessly.

Walking meditation is another form of meditation, which in recent years has been popularized by the Buddhist monk Thich Nhat Hanh. This form of medita-tion is often suited for active people who find it difficult to sit still. The goal is to focus your attention in the present by focusing on each step you take in tandem with your breathing. To enhance your experience, you can mentally repeat: *With each step I take I am fully present to my surroundings.* Over time, as you practice this form of meditation, don't be surprised if you find it becomes more difficult to hurry. The more you focus on the present, the less consequence time has, as you discover how profound even a simple act such as walking can be.

Gratitude

Most religious traditions prescribe specific prayers or grace before meals as a way of thanking God for our food and sustenance. As with other spiritual practices, there is something to be gained from these rituals, or they wouldn't have survived for thousands of years. A sense of gratitude for all the other areas of our lives can elicit similar life-enhancing benefits.

Gratitude has been described as the Great Attitude. Although most of us tend to take our lives for granted, they are in fact a gift, and every day that we are alive each of us receives many blessings. Even times of pain and adversity can be seen as opportunities for growth for which we can be grateful. By committing our-selves to becoming more aware of our blessings, we strengthen our connection with Spirit and are able to better recognize the wisdom and intelligence that un-derlies all of creation. Once we allow ourselves to appreciate the lessons presented during times of struggle or life crises, the brunt of the pain subsides and a state of inner peace follows. This is especially true of most chronic diseases, which can be

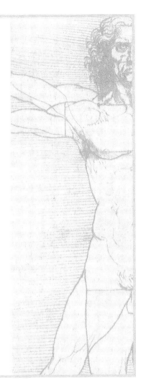

INTUITION

As you progress in your healing journey, eventually you will find yourself being guided by your intuition, which is often experienced as an "inner nudge" or a "still, quiet voice" speaking from within. If you are not already aware of your intuitive messages, most likely it is because your intuition is having a tough time competing for your attention. Most of the inner messages you hear come from your ego and tend to be loud, self-centered, and fear-based. Intuitive messages, by contrast, come from the heart and are usually more subtle, compassionate, and enlivening.

In order to develop your sense of intuition, you will need to slow down, eliminate distractions, and do a lot less talking. The methods provided in this chapter can help you to do so. Slow, relaxing walks are another helpful way to make contact with this inner guidance. The next step is learning to recognize when your intuition is truly speaking to you and when it is not. Learning to discern the difference requires practice. One useful method for determining whether the "voice" you hear is indeed your intuition is to notice how it feels. Often intuitive messages occur accompanied by feelings of excitement or an unequivocal sense that acting upon them is "the right thing to do." People who haven't learned to trust their intuition often experience doubts or fears immediately following such feelings. "How can I be

(continued on next page)

seen as external reflections of inner (emotional and/or spiritual) pain. Typically, when people choose to consciously focus on the positives in their lives and express gratitude for them, more positive things start to happen.

Gratitude can produce powerful feelings of joy and self-acceptance, and is an attitude that anyone can choose to have, just as you can choose to see the glass half full or half empty. By focusing on what you do have, instead of what you lack, you feel a sense of abundance that makes your problems seem much less acute, and you are better able to let go of negative thoughts and attitudes. This usually isn't easy to do, especially if you are feeling a great deal of fear or anger. But if you make the effort to release these painful emotions and to *choose the attitude of gratitude*, even for a moment, wonderful things can happen.

Like any habit, that of recognizing and acknowledging the gifts in your life requires practice. One simple way to begin feeling grateful is the following visualization taught by Rabbi Mordecai Twerski, the spiritual leader of Denver's Hassidic community. As soon as you wake up each morning, before you get out of bed, close your eyes and picture a person, scene, or situation that made you happy to be alive and for which you are still grateful. You never would have had that experience if you weren't alive, and by allowing yourself to reexperience it you open yourself up to the awareness that something equally wonderful can happen today.

(continued from previous page)

sure this is true?" "What if I'm wrong?" These and similar questions can quickly quash your inner guidance if you haven't learned to trust it.

To help you know if the messages you receive are in your best interest, experiment with the following exercise. Out loud, tell yourself something that you know to be true. As you do so, notice how you feel. Now state aloud something you know to be false. Again notice how you feel. Usually people practicing this exercise experience feelings of discomfort, confusion, even pain, in their bodies when they make the false statement, whereas they feel in alignment with the statement that is true. (Often the sensations occur in the area of the solar plexus, with false statements provoking queasy feelings or tension.)

Allowing yourself to be guided by your intuition is ultimately an act of faith. At first, learning to trust and act on the intuitive messages you receive will involve risk. The more trust you bring to your practice, however, the easier it will be to take action. Realize, too, that sometimes the results of following your intuition might be painful. Such times are not necessarily mistakes. They can be seen as lessons teaching you how to listen more effectively. Or they may be necessary to facilitate your growth and help you to better understand the higher purpose toward which Spirit is guiding you.

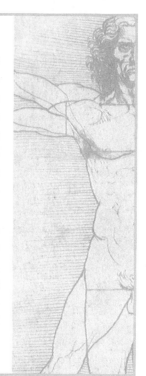

Create the habit of practicing this visualization each morning upon awakening and you will soon instill in yourself a new attitude of anticipation and appreciation for the day ahead.

Another way to cultivate feelings of gratitude is by making a *gratitude list*. This exercise is best performed before going to bed, as a way to detach from any concerns or problems you may have in order to appreciate the gifts and lessons that came your way during the day. Some people prefer to write out their list, others simply close their eyes and mentally review their day, making themselves aware of all the things that happened for which they feel grateful. Either way works well. Complete the exercise by praying silently, giving thanks for all that you experienced and learned that day.

By making gratitude a regular part of your daily experience, you set the stage for living more deeply connected to Spirit. In the process, your life will be transformed into an increasingly joyous adventure.

Spiritual Practices

Most of us have some sort of spiritual orientation, even if it is no more than rituals we were taught in childhood. Yet we often fail to realize how much some of these practices can contribute to our health. The ritual observance of Sabbath or

SPIRITUAL COUNSELORS

Due to the many uncertainties that can be part of the spiritual journey, you may consider working with a spiritual counselor, especially if you haven't been in the habit of listening to your intuition or need help in "tuning in" to Spirit. Just as you would visit a doctor to heal your physical body, or a psychotherapist to heal mental and emotional issues, spiritual counselors can help connect you to your spiritual core. The most common resources for spiritual counseling are priests, rabbis, ministers, and other clergy. Spiritual psychotherapists, medical intuitives, clairvoyants, and spiritual healers or shamans can also be of assistance. What these healers have in common is an ability to see beyond the boundaries of the five senses. Their services may include helping you to identify your life purpose, pointing out opportunities for your spiritual growth, or scanning your body's bioenergy field to diagnose the underlying cause of a particular health condition. Their primary value, however, lies in the assistance they can provide in helping you appreciate the meaning and lessons of your daily life.

Because of the lack of certification in these areas, to find a spiritual counselor you may need to rely on references from people you trust, experience some trial and error, and call upon your own intuition. Keep an open mind and see how you respond to the information provided. Some of these counselors are truly gifted and can provide you with information that can be a catalyst for transforming your life.

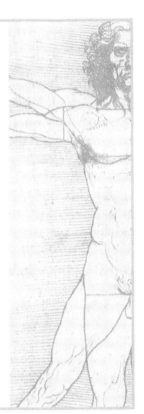

Sunday worship, for instance, can be an enormously healing experience. It is also a particularly good time to practice gratitude as you contemplate the blessings you share with those you love. Studies also reveal that those who regularly observe a weekly holy day tend to score higher in areas of optimism, stress management, and general well-being.

Fasting is another spiritual practice that is also healing. Not only can fasting have a cleansing effect on the body, eliminating toxins while giving the organs of digestion and assimilation a rest, it can also elicit a heightened feeling of spirituality and result in the healing of old emotional wounds. In his book *Live Better Longer*, Joseph Dispenza, director of the Parcells Center in Santa Fe, New Mexico, points out that fasting can purge the emotional body of old, toxic feelings, facilitate the release of psychological patterns that no longer work for you, and "open your mind and heart to new emotional, psychological, and spiritual sustenance." (The Parcells Center is based on the work of Hazel Parcells, Ph.D., a scientist and naturopathic physician who, at 41, cured herself of terminal tuberculosis using fasts and other natural methods. She went on to live a life of vibrant, robust health until she died peacefully in her sleep at age 106.)

If you are new to fasting, try a 24-hour fast, selecting a day when work and other responsibilities are limited and you won't be too active. Plan for some quiet time alone, and during the final two hours of the fast, drink six to eight glasses of water to help cleanse your body of toxins. (For more on fasting, see chapter 5.)

Gabriel Cousens, M.D., director of the Tree of Life Rejuvenation Center in Patagonia, Arizona, has had great success in treating a variety of diseases, including arthritis, diabetes, alcholism, and asthma with fasting and meditation.

The potential that spiritual practices have to heal is illustrated in the case of one of Dr. Anderson's patients, a 64-year-old woman named Lois, who had undergone the surgical removal of a very large, aggressive ovarian cancer. The procedure left her with a colostomy, and part of the original tumor was not removable, leaving hundreds of small metastases throughout her abdominal cavity. On Dr. Anderson's insistence, Lois agreed to consult with an oncologist, only to promptly reject his recommendation of chemotherapy, despite the fact that remnants of her tumor remained in her pelvis and abdomen. She was convinced that her condition would be cured by her own body with God's help, and returned to Dr. Anderson for aid in getting well. Although she undertook many initiatives, central to her program was her faith in the power of prayer and God. Each day she meditated for up to an hour and prayed numerous times.

Four months later, Lois was finally able to persuade her surgeon to remove the colostomy to restore her internal bowel function. During the course of a long and tedious surgery, hundreds of small, metastasized tumors appeared as before. Seven of them were biopsied. Three days later, the pathology report showed that their cancerous characteristics were gone. Lois fully recovered and resumed an active life focused around the activities she enjoyed and her continued prayers to God. Two years later, an operation to repair an abdominal hernia revealed that her abdomen and pelvis were completely normal, with no residual cancer anywhere. Though he has no way of proving it, Dr. Anderson remains convinced that Lois's daily prayers and meditations were somehow central to her recovery.

Finding Spirit in Nature

Nowhere is the creative power of Spirit more visible than in nature. It is there that we most directly experience life's four elemental forms of energy: earth, water, fire, and air. Earth is matter in its deepest form; water represents the receptive yielding principle; fire is the transformational energy that causes matter to change form; and air is the resultant blend of these other three elements into a subtler vibration of life force energy. In our bodies, earth is cellular matter, water is blood and circulation, fire is metabolism and energy production, and air is oxygen, the nutrient most essential for our sustenance. By regularly exposing yourself to nature's four elements—ideally on a daily basis—you will expand your awareness of how each of them is uniquely embodied within you. Here are ways for you to do so.

Earth. Spend as much time as possible outdoors in close contact with the earth. Walking is a wonderful way to do this, as are outdoor sports, bike rides in a park, and gardening. When you can, also visit the beach, woods, and mountains, and take time to notice the beauty surrounding you. The more time you spend immersed in nature, the more aware you will become of life's natural rhythms, and the ways the earth retains and radiates energy.

Most of us, however, live in urban settings and are relatively detached from the natural world. Making the effort to spend time in nature can go a long way toward restoring more balance in your life, while deepening your connection with Spirit at the same time.

Water. One of the most visible forms of Spirit in nature is the flow of water as it follows the contours of the earth. Water is a receptive form of energy and is affected by the forces acting on it. Rivers flow, for example, because of the gravitational pull caused by the gradient of the landscape. The action of water tumbling over rocks also releases a more subtle energy in the form of negative ions, which can contribute to feelings of well-being. Swimming in the ocean, lakes, or rivers provides invaluable exposure to this special form of energy. Soaking in a mineral hot spring can also provide therapeutic benefits for a variety of ailments, as well as being one of life's great pleasures.

A healthy routine that anyone can adopt is bathing in warm water at least once a day. For added benefit, practice conscious breathing while you enjoy a soak in the tub. This is a very effective way to connect with your body's bioenergy field and can help heal mental and emotional upset.

Fire. Throughout the Bible and other sacred scriptures, the dominant symbols of the divine essence in human beings is fire and light, such as the tale of Moses speaking to God in the burning bush, or the transfiguration of Jesus on the mountaintop before his closest apostles. Candlelight is also common as a tool for spiritual focus in most religions. Anyone who has experienced the pleasures of an open campfire can attest to the healing properties of fire. According to Leonard Orr, the founder of Rebirthing, spending time before an open fire, including a fireplace, cleanses the bioenergy field of negative energies and can be a powerful aid in curing physical disease. Orr recommends spending a few hours each day before fire for people who want to experience such benefits.

Fire is also an important component of the vision quests employed by Native Americans as a means of connecting to Spirit and discerning their life purpose. The ultimate source of fire energy is the sun, which provides healing and creative energy that directly or indirectly gives life to all living organisms. Regular exposure to sunlight has been linked to a variety of mental and emotional benefits, while depression, anxiety, and other mental dis-ease can occur when we are deprived of the sun's healing rays. Time spent daily in the sun is a very healthy practice, as long as appropriate precautions are taken, including sunscreen, hats, and long sleeves and pants when needed.

Air. Of the four elements, air is perhaps the closest expression of Spirit, so much so that the ancient Greeks equated Spirit (*pneuma*) with the wind. The most potent method of imbuing yourself with the life force energy of air is through the conscious breathing methods outlined in chapter 5. A daily practice of these methods can significantly energize you, open you up to new levels of creativity and productivity, and make you more aware of Spirit's guidance and power flowing through you.

SOCIAL HEALTH

No man is an island.

JOHN DONNE

COMPONENTS OF OPTIMAL SOCIAL HEALTH
Intimacy with a spouse or partner, relative, or close friend
Forgiveness
Sense of belonging to a support group or community
Touch and/or physical intimacy on a daily basis
Selflessness and altruism

Our relationship with others is the crucible that most determines how spiritually healthy we are. Optimal *social health* consists of a strong positive connection to others in community and family, and intimacy with one or more people. It is often much easier to feel our connection with Spirit during moments of solitude than it is to express that connection through our interactions with others. At the same time, our relationships offer us the greatest opportunities for spiritual growth and for learning how to receive and impart unconditional love. *True spiritual health is a balance between the autonomy of the self and intimacy with others.*

The importance of social relationships with respect to health is documented in a growing number of studies demonstrating the benefits of the diversity and depth of connection to community, family, and spouse. Lack of healthy social relationships is a common denominator among patients with heart disease, particularly when accompanied by feelings of hostility and a sense of isolation. Conversely, the longevity of terminal cancer patients with long-term survival rates has been attributed to a relatively high degree of social involvement. One of the most convincing studies highlighting the importance of community showed that Hispanics, despite poverty, lack of health insurance, and poor access to medical care, are surprisingly less likely than whites to die of major chronic diseases, including all forms of cancer, heart disease, and respiratory ailments. Further, with the exception of diabetes, liver disease, and homicide, their overall health outlook is significantly better than for whites. Some health experts, including former Surgeon General Coello Novello, the first Latina to serve in that post, postulate that the reason for this stems from Hispanic culture, which promotes strong family values and frowns on health risks such as drinking and smoking. Based on a growing number of relationship studies, researchers have concluded that *social isolation is statistically just as dangerous as smoking, high blood pressure, high cholesterol, obesity, or lack of exercise.*

The primary opportunities available to each of us for improving our social health include forgiveness, friendships, selfless acts and altruism, support groups, and especially marriage, committed relationships, and parenting.

Forgiveness

To err is human; to forgive, divine. ALEXANDER POPE

Intimate relationships and unconditional love cannot exist without forgiveness. How often do you blame yourself for your past actions and mistakes? How often do you blame others for your own problems, stress, or slights (both real and imagined) against you? Forgiveness cancels the demands that you or others *should* have done things differently. Hanging on to these demands changes nothing but keeps us under stress. Refusing to forgive yourself or others keeps you locked into limiting patterns from your past, unable to mobilize the creative power in your life here and now.

The next time you find yourself blaming others, physically point your index finger at them or their images and take a look at where the other three fingers of your hand are pointed. Right back at you! Forgiveness, therefore, begins with accepting responsibility for the role you play in shaping your life's experiences. Only after you begin to forgive yourself can you truly forgive others.

A key first step in your journey of forgiveness is the recognition that you are always doing the best you can at any given moment, in accordance with your awareness at the time. This is true of everyone else as well. All of us make mistakes, and all of us ideally learn from them. You may even choose to believe that there are no mistakes, only lessons. In that moment, your action or behavior was based on past experience, environment, and heredity. You can, however, consciously choose to be different in the future. To continue to blame yourself or someone else for something that occurred in the past is energy depleting and keeps you from moving forward with your life.

Forgiving yourself may be your greatest challenge. No doubt there are a number of things in your past that you regret or for which you feel shame. But wouldn't it be healthier to look at what you can learn from your mistake or painful lesson so that it's not repeated; forgive yourself unconditionally for not knowing more or not performing well enough; and be grateful for this opportunity to learn to do better or change your behavior? A tennis player who misses a shot he thinks he should have made will lose his confidence and ultimately his match if he doesn't quickly recognize what he did wrong, forgive himself, and move on to play the next point. Similarly, we lose the ability to focus and to do as well as we know we are capable of in the present if we do not forgive ourselves and let go of the past.

The more you are able to do this for yourself, the better you will be able to forgive others. *Remember that you are forgiving the actor, not the action.* You are not condoning cruelty, insensitivity, or incompetence; you are forgiving the offending person. By doing so, you are freeing yourself to move out of the past into the healing present. Anger is the problem, forgiveness is the solution.

Bear in mind that the people you decide to forgive may not choose to accept your forgiveness. Though their refusal to do so can be hurtful, their choice should be respected. What matters is that you are taking the step to heal the relationship. The act of forgiveness takes place within your own psyche, and the person you are forgiving may therefore be totally unaware of your action. Or you may be forgiving someone who is deceased. Be realistic and don't set your sights too high—begin with someone who has been critical of you or guilty of another relatively minor offense. Forgiving others does not necessarily mean that your relationship with them will change, but forgiving them will enable you to feel a greater sense of wholeness. Although your relationship with the people you forgive may remain the same on the surface, it doesn't mean that healing hasn't taken place. You will know it when you feel it.

Friendship

A 1997 study conducted at Carnegie Mellon University in Pittsburgh found that people with a greater diversity of relationships were less likely to get colds. Those with six or more social ties (family, friends, coworkers, neighbors, etc.) were four times *less* susceptible to colds than those with one to three types of relationships. Researchers found that it was not the amount of people in the social network that was the important factor, but the diversity. To varying degrees, most of these types of relationships can be called *friendships*.

As children and teenagers, most of us had a number of friends with whom we enjoyed sharing the day's adventures. Our friends helped us meet such challenges as each new year at school, sports, puberty, dating, family problems, and the existential concerns through which all of us passed during our journey into adulthood. Between kindergarten and college, sustaining friendships was made easier by the fact that our friends provided us with a sense of belonging, a feeling of "being in this together," and offered us a forum in which to mutually discuss the problems and issues we faced at the time. Because of such friendships, many people regard the times they spent in high school and college as the happiest days of their lives. Once past college, as they have entered the workforce, got married, and juggled the responsibilities of their careers and families, a large segment of people in our society have lost track of their friends from the past and have not replaced them with new friends.

While most adults enjoy the company of neighbors, coworkers, and other acquaintances, by the time we reach our thirties, studies reveal, those of us who still have a best friend in whom we can confide are exceptionally rare. This is particularly true of men, who, because of this lack of a confidant, experience feelings of isolation and absence of support, no matter how fulfilled they may otherwise be in their personal lives and careers.

If you find yourself in need of a good friend, realize that it's never too late to rekindle old friendships or to make new ones. All that is required is a willingness to take risks and make the effort. Having a close friend you can talk to from your heart can provide many additional blessings in your life and deepen your connection with Spirit.

Selfless Acts and Altruism

Remember a time when you stopped to spontaneously help someone, either a friend or total stranger. Such selfless acts of giving go to the essence of Spirit, which is always with us supporting our lives while asking for nothing in return. Sharing with others your time, help, and special gifts and talents in ways that benefit them provides you with perhaps the most powerful means of engaging and expressing Spirit and enhancing social health. The opportunities for sharing are abundant and might include donating clothes or money to worthy charities, volunteering time at a homeless shelter, soup kitchen, or afterschool tutoring program, or simply setting aside our own tasks and concerns to address the needs of our spouses or children. (There is a great deal of truth in the adage "Charity begins at home.") Another form of sharing that is regaining popularity is *tithing*. Dating back to biblical times, tithing is the practice of donating a certain percentage (usually 5 to 10 percent) of one's yearly income to charity. Interestingly, many people who adopt the practice of tithing also find that their incomes actually begin to increase, although that should not be your motivation for doing so. However you choose to perform selfless acts, remember that the truest form of giving is one that does not call attention to the giver. As Jesus instructed in the Gospel of Matthew, "When you give to the needy, do not announce it with trumpets." The purpose of sharing is *to share*, not to acquire praise or honors. Sharing selflessly will deepen your awareness of how abundantly Spirit is giving to you.

The late Hans Selye, a pioneer in modern stress research, thought that by helping people you earn their gratitude and affection and that the warmth that results protects against stress. Today, Selye's belief is borne out by mounting evidence that selfless acts not only feel good but are healthy. Epidemiologist James

House and his colleagues at the University of Michigan's Survey Research Center studied more than 2,700 men in Tecumseh, Michigan, for almost 14 years to see how social relationships affected mortality rates. Those who did regular volunteer work had death rates two and one-half times lower than those who didn't. It may well be that the highest form of selfishness is selflessness. When we freely choose to help others, we seem to get as much, or more, than what we give.

The closer our contact with those we help, the greater the benefits seem to be. Most of us need to feel that we matter to someone, a need that volunteer work can fulfill. There are a growing number of people requiring help in our society, including the homeless, the elderly, the hungry, runaways, orphans, and the illiterate, and there are many ways to help them. Choose to do so in the way that most compels you, but recognize that altruism works best when it comes from the heart and is not calculated as a means to receive something in return.

Support Groups

As a society we are plagued by social ills, most notably divorce rates that top 50 percent, a general sentiment of feeling overworked, dual-career marriages, an increasing number of single-parent families, and a generation of children more adrift and alone than any that has preceded them. At the same time, a movement is afoot in America toward a greater sense of community in response to the silent epidemic of isolation that affects so many of us; there has been a significant increase in support groups for those sharing common values, experiences, and goals. Support groups for couples, divorcees, single parents, men, women, people with an illness in common (especially cancer), and a large number of people recovering from alcohol and drug addiction, and other addictions, are gathering all over the country. Many of them are affiliated with a church or synagogue, with the added purpose of enhancing spiritual growth. They meet regularly—every week, every other week, or every month—and the participants by and large report that they benefit from the social connection they find there. If you would like to participate in such a group, most likely you can find them in your local Yellow Pages, or you can contact organizations such as your local United Way, Catholic Charities, or AA group. Many communities also have support groups devoted to specific diseases. Such groups can also be found on the Internet.

Recent research also verifies that support groups can play an important role in helping people with chronic disease. David Spiegel, M.D., conducted a study at Stanford University School of Medicine on women with metastatic breast cancer. All the women received chemotherapy or radiation therapy. Half of them were in a support group that met weekly for one year. These women lived twice as long as those who were not in a support group, and three of them were still alive ten years later.

Committed Relationships and Marriage

Healthy committed relationships promote physical, emotional, and especially spiritual well-being through the experience of unconditional love. The model for all committed relationships is marriage, usually the most challenging as well as most rewarding of all interpersonal relationships. It is potentially our most powerful spiritual practice. If humanity's fundamental moral principle is to "love thy neighbor as thyself," its practice begins not with the person living next door but with the neighbor with whom we share our bed.

Regardless of who your partner may be or how long you have been involved with him or her, the key to all committed relationships is *intimacy*. Think of intimacy as *into-me-see*. As you develop the skills for seeing into, and learning to appreciate, yourself, you have the opportunity to also "see into" your partner and to allow your partner to see into you. Once a commitment is made, the relationship becomes greater than the sum of its parts, allowing both partners to flourish and realize their full potential as human beings. The transformation that can occur in marriage and other committed relationships is primarily a result of letting go of judgment. As you do so, you will realize that in giving more to the relationship you are ultimately giving to yourself. Studies have shown that you might otherwise be contributing to making yourself and your partner sick. Marital conflict lowers immune function, especially in women, according to researchers at Ohio State University.

Hallmarks of a healthy committed relationship include having a shared vision, attentive listening to each other, the freedom to make requests so that both partners can better ensure that their needs are met, and regular intervals of fun and recreation together. Discussion of these practices follows. If you are interested in making a deeper commitment to your relationship, you might also consider working with a good marriage counselor or other relationship teacher.

Shared vision. A vision that you share with your partner is a way of defining your mutual goals and focusing your energy on their attainment. Lack of a vision can cause your relationship to lose direction or become stagnant. One simple but effective way to create a shared vision with your spouse or partner is to take time to individually list your relationship goals (keep them positive, short, descriptive, specific), prioritizing them in numerical order. Then begin combining lists, starting with the goals that have the highest value and alternating between the two lists to form a composite vision that you and your partner are both comfortable with. The resulting *mutual relationship vision* can help keep you and your partner working together toward your common goals, while reducing conflict and enhancing your relationship.

Attentive listening. Most of us are poor listeners. We *hear* what is being said, but we don't always *listen* to it. This is because hearing can be unconscious while listening requires conscious effort. Since communication is the foundation of any relationship, and listening is a critical aspect of effective communication, it is important to get in the habit of consciously paying attention to what your partner tells you *without responding immediately.* The practice of listening can greatly enhance both intimacy and autonomy. This type of listening can be practiced as a "listening exercise." Schedule an uninterrupted 40-minute block of time in which both you and your partner speak for 20 minutes while the other person listens *without responding.* Talk only about yourself and how you're feeling, without blaming or talking about your relationship issues. There is no discussion following the exercise.

Attentive listening makes it possible for both partners to be able to talk freely and express thoughts and feelings without worrying about judgment or criticism. Focusing on what your partner is saying requires you to empty your mind of your own thoughts and concerns as you listen, thereby minimizing negative reactions. This exercise allows for a balance between intimacy and autonomy, a critical component of healthy relationships. Cultivating the habit of attentive listening will help you and your partner create a safe environment for expressing your feelings, allowing you to be more vulnerable and open with each other, which is extremely valuable for building trust, understanding, and deeper, even exhilarating, feelings of intimacy.

Requests. By committing to another person, you enter into a relationship in which you have promised to give and receive love. But since each of us is different, what feels like love to one person might not even be noticed by another. Most of us attempt to love our partners in ways that feel like love to *us* and are surprised when they do not react as we would. A good method for eliminating this problem is simply to tell each other what feels good to you and what you want.

It can be quite a revelation when someone you thought you knew well tells you what they really *need* from you. We often expect our partners to be able to read our minds, but we really can't know what each other wants unless we are told. Refrain from general statements such as "Love me" or "Be nice to me." Making specific requests like "I would like you to buy me flowers once a week" or "I would like you to cook dinner once a week" will significantly improve the likelihood that you will get what you need. When you do, be sure to thank your partner for complying with your request. This is extremely important, since your request is usually not an easy or natural thing for your partner to do. Otherwise you probably wouldn't have had to ask for it in the first place.

Having fun together. Life's daily pressures and responsibilities make it difficult to remember to have fun. For many couples, the glue that reinforces their relationship is the memory of the enjoyment they shared during their courtship and early years together. Setting aside time that you and your partner can spend in recreation together is an important way to *re-create* the joy and spontaneity that first brought you together. To rekindle some of that excitement and minimize the risk of boring routines, it helps to schedule fun activities together on a regular basis. Plan to spend at least half a day each week together away from home, taking turns each time to choose your activity. Getting out of the house, alone together, can help you focus attention on each other. Although this is more difficult to do if you have young children, it is still possible to plan an exciting evening at home after they go to bed. Choose something neither of you has tried before to add another dimension of adventure to your play, and if you can manage it, plan several weekends per year out of town. This can be especially rewarding if a real vacation isn't feasible. Having fun regularly with the person you love is refreshing and invigorating and can help ensure that your relationship remains healthy and fulfilling.

Parenting

Parenting is easily one of life's most enriching experiences, and at the same time, one of our most challenging jobs. Through their children, parents have the opportunity to reconnect with play, to feel more in touch with their own "inner child," to experience selflessness, and to learn how to love unconditionally. Those of us who are parents are also provided with a wonderful forum for practicing forgiveness, trust, acceptance of ourselves and others, self-awareness, and most of all, patience (as any parent of a teenager well knows). Perhaps the greatest human expression of love is that of parents for their children.

Unfortunately, in our society parenting isn't always consciously approached. If you are already a parent, however, it is not too late to meet your parental obligations more consciously than you may currently be doing. One useful guideline is to regularly ask yourself: *Will this (action, response, activity, demand) of mine help my child's self-esteem?* The same principle holds true in parenting as it does in marriage: *To love another is to help that person better love him- or herself.* This commitment not only will affect your child's happiness in the present, but will significantly impact his or her future health. In the landmark Harvard Mastery of Stress Study, college students rated their parents on their level of parental caring. Thirty-five years later, 87 percent of those who rated both parents low on parental love suffered from a chronic illness, whereas only 25 percent of those who rated both parents high in caring had a disease.

In the field of family therapy, the family is usually seen as a "system." This view holds that if a family member's behavior is harmful to himself or others, the

SEX

Of all the major world religions, the Judeo-Christian tradition is the only one that does not commonly recognize the potential that sex has as a pathway to Spirit. Other religions, including Hinduism, Buddhism, Islam, and Taoism, as well as the spiritual traditions of Africa and the Amerindians, freely acknowledge that sex, properly entered into, can be a powerful spiritual experience capable of transforming consciousness and enhancing physical and emotional health. In the West, perhaps the most well-known of these teachings on sex is *tantra*. This is an ancient system of sexual and sensual techniques for consciously controlling the mind, increasing life force energy, and tapping into Spirit. Tantra's erotic practices include specific positions, breath, and visualization to heighten sexual energy and move it upward along the spine in order to create rapturous waves of blissful energy that can ultimately lead to enlightenment. Many mystic writings, such as the verse of the Sufi poet-saint Rumi, also refer to the Divine using the language of sex and romantic love, often equating God with the Beloved while yearning to experience union with the Absolute.

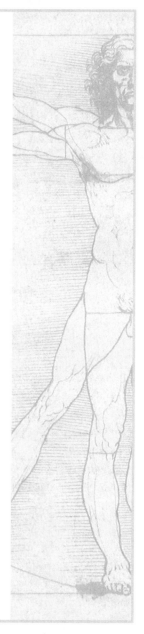

To experience sex from this exalted perspective requires expanding your focus beyond physical gratification and genital orgasm into an experience of yourself and your spouse or lover as expressions of Spirit-in-the-flesh. Adopting this attitude leaves you extremely vulnerable and simultaneously in touch with your own divine power. Lovemaking in this state is free of the machinations of ego and proceeds slowly, gently, and consciously, ensuring that the needs of both partners are always met before moving on to the next cycle of pleasure and awareness. Couples who master this approach are able to remain in a state of heightened excitation for several hours, prolong and intensify orgasm, and experience total body orgasms. Among the experiences they report are a continuous flow of energy throughout their bodies, a joined climax of body and soul, the sensation of being united with the cosmos, and afterward being refreshed and revitalized. The primary goal of "spiritual sex" isn't prolonged orgasm, however, but an experience of being more deeply connected with the person you love, and through that connectedness, an awareness of your integral role within the whole of creation. Not everyone will feel the need to master, or even explore, a tantric approach to sex, yet all of us can benefit from more conscious lovemaking. Of all the spiritual practices, it is certainly the most pleasurable. (To learn more about the tantric approach to sex, see *The Art of Sexual Ecstasy* by Margo Anand.)

problem and the solution lie not only within the individual but within the entire family system. This perspective encourages parents to examine their roles and the responsibility they share with their child for his or her problem. Often a child's crisis serves as a mirror reflecting an imbalance in his or her individual system as well as in the family system as a whole. One of the significant advantages of family therapy is that change often occurs more rapidly than in individual psychotherapy. In much the same way that holistic medicine treats the entire person, not simply physical symptoms, the family systems approach recognizes the need for family therapy when any family member is suffering. If this is a situation that applies to your family, family counseling is strongly recommended. The family systems approach is practiced predominantly by social workers.

Good parenting requires both *time* and *consistency* in order to impart to your children the values you would like to instill in them. Putting in time as a parent includes being with them on a regular basis and making an effort to get to know them better. What are their talents? What do they enjoy doing? What are they thinking about and how do they feel? Learning the answers to such questions can pay big dividends for both you and your children. In fostering their growth as individuals, it is essential to give them greater power and responsibility by allowing them to make some of their own decisions. By doing so you will also help them gain confidence and trust, both in themselves and in you.

Other helpful ways to spend time as a family are to worship together each week at church or synagogue, and to designate a regularly scheduled time during the weekend for a fun activity. Take turns allowing each member to choose the activity for the day. The value of such play cannot be overemphasized. Having fun together as a family strengthens the bonds of love between each family member and defuses whatever stress or other problems may have built up during the week. Even if you cannot be with your children daily (due to being away on business or divorce, for instance), spending consistent time with them on a regular basis will help them experience the world and live their lives with the security, confidence, and caring that comes from their knowing that you love them. Despite all of its inherent struggles and perils, parenting is first and foremost an incredible gift. Appreciating that gift by regularly interacting with your children is one of the most potent means for creating community and fostering both spiritual and social healing that you will ever have.

SUMMARY

Your spiritual well-being is ultimately the most important aspect of your ability to care for yourself. It is also the dimension of holistic medicine that is most often neglected in our society. Becoming spiritually healthy is a process of *diminishing fear and increasing love while developing an awareness of Spirit and allowing it to guide you to a deeper connection to other human beings.* This infinite source of compassionate and forgiving transcendent power is the essence of all life on earth and is the spark of life force energy within each of us. The most direct path to becoming spiritually healthy is learning to love yourself. As you do, you will appreciate the greater meaning and purpose of your life, experience gratitude for your many blessings, and become highly attuned to and trusting of your intuition. As you move beyond the confining restraints of your ego, you will become a more loving friend, spouse or committed partner, parent, and member of your community. In short, you will achieve the goal of holistic medicine—*to become whole.*

5

Action Steps

The journey of a thousand miles begins with the first step.
LAO TZU

THE ROAD TO OPTIMAL well-being is a journey without short cuts. Reversing disease and improving health requires commitment, time, and a willingness to change. Nonetheless, there are measures that you can take to begin to feel better *now*. Exercises and activities follow, arranged by category (body, mind and spirit), that anyone can easily use to enhance the holistic health program outlined in chapters 2, 3 and 4. Think of these measures as *action steps* that are meant to be practiced daily in order to help you establish healthy habits. While it is not necessary to incorporate all of them into your lifestyle, the more of them that you practice, the more quickly you will begin to feel better. Initially you may find it easiest to select one or two practices from each category, adding new ones from each list as your original choices become more a part of your daily routine. Attempting to make too many changes at the same time can lead to discouragement and loss of commitment. Do them at your own pace, and let your intuition guide you to the ones that will offer you the most immediate benefit.

BODY

Brush your teeth and floss your gums. Proper dental care has grown more important in recent years, due to studies showing that dental plaque may contribute to a number of disease conditions, including heart disease, stroke, and diabetes. This occurs as a result of oral bacteria, over time, entering the bloodstream, traveling throughout the body, and seeding infection elsewhere. In addition, pregnant women with gum disease have up to an 800 percent increased risk of giving birth to premature, low-weight babies, compared to women whose gums are healthy. The easiest preventive measure to safeguard against plaque buildup is to floss every day and brush your teeth after each meal, and have regular dental checkups to ensure against gingivitis and other forms of gum disease.

Take a walk. Walking is one of the most complete forms of exercise, offering many health benefits without much strain or risk of injury. Get in the habit of walking at least one or two miles each day. Walking helps to burn calories, provides an aerobic workout (if done briskly), and contributes to increased oxygenation and bloodstream circulation. It's also an effective way to relieve stress and provides a useful break from your daily responsibilities. Ideally, it is best to walk outdoors in a peaceful, sunny, and nonpolluted environment, such as a park, a beach, or neighborhood sidewalks. If your location or inclement weather make this impractical, you might consider walking a few laps around your local mall. Many people find that taking a walk after their evening meal improves sleep, in addition to burning calories. Other ways to incorporate walking into your daily routine are to use the stairs instead of the elevator or escalator, to walk to appointments and errands that are within easy distance, or to buy a treadmill and position it in front of your TV.

Stretch. Practice one or two positions of limbering stretching activity at least once a day. Over time, gradually work up to five stretching exercises each day, for a period of 10 to 20 minutes. Both *yoga* and *t'ai chi* offer effective systems of stretching activity, combined with mild to moderate aerobic breathing. Qualified instructors of both disciplines are now available in most communities.

Practice abdominal breathing and breathe healthy air. Breathing through the abdomen instead of through the chest is a simple yet powerful way to improve energy and flow of oxygen, enhance digestion, relieve stomach pain and flatulence, and diminish stress. Since most of us rarely breathe through our bellies, learning to do so at first may seem odd. Yet abdominal breathing is easy to do. Just direct your breath in and out through your belly. If you do so correctly, your chest will not move. You can easily check this by placing one hand on your belly and the other on your chest. As you breathe, the lower hand should move, while the hand on your chest should remain motionless.

Don't get discouraged if you are unable to accomplish this on your first try. Make it a practice to spend a few minutes each day breathing abdominally (working up to 20 to 30 minutes a day is recommended), along with regular brief sessions whenever you notice yourself feeling tense or irritable. Abdominal breathing can also be performed in conjunction with meditation. (see below.)

Do your best to breathe clean, moist air, rich in negative ions and oxygen, both at home and at work. Refer to the environmental health section in chapter 2 and the holistic treatment and prevention of chronic sinusitis in chapter 6.

Get a good night's sleep. At the beginning of the twentieth century, Americans went to bed earlier and slept longer (nine hours on average) than we do today. In fact, lack of sleep is now epidemic in the United States, with as many as 60 million Americans suffering from insomnia at some point in their lives. By getting eight hours of restful sleep every night, you allow your body to more effectively cope with the numerous stressors of modern life, while also having time to effectively carry out the various repair mechanisms that occur while you're sleeping. To get the most from sleep, make it a point to go to bed each night at the same time, ideally about 10 P.M. To allow your body to get the amount of sleep it needs, stop using an alarm clock. (For other sleep recommendations, see the insomnia section in chapter 7.

Diet and nutrition. Begin to incorporate the dietary recommendations outlined in chapter 2, along with taking a multivitamin and mineral supplement. Also be sure to drink plenty of filtered water.

Baths and showers. Although often overlooked as a tool for health, your bathtub can become an important part of your personal health program. Baths are not only soothing, they also are capable of providing relief for physical pain and can improve digestive irregularities and ease respiratory congestion. Hot baths stimulate the immune system, promote detoxification through perspiration, and ease stress. To further promote detoxification, add one cup of apple cider vinegar to your bath and soak for at least ten minutes. Cold baths can be effective in reducing inflammation and fever and for toning muscles and relieving fatigue.

Showering can also be an effective self-care tool. If your nose is congested or you have a sinus problem, increase the water temperature as you shower as much as you can tolerate and let the hot water strike your face, especially around your nose and sinuses. Moving your face from side to side or in a circular motion will enable you to tolerate the hot water longer.

As a general immune stimulant, end a hot shower by switching to cold water, allowing it to strike the midpoint of your chest for about a minute. This technique can stimulate the thymus gland, an essential part of the immune system located in your chest cavity directly behind the breastbone.

Fasting. Because of the proliferation of toxins in our air, drinking water, and food, you would probably benefit from detoxifying your body as part of your optimal health program. Fasting is an effective method of detoxification. Doing a fast will allow your internal organs to rejuvenate themselves and to better utilize the nutrients from food and supplementation. This in turn leads to increased energy and a more balanced emotional state and can also contribute to greater spiritual awareness as your focus shifts away from physical concerns. One method is to fast once a week for 24 hours, either on water, vegetable juices, or fruit. Select a day when work and family responsibilities are limited and you won't be too active. Plan to spend at least part of your fast in quiet time alone. During the final two hours of the fast drink six to eight glasses of water, which will help you flush your body of toxins.

A milder form of fasting is to drink only fresh juices made from organic fruits and vegetables. These juices are easily assimilated by the body and supply a variety of nutrients while stimulating the body to release wastes. Be sure to consume only juice that is freshly made, not store-bought, since commmercially processed juices will not provide the same benefit. Another option is to do a fruit fast, in which you eat only fresh organic fruits during the day. If you have never undergone a fast before, you may wish to consult your physician before undertaking one.

After you have fasted once or twice, notice how you feel. If you think your fast was beneficial, continue fasting on a regular weekly basis. You'll be surprised at how much easier fasting becomes with each subsequent fast.

Kegel exercise, and contractions. According to Chinese medicine, one's health is directly related to the health of the sexual organs. A simple and effective way to ensure the health of your sex organs is the daily practice of Kegel exercises, which contract the *pubococcygeous* (PC) muscle located midway between the anus and genitals. (To locate your PC muscle, stop your flow of urine in midstream. The muscle you contract is the PC.) Regular exercise of the PC both strengthens the sex organs, and enhances sexual pleasure. For women, it strengthens the vaginal muscles, and for men, it may help to reduce an enlarged prostate. If the PC is contracted just prior to ejaculation, orgasm can be delayed and prolonged.

This exercise can be performed anywhere at any time. Start by doing 15 PC contractions daily, then increase the repetitions to the point where your PC muscle tires. Contraction and relaxation should be about the same duration—two to four seconds. As your PC muscle strengthens, you can increase the length of each contraction and also combine the exercise with abdominal breathing (contracting the PC muscle with each inhalation).

The Body Scan. An easily mastered skill that can help you to quickly become more in touch with your body is the Body Scan. To perform this exercise, sit comfortably in a chair and close your eyes, then begin to breathe gently in and out through your abdomen. As you do, mentally scan your body from one end to the other. (It doesn't matter if you begin at the top of your head or at the bottom of your feet.) Don't be concerned with timing or counting breaths. The object of the Body Scan is to pay close attention to the muscles, joints, and organs of each area of your body in order to identify and release any tightness or pain that might be present within them. As you locate each problem area, visualize your breath as a wave of healing energy that you are directing to that area to promote relaxation. When you finish scanning your entire body, place your attention on your lower abdomen and continue breathing for a minute more. Doing so will help you be more fully present in the moment, allowing you to become more centered and better able to cope with stress-filled situations.

The Body Scan is best done when you have an adequate amount of time to devote to it. Performing it just before you go to bed can be especially beneficial, since it very effectively promotes sleep. Be sure to breathe at least two or three times for each area of your body that you scan before moving on to the next one. Spend even more time on the areas in which you detect discomfort, not moving on until you are able to sense some relaxation occurring in the area in question. It's not uncommon to spend half an hour or more performing this exercise, but you'll soon discover that the relaxed state that results makes the time commitment well worth it. Moreover, by performing the Body Scan regularly, you will become better able to detect the onset of dis-ease in your body before it manifests as a more serious problem.

MIND

Goals and affirmations. Make a list of your goals, desires, and objectives in every realm of your life (physical, environmental, mental, emotional, spiritual, and social), listing everything that you'd like to see in your life as long as you believe it is even remotely possible. When your list is complete, arrange each section according to time, beginning with goals you wish to accomplish today, this week, this month, this year, and five years from now. Knowing your specific goals makes it easier to attain them and provides you with a focus and game plan for succeeding. Without this clarity and direction, our desires often go unmet or are delayed, creating feelings of frustration and disappointment.

To further help you achieve your goals, write them in the form of affirmations and repeat them regularly, either orally or in writing (doing both is best); or record them onto a cassette and play them back daily. Be sure you state them in the present tense, and each time you repeat them, visualize or feel your goal *as if it is already happening.* (For more on goals and affirmations, see chapter 3.)

Operate from choice. Recognize that you are a unique individual capable of choosing your own beliefs, attitudes, and emotions according to what feels right for you. Happiness and optimism (the expectation that things will work out well) are both attitudes found in most healthy people, and those that you can *choose* for yourself. The more conscious you become of your ability to choose, the more you will realize how powerfully you can affect your state of physical, mental, and spiritual well-being. So why not choose how you want to feel and create a life in harmony with your own desires instead of reacting to circumstance or societal pressures? By doing so you will become much more aware of the options for further growth that exist in your present life experiences.

Humor. Make it a habit to look for more humor and opportunities for laughter in your life. Lighten up and take life less seriously. Living is an adventure. Have fun and laugh several times a day.

Work. Find a job that you passionately enjoy and that utilizes your unique talents. Even if your current job is less than your ideal, you can still find ways to make it more pleasant and fulfilling. Your attitude is critical in this situation. So too is understanding how to use your talents to best meet your work's responsibilities, while eliminating those aspects of the job you most dislike. As you recognize and appreciate how your greatest talents contribute to your job, the more joy and satisfaction you will derive from it. Practice congratulating yourself for a "job well done."

Leisure time and play. A major source of stress in modern-day life is the fact that so many of us fail to take relaxation breaks on a regular basis. Give yourself permission to play. Balance planning and goal-setting with spontaneity, while taking time to experience the joys of "doing nothing" and just "being." Make a commitment to a hobby, a musical instrument, or time in nature. Another option is to select a sport, dance, game, or other activity that requires you to move your body. Practice it for an hour at least three times a week. If you have young children at home, then you've already found the perfect playmates, and a simple and wonderful way to become more childlike.

Twenty connected breaths. This technique was developed by Leonard Orr, the founder of Rebirthing or Intuitive Energy Breathing. Orr maintains that learning to breathe with awareness without pausing between the inhale and the exhale can result in many physical, psychological, and spiritual improvements. It can also enhance the quality of your thoughts and release limiting and distorted beliefs. In this exercise, you may notice a tingling sensation in all or part of your body. For some, this can be uncomfortable at first, but the feelings will quickly become pleasurable if you allow yourself to simply keep breathing. The exercise is performed as follows.

Once a day, preferably upon arising or before going to bed, take four short breaths into the chest with your mouth closed, remembering not to pause between the inhale and the exhale. Do not force the breath, especially on the exhale, which should simply release of its own accord. On the fifth breath, inhale and exhale deeply and fully. These five breaths together count as one cycle. Repeat three more times for a total of four cycles and 20 connected breaths.

Breathing in this manner can sometimes bring up repressed feelings and unpleasant thoughts. If you find they make you uncomfortable, you may wish to receive deeper instruction in Rebirthing from a trained Rebirther. For information on Rebirthing and where to find a Rebirther in your area, contact Rebirth International, P.O. Box 118, Walton, NY 13856, (607) 865-8254; fax (607) 865-8247.

The One Minute Drill and The Quiet Five. The following exercises are very effective ways of relieving stress and providing a boost in energy. *The One-Minute Drill:* Sit in a chair without armrests, with your feet flat on the floor, your back straight, and your eyes partially or entirely closed to avoid distraction. Place your hands palm down on your thighs, or lay them on your lap, one over the other.

Now slowly inhale and exhale through your nose, breathing abdominally. Your breath should first expand your abdominal cavity, then fill your chest. To stay focused on your breath, count each cycle of respiration. Stay in a comfortable rhythm without straining. Practice this exercise at least once per day. Doing so will provide you with a simple tool to quickly and easily diminish tension and promote deeper relaxation.

The Quiet Five: Seat yourself as in the One-Minute Drill. You will again breathe abdominally, but this time for five minutes and in a different rhythm. Inhale through your nose for a count of eight, then hold your breath for a count of four. Exhale through your nose for a count of eight, then again hold your breath for a count of four. Then repeat this cycle, continuing to breathe in this pattern for five minutes. By focusing on your count, you can more easily let go of your thoughts and concerns. On a cellular level, the Quiet Five can oxygenate and recharge your entire body, while also inducing deep relaxation and peace of mind.

Journaling and dreamwork. Keeping a journal or keeping a dream diary are other effective ways of becoming more aware of your thoughts, beliefs, and emotions. Both methods can also help you to better connect with your intuition and receive guidance and solutions to life challenges you may be facing. For more on these methods, see chapter 3.

The Body-Emotional Scan. This exercise is highly effective in helping you identify your feelings. To perform the Body-Emotional Scan, begin with a few minutes of abdominal breathing with your eyes closed. Then spend 10 to 15 minutes doing a Body Scan (see page 87), identifying the places in your body that are tense, constricted, or painful. Once you have identified a specific physical sensation, allow yourself to imagine an experience that you associate with that sensation while you continue breathing abdominally. (For example, neck and shoulder tightness might be associated with a stressful situation at work.) The inner image that results can be either actual or imaginary. What is important is that you are able to identify what the experience might be. Once you do, relate that experience to a specific emotion—anger, fear, sorrow, loss, grief, humiliation, and so on. Whatever the emotion, it is probably contributing to your physical pain or discomfort. Ask yourself what beliefs are associated with the emotion you've uncovered, and how your behavior is affected by them. (Using the preceding example, you've been told by your boss to meet an unreasonable deadline, and your belief might be "I'll lose my job if I don't comply." The associated emotions are both anger and fear.) Then ask yourself how these emotions and beliefs that are contributing to your pain might be benefiting you. (Motivating you to work harder.) What is your physical and emotional pain preventing you from doing? (Relaxing, exercising, taking time off.) What is it helping you to gain? (A possible raise or promotion.)

Regular practice of the Body-Emotional Scan will make it easier for you to discover feelings and beliefs that are unconscious or that you have denied. Once you identify these underlying triggers, you can choose to change your current behavior patterns stemming from these emotions, and limiting, negative, or critical beliefs. But first it is essential that you reexperience these feelings—by crying, venting anger, and so on—in a safe context so that you can discharge their energies and release them from your bodymind. See chapter 3 for more information that can help you do so.

SPIRIT

Prayer. Pray daily in whatever manner feels most comfortable to you. Spending a few moments in prayer as you start the day and before you go to bed is an excellent way to maintain your connection to Spirit, *that power that is both within you and transcends you.* If you are so inclined, you can gain added benefit by affiliating with your local church or temple and participating in a spiritual community through a structured weekly observance of honoring God.

Meditation. Meditate for at least five minutes twice a day, choosing a time when you will be comfortably seated in a quiet surrounding, and beginning with conscious breathing. Once you are centered and deeply relaxed, you can proceed by simply focusing your attention on a spiritual thought or phrase ("Love," "Peace") while breathing gently, deeply, and fully. As you become more comfortable with your meditation practice, gradually build up to two 20-minute periods each day. If you need more assistance, many communities now provide formal training in meditation techniques.

Gratitude. Begin your day by visualizing a scene that makes you feel happy to be alive. Don't take life for granted; there are numerous blessings for which you can be grateful. Take a few seconds each day to acknowledge them. Also focus on what you have, not on what you lack.

Forgiveness. Remember that you are a human being with imperfections, weaknesses, and flaws, like everyone else. Learn to accept your mistakes and forgive yourself for them, cancelling the demands that you "should have" behaved differently. Do the same with others, *forgiving the person, not the action.* Recognize your limitations, and also give yourself credit for all that you've achieved in spite of them. Doing so will allow you to be more accepting of yourself and others.

Meaning, purpose, and intuition. Take time to reflect on what your life is about, where you are heading, what you most enjoy, and what feels most meaningful to you. This will help clarify your sense of purpose and provide you with greater opportunities to share your unique gifts with others. Your intuition, or inner voice, is your best guide in this process. Take time to listen to it and be willing to take risks as it guides you toward your most valuable lessons.

Eye contact. "The eyes are the windows to the soul." There is more truth to this adage than most of us realize. To deepen your awareness of yourself as a spiritual being, make a practice of looking at yourself in the mirror for five minutes every day. This powerful exercise can help you to better appreciate and love who you see. It works best to look into your left eye, which is connected to the more "receptive" right side of your brain. You might also experiment with smiling as you do this exercise. This is a fun and effective way to see yourself as a lovable person, deserving of the highest good. Making use of affirmations while staring at your reflection is also beneficial. (For more on affirmations, see chapter 3.) The more you practice this exercise, the more you will also notice the eyes of others and recognize their own spiritual nature. This can enhance the quality of your relationships.

Touch. Touch is both an effective form of healing, and perhaps the most powerful and direct means we have for conveying and receiving love. Biblically, the spiritual dimension of touch is illustrated in the healing practice of the "laying on of hands." Numerous studies now attest to the healing power of touch, yet in comparison to other countries we in the United States are a "touch averse" society. In order to be healthy, we need to consciously make touch a more frequent occurrence in our lives, recognizing that touch is a gift we can give ourselves and each other every day.

Two of the easiest ways of learning how to accept touch are *self-touch* and *hugging*. Self-touch can be as simple as giving yourself a foot massage or kneading your shoulders. Instead of engaging in such activities mechanically, focus on what you are doing and be attentive. Touching yourself gently and compassionately is another way of bringing the gift of touch into your life. It can also help you become centered during times of prayer or meditation. A number of polls indicate that most people, especially women, are not satisfied with their physical bodies. Self-touch is a wonderful way to learn to accept your body and to appreciate what an awe-inspiring gift it really is.

Hugging and being hugged is another simple, yet powerful, means of connecting with Spirit. Here, too, it pays to be more aware. It's not uncommon for people to unconsciously pull away from a hug before the embrace is completed. Most are not aware of the healing benefits of hugging, and many are uncomfortable with the physical closeness. The next time you receive a hug, allow yourself to fully partake of it. Often simply breathing deeply and freely can assist you in doing so. Notice the difference in how you feel before, during, and after your embrace. Hugging is a good way to raise one's spirits, increase feelings of security, and instill warmth and well-being. Try to make it a practice to give and receive several hugs each day with your family and friends. Hand-holding or a friendly pat on the back are also ways that you can receive and convey the benefits of touch. Petting and holding household pets and stroking domestic animals such as horses can bring similar benefits.

Listening exercise. Attentive listening can be a very powerful method for enhancing intimacy in a committed relationship. Refer to chapter 4 for more detailed information.

Support groups. Support groups comprised of people who meet regularly to share and explore common values, beliefs, problems, or common ailments can be an effective tool you can use to strengthen your sense of community and enhance your spiritual growth. Perhaps the easiest way to become involved in such a group is to organize it yourself, inviting family members, friends, and coworkers who share a common interest. For the greatest benefit, try to meet together at least once a week.

Altruism. Helping others through donations of your time and resources is not only spiritually rewarding but also pleasurable and is capable of boosting your immune system. Helping others with genuine goodwill produces strong feelings of connection, a sense of unity, and the recognition that in giving to others you are ultimately giving to yourself. It is also a potent antidote for the negative effects of self-involvement. Learn to recognize your opportunities for altruism and take advantage of them.

Relationships. Your role as a lover, spouse, parent and/or friend provides you with the most powerful opportunities for spiritual growth on a daily basis. Make a commitment to become more conscious in all your relationships, and especially those with whom you are most intimate. There is a divine spark, a lifeforce energy, residing within each of us. And it is in those whom we love the most that we can best appreciate that energy. By honoring that spark in your loved ones, you help them become more of who and what they are—*human embodiments of Spirit.* In return, they help you to do the same. Don't take your relationships for granted. Instead cultivate wonder and gratitude for all the gifts you are able to share with your loved ones. Doing so will reward you with the greatest health benefit of all—*the gift of unconditional Love.*

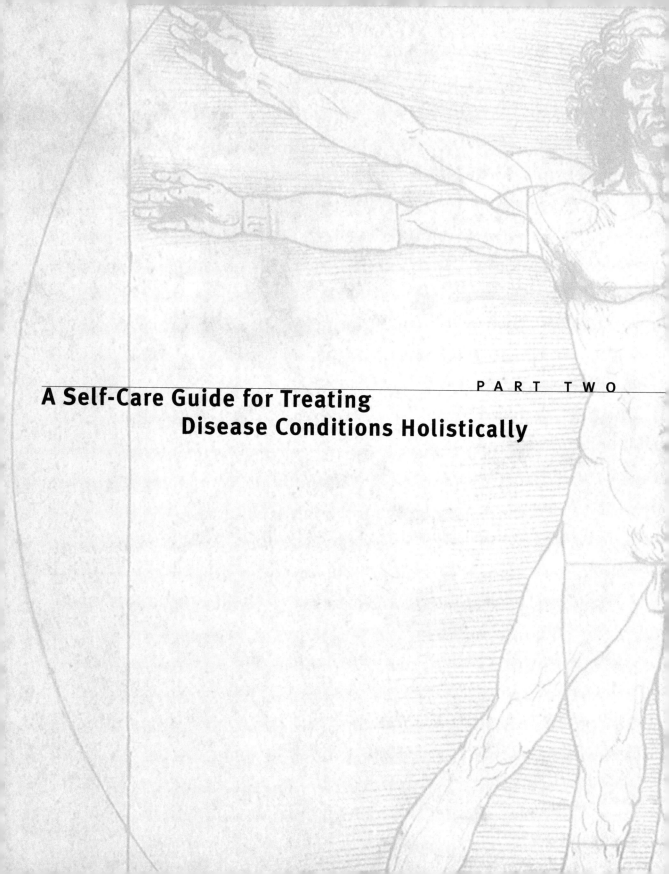

PART TWO

A Self-Care Guide for Treating
Disease Conditions Holistically

Introduction
How to Use Part Two

A comprehensive guide to therapeutic options for treating specific chronic diseases is contained in the chapters that follow. Holistic self-care treatments are outlined for preventing and treating over 60 of the most common chronic diseases in America today. (The acute ailments—colds, influenza, otitis media, and diarrhea—are also included.) Our recommendations are based on the successful approaches that we and our holistic medical colleagues use to treat these conditions in our clinical practice. By following these recommendations, over time you will experience considerable improvement in your condition, with great potential for freeing yourself of disease and feeling healthier than you've ever been before. Bear in mind, however, that true healing is far more than simply the absence of illness.

The most effective way to cure any chronic illness is to heal your life, not just repair your physical dysfunction. Therefore, we *strongly advise* that you use the tools and information provided in Part I in conjunction with the recommendations that follow. The material in chapters 2 through 5 is the foundation on which the holistic treatments in Part II are built. By combining the focus on optimal health of Part I with the information in Part II, you will be nurturing your body, mind, and spirit while at the same time treating your particular disease and its related symptoms. This comprehensive focus on healing all the life issues that may be contributing to your illness lies at the heart of holistic medicine.

The diseases listed in Part II are arranged and grouped by category. For example, *diarrhea, constipation, Crohn's disease, ulcerative colitis, diverticulosis and diverticulitis, peptic ulcer, cholecystitis (gallbladder), hemorrhoids,* and *parasites* are included in chapter 11, "Gastrointestinal Disease." That's because all these conditions affect the gastrointestinal tract and share similar causes and risk factors, as well as many of the same holistic recommendations. Most of the discussions of disease conditions in Part II include the following elements:

- Prevalence

- Anatomy and physiology

- Symptoms and diagnosis

- Conventional medical treatment

- Risk factors and causes

- Holistic medical treatment and prevention, with specific recommendations for body, mind, and spirit (including *diet*, *nutritional supplements*, *herbs*, and specific *physical*, *psychological*, and *bioenergetic therapies*)

If you suffer from a gastrointestinal condition, practice the recommendations provided in Part I, and use the specific therapies outlined in chapter 11. Your regimen from Part I will start to strengthen your immune system and increase your awareness of the physical, environmental, mental, emotional, spiritual, and social factors that may be contributing to your disease. The specific approaches in Part II will then enable you to begin to reverse them. *Treatment of all chronic diseases should include a healthy diet, regular exercise, affirmations, visualizations, emotional work, intimate relationships, and prayer or meditation.* In addition, building positive attitudes and belief systems in body, mind, and spirit are essential in helping to reverse the symptoms of disease and to create optimal health.

WORKING WITH YOUR PHYSICIAN

Although this book is a self-care guide to optimal wellness, we recognize that many people will read it while under the care of a physician. We recommend that you use the suggested therapies in Part II as a *complement* to the medical treatment you may already be receiving. You may also want to inform your doctor that you are doing so, and give him or her an opportunity to learn another treatment option. Nothing in Part II contradicts conventional medical treatment, and *proper drug use under the guidance of your physician can be used safely in conjunction with the holistic therapies we provide, unless specifically stated.* Holistic physicians recognize that conventional medical treatment (primarily drugs and surgery) plays an important role in treating disease. For this reason, we have included descriptions of the most common and appropriate conventional medications for each disease condition in our treatment recommendations.

WORKING ON YOUR OWN

If you are not already under a physician's care, you might try starting with the holistic therapies on your own, unless otherwise indicated, and see how you feel after a month or two, before deciding to use conventional treatment or finding a holistic physician. And if you have been treated conventionally and conclude, after careful consideration and consultation with your physician, that the liabilities of the conventional treatment (such as toxic side effects) outweigh their potential benefits, then commit solely to the holistic approaches in both Parts I and II or take steps to find a holistic physician. One of the advantages of holistic medicine is that its combined use of complementary and conventional therapies often makes it possible to use lower dosages of medications to good effect, thereby minimizing harmful side effects.

HOLISTIC PHYSICIANS

If you are suffering from a chronic disease or trying to improve the quality of your life, you may want the support of a holistic physician. You can find one in your area by contacting the American Holistic Medical Association (AHMA) at (703) 556-9728, or visiting their Website, at www.holisticmedicine.org., to obtain their *Physician Referral Directory.* This list includes both physician members (M.D.s and D.O.s) and associate members (holistic practitioners other than M.D.s and D.O.s) of the AHMA.

PROFESSIONAL COMPLEMENTARY THERAPIES

The discipline of holistic medicine includes the prudent use of both conventional Western medicine and professional care alternatives, such as *ayurveda, acupuncture, behavioral medicine, Chinese medicine, chiropractic, energy medicine, environmental medicine, homeopathy, naturopathic medicine, nutritional medicine,* and *osteopathic medicine.* The chapters in Part II include mention of those therapies that have been scientifically verified as appropriate professional care treatments for each disease condition we cover. To learn more about these therapies, see the appendix, which provides an overview of what they are and how they work, and the Resources guide, which lists the primary organizations that oversee each of these therapies and provide listings of practitioners nationwide.

CHARTING YOUR PROGRESS

One way to monitor the progress of your holistic treatment program is to evaluate your physical symptoms on a weekly basis in a chart. Start with a list similar to the Symptom Chart for respiratory disease shown on page 101. This sample chart lists the most common symptoms you might experience if you suffer from chronic sinusitis, allergies, chronic bronchitis, or asthma. Whatever your particular ailment, list its most frequent symptoms in the left-hand column of your chart and rank them from one (worst) to ten (best or no symptom) on a weekly basis. You can also uncover possible emotional factors that are contributing to your condition by similarly ranking your emotional stress level each week. You should be able to graphically correlate higher stress with worsening physical symptoms. Also keep track of the medications, herbs, nutritional supplements, and other remedies you are using at the bottom of the chart. NOTE: *The vitamins, herbs, and supplements recommended in Part II are available in most health food stores. The suggested dosages are based on those coauthors Rob Ivker and Bob Anderson have used extensively in their clinical practice and on the recommendations of their colleagues Steve Morris, N.D. (Mukilteo, WA) and Todd Nelson, N.D. (Denver, CO). These dosages may differ from the suggestions of your own personal holistic physician.*

By using your symptom chart you can more easily evaluate your progress, and better determine what works for you and what doesn't. (Remember that each of us is a unique individual, with specific needs and requirements in order to be healthy.) As you practice using this chart you'll become quite adept at the early recognition of emotional factors that aggravate your condition, and you'll be able to quickly respond with an effective therapy. The better you become at listening attentively to your body and mind, the more effectively you will be able to *prevent* recurrences of your illness. This art, science, and discipline is the basis of the practice of both holistic and preventive medicine. As you continue your training you will develop into a highly skilled self-healer. Although you may be starting out suffering with a chronic disease, remember that the greater your *enjoyment* of this life-changing challenge, the better your results will be.

SYMPTOM CHART–RESPIRATORY DISEASE

Began Thriving Program on _____   Rate Symptoms from 1 (worst) to 10 (best = normal)

Symptom	Begin	End Week 1	End Week 2	End Week 3	End Week 4	End Week 5	End Week 6	End Week 7	End Week 8	End Week 9	End Week 10	End Week 11	End Week 12
Head Congestion (fullness)													
Nasal Congestion (stuffy nose)													
Postnasal Drip													
Headache													
Yellow/Green Mucus (from nose)													
Yellow/Green Mucus (back of throat)													
Sneezing													
Itching: Nose, Throat													
Ear Congestion (ears plugged up)													
Sore Throat													
Swollen Glands (in neck)													
Cough—dry													
Cough—wet/mucusy													
Shortness of Breath													
Wheezing													
Fatigue (rate energy level)													
Average # of hours sleep													

Emotional Stress

Work													
Family													
Other													

Medications

Vitamins, Herbs, Supplements

6

Respiratory Disease

Chronic Sinusitis

Allergic Rhinitis (Allergies or
Hay Fever)

Chronic Bronchitis

Asthma

Colds

Influenza

Otitis Media (Middle Ear Infection)

Prevalence

THE MOST COMMON group of diseases afflicting Americans are those of the nose, sinuses, and lungs—the respiratory tract. Its job is breathing, which we do about 22,000 times a day, inhaling a pint of air 15 times a minute. Often the air we breathe is laden with viruses, bacteria, mold, pollen, smoke, dust, animal dander, and a variety of pollutants. This direct and prolonged exposure is the chief cause for the prevalence of respiratory diseases.

As a result of the environmental plague of air pollution, most urban dwellers are breathing unhealthy air. The nose, sinuses, and lungs are relentlessly assaulted by a barrage of pollutants. The EPA says that 60 percent of Americans live in areas where breathing is a risk to one's health. A 1993 study performed by the EPA and the Harvard School of Public Health reported that 50 to 60 thousand deaths a year are caused by particulate air pollution. A subsequent study in 1995 bolstered the earlier findings while concluding that people who live in highly polluted cities die earlier (15 percent, or about ten years sooner) than they would were they breathing healthier air.

Air pollution has become such a significant health hazard that four of America's most common *chronic* diseases are now respiratory ailments: chronic sinusitis (no. 1), allergies (no. 5), chronic bronchitis (no. 8), and asthma (no. 9). *Ninety-two million of us, or one out of every three people, suffers from at least one of these respiratory diseases.* Acute sinusitis (sinus infection) may have already replaced the common cold (the most common respiratory tract infection) as our nation's most prevalent acute illness. In a study performed at the University of Virginia in 1993, students who thought they had a *cold* were evaluated with CT scans—the most accurate diagnostic test for sinusitis. The scans revealed that 87 percent did not have a simple cold but in fact had a *sinus infection.*

Anatomy and Physiology

The Respiratory Tract

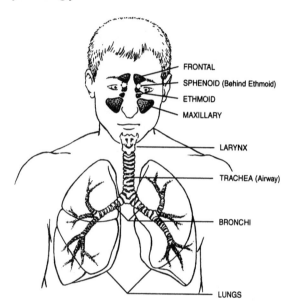

The nose and sinuses serve as the body's *primary air filter and protector of the lungs.* The respiratory tract works ceaselessly to provide every cell in the body with an adequate supply of oxygen and to expel carbon dioxide. To accomplish this, the average person inhales about 22,000 pints of air per day. Nothing is more important to optimal physical well-being than the quality of our air and our ability to breathe it. During the past 20 years, both of these critical aspects of health have drastically diminished.

The Respiratory Tract Lining,
Healthy

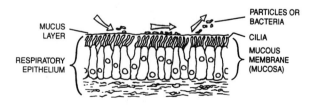

The outermost lining of the entire respiratory tract is one continuous tissue, called the *respiratory epithelium*, that extends from just inside the nostrils to the alveolar sacs in the lungs. The outer layer of this tissue is called the mucous membrane or mucosa. Like an extension of the skin covering the external surface of your entire body, this membrane is a connected porous protective shield for the air portal of your body. It serves as your first line of defense against bacteria, viruses, pollen, animal dander, cigarette smoke, dust, chemicals, automobile exhaust, and any other potentially harmful air pollutants. With a protective capability and breathability far beyond that of Gore-Tex or any similar high-tech material, this membrane also has the job of humidifying dry air and warming cold or cooling hot air. The bulk of the job of filtering, humidifying, and regulating temperature occurs in the nose and sinuses—the entrance and vestibule of the respiratory tract. If the mucous membrane breaks down, the immediate consequence might be a cold or sinus infection. Since the lungs are the site of oxygen/carbon dioxide exchange, they need the protection provided by the nose and sinuses to do their best in carrying out this vital life-giving function. Unfortunately, the frontline nose/sinus defense is losing the battle to the massive assault by a barrage of air pollutants.

The Respiratory Tract Lining,
Chronic Inflammation

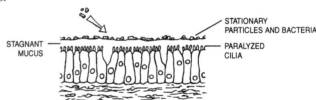

Risk Factors and Causes of Respiratory Disease

Air pollution appears to be the leading cause of America's first environmental epidemic—respiratory disease. Every chronic respiratory condition is impacted by air quality, and as was pointed out in chapter 2, the condition of our air—both indoor and outdoor—is deteriorating. *Particulates* have been identified as the most unhealthy outdoor pollutant. They are tiny particles of dust, sand, cinders, soot, smoke, and liquid droplets found in the atmosphere. They come from a variety of sources, including roads, farm fields, construction sites, factories, power plants, fireplaces, wood-burning stoves, windblown dust, and diesel and car exhaust. While our mucous membranes are overloaded with too much to filter, they are also being injured, irritated, and abraded by the pollutants themselves. Imagine rubbing a piece of fine sandpaper across the back of your hand 22,000 times per day! Can you picture the condition of your skin and how difficult it would be for that skin surface to ever heal? That is comparable to the assault your mucous membranes are subjected to daily merely from the act of breathing. The longer

INDOOR AIR POLLUTANTS

Automotive Fumes

Sources include outdoor traffic, outdoor parking lots, and outdoor loading and unloading spaces, as well as indoor garages

Chemicals and Chemical Solutions

(Chemicals that affect indoor air quality are those associated with a building's architecture, the interior, artifacts, and maintenance)

Fungicides and pesticides in carpet-cleaning residues and sprays; formaldehyde used in the manufacture of insulation, plywood, fiberboard, furniture, and wood paneling; toxic solvents in oil-based paints, finishes, and wall sealants; aerosol sprays; office equipment chemicals, especially photocopiers and computers; and chemicals from dry cleaning.

Combustion Products

Tobacco smoke (from all of the available scientific data, tobacco smoke is the most unhealthy indoor air pollutant)

Coal- or wood-burning fireplaces and stoves

Fuel-combustion gases from gas-fired appliances such as ranges, clothes dryers, water heaters, and fireplaces (they produce nitrogen dioxide, carbon monoxide, nitrous oxides, sulfur oxides, hydrocarbons, and formaldehyde)

Ion Depletion or Imbalance

Too few negative ions, especially in airplanes and in sealed buildings

Excess of positive ions over negative ions (primarily from computer and TV screens)

Microorganisms

(Primarily from humidifiers, air conditioners, and any other building components affected by excessive moisture)

Bacteria

Viruses

Molds

Dust mites (usually found in humid areas)

Particulates

Dust

Pollen

Animal dander

Particles (frayed materials)

Asbestos

Pesticides, herbicides, fungicides

Radionuclides

Radon, a radioactive gas emitted from the earth that enters homes primarily through basements, crawl spaces, and water supply, especially from wells (it can attach to the particulates of cigarette smoke, dust particles, and natural aerosols)

---

this insidious barrage of pollution persists, the greater the irritation of the membranes, and the higher the risk of subsequent inflammation and swelling.

In addition to the chronic irritation from pollution, severe or persistent swelling of the membranes, usually resulting from colds and/or allergies, can easily block the openings of the sinus ducts that drain into the nose. This can often lead to a sinus infection, or acute sinusitis. In people with weak or hyperreactive lungs, the sinusitis might in turn precipitate acute bronchitis or an asthma attack.

People suffering from allergies and/or chronic sinusitis have ongoing diminished protection of the lungs and increased vulnerability of its mucous membrane to *cigarette smoke* and any other air pollutant. The inflammation and swelling that might ensue in the lungs can then cause narrowing of the airways and excessive mucus, which can in turn create a greater susceptibility to the onset of both asthma and bronchitis. The EPA has concluded that air pollution—both indoor and outdoor—is the primary cause for the nearly 50 percent increase in the incidence of asthma, chronic bronchitis, and emphysema over the past decade.

In addition to air pollution and cigarette smoke, the other significant risk factors for causing respiratory disease are:

- Diminished immune function
- Emotional stress
- Food allergy and sensitivity
- Genetics

CHRONIC SINUSITIS

Symptoms and Diagnosis

Acute sinusitis is an infection or inflammation of one or more of the eight sinus cavities. It usually begins as a cold and is accompanied by most or all of the four primary symptoms of *head congestion, headache or facial pain, green/yellow mucus (often postnasal), and fatigue.* (Since *acute sinusitis* is so often confused with a cold or allergies, please refer to the list of symptoms that follows to differentiate between them.) If this problem recurs three or more times within six months, or never goes away completely, then it is *chronic sinusitis.*

The definitive medical diagnosis of sinusitis is determined with a CT scan of the sinuses. This is a costly procedure and is usually not necessary.

Conventional Medical Treatment

Most people with sinus infections will first visit their primary care physician—family doctor, internist, or gynecologist—for treatment. In almost every instance that consists of a prescription for a broad-spectrum *antibiotic.* Amoxicillin is most often the first choice. If after ten days to two weeks the infection has not cleared, then a more powerful drug is prescribed.

Second-Step Antibiotics for Sinus Infections—after Amoxicillin Best drugs for killing both Streptococcus pneumoniae and Hemophilus influenza (the most

DIAGNOSING AND RECOGNIZING THE SYMPTOMS OF
COLDS, SINUSITIS, AND ALLERGIES

Primary symptoms—almost always present

Secondary symptoms—frequent but less often present

The Common Cold

Primary

- Preceded by high stress; too much going on at once

- Preceded by a sore throat

- Nasal congestion

- Runny nose

- Thin, clear/white nasal mucus

- Fatigue

- Mild muscle aching

- Lasts for four to seven days

Secondary

- Headache

- Sore throat

- Cough

- Low-grade fever

Sinus Infection (Acute Sinusitis)

Primary

- Preceded by the common cold

- Preceded by unexpressed anger

- Head congestion (facial or head fullness)

- Head or facial pain (headache, cheek, tooth, or eye pain)

- Thick green/yellow nasal or especially postnasal mucus drainage (down back of throat)

- Extreme fatigue

- Lasts for two or more weeks

Secondary

- Preceded by allergies or by prolonged exposure to air pollution, smoke, or toxic fumes

- Fever

- Sore throat

- Cough

- Hoarseness

- Nasal congestion

- Lasts for several months

Allergies, Hay Fever, or Allergic Rhinitis

Primary

- Preceded by personal or family history of allergies, eczema, or asthma

- Intermittent symptoms: either seasonal (pollen), food-related, environmentally or emotionally triggered

- Positive allergy skin tests

- Thin, clear/white nasal mucus

- Nasal congestion

- Sneezing

- Itching of nose, eyes, or throat

- Symptoms relieved with antihistamines, food elimination, environmental clearing, or stress reduction

Secondary

- Persistent or perennial symptoms

- Postnasal drip with intermittent sore throat, cough, or hoarseness

- Wheezing, difficulty breathing

- Skin rash

- Allergic "shiners" (dark circles under eyes)

common bacteria causing sinusitis) (Drugs are listed in order of efficacy; those on the same line are roughly equivalent):

Augmentin

Ceclor, Ceftin, Lorabid

Biaxin

Bactrim, Septra, Cotrim

Vibramycin, Vibra-Tabs

Best for killing *Staphylococci*:

Augmentin

Ceclor, Ceftin, Lorabid

Duricef, Ultracef, Keflex, Cefanex, Anspor, Velosef

Bactrim, Septra

In addition to antibiotics, doctors often prescribe a *decongestant* or recommend an over-the-counter (OTC) alternative. The most common ingredients in both choices are pseudoephedrine, phenylpropanolamine, and phenylephrine. Each works in much the same way to shrink swollen mucous membranes and reduce nasal and sinus congestion. These should be avoided if you have high blood pressure. They can also cause insomnia.

If head and nasal congestion are severe, a *nasal decongestant spray* might be recommended. There are a number of OTC sprays from which to choose, including Afrin, Dristan, Sinex, Neosynephrine, and Vicks. These should be used with great caution and only for three days at most. They can easily become addictive! They produce what is called a rebound effect, which means that as their decongestant effect wears off and the head and nasal congestion return, the feeling of stuffiness is often worse than it was before using the spray. This elicits a strong desire to spray again, and a vicious cycle begins. Be careful with these sprays.

Depending on the symptoms accompanying the sinus infection, such as headache, cough, or sore throat, other OTC drug recommendations might include analgesics (pain relievers), expectorants (thin the mucus), antitussives (cough suppressants), or combinations of all three with decongestants.

If repeated courses of antibiotic are not successful in treating the sinus infection (an increasingly more common occurrence), then *surgery* is often recommended. Through the use of the endoscope (a tiny telescope inserted into the nasal cavity), sinus surgery has improved dramatically over the past decade. *Endoscopic surgery* usually involves the enlarging of the ostia, the sinus drainage ducts, so the sinuses will be able to drain more effectively. The number of sinus surgeries has quickly risen to more than three hundred thousand procedures per year, costing anywhere from $3,000 to $10,000. Unfortunately, surgery is still a long way from being a guaranteed cure for chronic sinusitis. Most people experience short-term improvement, for six months to one year, then begin the cycle of sinus infections and antibiotics over again. The surgery is usually successful when it eliminates one or more of the obstructive causes of sinusitis, such as polyps, cysts, an enlarged or distorted nasal turbinate (turbinate hypertrophy), or a deviated septum. But even in these cases, the surgery is still treating the symptom, not the cause. What is responsible for stimulating the growth of the polyps, cysts, or swollen turbinates in nasal mucous membranes to such an extent that a congenitally deviated septum is now all of a sudden obstructing the sinus from draining? (A deviated septum is most often the reason that surgery is performed.) Most ear, nose, and throat (ENT) surgeons claim that there is no known cause for these phenomena. They just happen. Until conventional medicine addresses the multiple causes of chronic sinusitis, this symptom-focused treatment means the ailment will remain largely incurable, with the prognosis: "You're going to have to learn to live with it."

Risk Factors and Causes

The leading causes of *chronic sinusitis* are:

- *Air pollution*—indoor and outdoor
- *Cigarette smoke*
- *Overuse of antibiotics*—causing antibiotic-resistant bacteria and yeast (candida) overgrowth
- Emotional stress—especially *repressed anger and sadness* ("unshed tears")
- Dry air
- Cold air
- Allergies—pollen, animal dander, mold, and food (wheat and dairy products are most common)
- Occupational hazards—especially for auto mechanics, construction workers, and airport and airline personnel
- Dental problems—especially with the upper teeth

The first four risk factors on this list are the most significant. Although antibiotics are the mainstay of conventional medical treatment for sinusitis, they are not absolutely necessary to successfully treat sinus infections. Unfortunately they have been overused and in many cases prescribed so indiscriminately that we are now seeing a growing number of *antibiotic-resistant bacteria,* called supergerms. Besides the prescriptions, our diets are filled with antibiotic-laden meat and dairy products. Many of the people suffering from chronic sinusitis are still sick because their sinuses are infected with antibiotic-resistant bacteria.

Another problem resulting from antibiotics is that they also tend to destroy the friendly bacteria in our digestive tract, allowing *overgrowth of yeast or candida* organisms. The subsequent infection of the sinuses by candida may be creating another epidemic. People infected with candida often have the most severe cases of chronic sinusitis. Not only can this problem weaken the immune system, but it can also cause a multitude of food and mold allergies that further aggravate the sinusitis.

As with every chronic disease, *repressed emotions* contribute to weakening the immune system. Many patients with chronic sinusitis are high achievers and perfectionists, and not infrequently, first children. They often have a strong need for control. *Anger* often results from their perception of mistakes made by themselves or others or from a perceived loss of control. Repressed anger may be the single most significant risk factor in triggering a sinus infection. A deep sadness may also exist in the majority of these patients. The many tears that have not been shed can result in congestion of the tear glands that surround the eyes and that are in close proximity to the sinuses as well. Perhaps this swelling and congestion is also a contributor to congested sinuses.

ALLERGIES
(Allergic Rhinitis or Hay Fever)

Physiology

The response to allergens such as pollen or mold triggers a strong immune response in the mucous membrane lining the nose. Substances known as IgEs flood the nasal lining, along with eosinophils (a type of white blood cell) and a tremendous release of inflammatory cells such as histamine, prostaglandins, and leukotrienes. This dramatic response results in the swelling, dripping, and itching of the mucous membrane.

Symptoms and Diagnosis

See the list under chronic sinusitis for a complete list of symptoms.

Conventional Medical Treatment

Besides removing the offending allergen, the conventional medical treatment consists of *medication* and *allergy desensitization injections* ("allergy shots").

Eliminating the allergen is usually a bit of a challenge. Avoiding allergenic foods can be relatively simple, but getting rid of the family pet, if you're allergic to cats, or escaping from pollen is much more difficult.

You can minimize pollen exposure by taking refuge in sealed, air-conditioned office buildings and houses, where filters cleanse most of the offending pollen from incoming air. For those allergy sufferers unconcerned with domestic decor, the National Institutes of Health (NIH) recommends the following: Remove carpeting, upholstered furniture, heavy curtains, venetian blinds, fuzzy wool blankets, and comforters stuffed with wool or feathers. Empty the room, scrub all surfaces and everything that is to be returned to it, and thereafter thoroughly clean the room every week. If replacing curtains, hang some that are lightweight and can be laundered weekly. Replace the upholstered chairs with wooden or metal ones that can be scrubbed, and keep clothing in plastic zippered bags and shoes in closed boxes off the floor.

For temporary relief of mild allergies, doctors usually prescribe *antihistamines*. For years these drugs almost always caused drowsiness, but now there are a few that *usually* do not have this inconvenient side effect. Claritin, Allegra, and Zyrtec are all nonsedating prescription options. There are a number of OTC antihistamines (most will cause some drowsiness), formulated either alone or in combination with decongestants.

Many allergy sufferers also derive significant benefit from the antiallergic and anti-inflammatory effects of the prescription *corticosteroid nasal sprays*, such as Beconase, Vancenase, Nasalide, and Nasacort. Cromolyn sodium has a similar action and is available as a nasal spray (Nasalcrom) and as an eye drop (Opticrom). A seasonal pollen allergy sufferer, especially one who is also prone to sinus infections, should use the spray on a maintenance schedule throughout most of the allergy season, about one to two months. Long-term use of these cortisone sprays, beyond three months, can cause chronic irritation, inflammation, and increased mucus secretion.

If you are not satisfied with the symptomatic relief you have received from antihistamines and steroid nasal sprays, your next step will often be a visit to an allergist. Depending upon the results of a battery of *allergy skin tests*, you might then be considered a candidate for allergy *desensitization injections*. These shots, containing very small amounts of the offending allergen(s), will often be given a few days apart early on and will progress to monthly injections that could last for several years. People with severe pollen allergy seem to benefit most from this course of treatment, while those with mold, dust mite, and animal dander allergies do not fare as well. Why the shots do and sometimes don't work remains a mystery. Whether or not they do, however, they are consistently an expensive treatment option.

Conventional medicine continues to develop better diagnostic tools and more effective medications to both identify the allergen and nullify its effects. But a guaranteed or permanent cure for the sneezing and stuffy and drippy nose of allergic rhinitis is still a long way off.

Risk Factors and Causes

Possibly even more than chronic sinusitis, allergic rhinitis has a strong *genetic* component. Often at least one parent or a sibling has had a history of allergies or hay fever, eczema, or asthma. However, *airborne allergens* (pollen, mold, animal dander, dust mites, chemical exposures, etc.) together with *emotional factors* are the primary *triggers* precipitating the allergy symptoms. Polluted, dry, and cold air can act as an irritant that over the years can cause the nasal mucous membrane to become extremely sensitive and hyperreactive to pollen, mold, dander, dust, and smoke, and so on. The *foods* that most commonly cause nasal allergies are: *cow's milk* and all dairy products, wheat or any grain, chocolate, corn, white sugar, soy, yeast (brewer's and baker's), oranges, tomatoes, bell peppers, white potatoes, eggs, fish, shellfish, cocoa, onions, nuts, garlic, peanuts, black pepper, red meat, aspirin, artificial food coloring, coffee, black tea, beer, wine, and champagne. Milk is by far the most common food allergen contributing to hay fever. In most cases it is the cumulative effect of milk, pollen, mold, and pollution that causes the severe allergic reaction. It is the protein in milk, not the fat, which is the offending allergen. Therefore, low fat, skim, and acidophilus-enriched milk, as well as ice cream, can all be a problem. In aged cheese, cottage cheese, and yogurt, the protein is partially broken down and is usually not as serious a potential allergen.

The emotion most often identified in allergy patients is *fear.* It is probably more important to determine who or what situation or circumstance in your life you are "allergic" to (are afraid of or feeling insecure about) than what food or airborne allergen is causing your symptoms. The next time you have a sneezing spell, pay attention to the thoughts, mental images, and feelings that immediately preceded the onset of your symptoms. Your sneezing, itching, and congestion can become an emotional barometer that helps you to identify the deeper and hidden causes of allergic rhinitis.

CONDITION CHRONIC BRONCHITIS

Symptoms and Diagnosis

Bronchitis can be either an infection (acute bronchitis) or an inflammation (chronic bronchitis) of the bronchi, the two large tubes that branch off into the lungs from the windpipe or trachea. The typical person suffering from chronic bronchitis is a *smoker* over the age of 45. Acute bronchitis often occurs in conjunction with acute sinusitis, an infection called sinobronchitis. This results from the postnasal drainage of infected mucus from the sinuses into the lungs. The primary symptom of *acute bronchitis* is a persistent (day and night), deep, wet, and green/yellow mucousy cough. In *chronic bronchitis*, excessive mucus is secreted from the inflamed respiratory mucosa lining the bronchi. According to the American Lung Association, to qualify as chronic bronchitis, there must be a cough that produces thick white or gray mucus for at least three months, and the cough must recur for at least two consecutive years. In addition, there may be shortness of breath and wheezing, similar to the breathing problems experienced by people with asthma. Other frequent symptoms of chronic bronchitis include:

- Difficulty breathing
- Frequent episodes of acute bronchitis
- Weakness
- Weight loss

Conventional Medical Treatment

Just as with acute sinusitis, the treatment for acute bronchitis is an *antibiotic*. However, the first choice may be erythromycin, or its newer and stronger derivatives Zithromax and Biaxin. The basic conventional medical treatment for chronic bronchitis begins with *stopping smoking;* otherwise there can be no effective treatment.

The primary objective is to open and drain the bronchi of its thick and/or infected mucus. *Steam* can be helpful. Steaming in the shower, steam room, or with a device called a steam inhaler (available in many pharmacies) is recommended at least once a day. This should be followed by *postural drainage* to loosen and remove the trapped mucus blocking the airways.

Drinking plenty of water daily; avoiding the use of cough suppressants; regular use of a humidifier that puts out warm moisture; and avoiding highly polluted, cold, or dry air will also help to thin and loosen the mucus. If you must be in an area where there is highly polluted air or strong fumes, wear a special protective mask over your nose and mouth. Some pharmacies and bike shops sell them. There is also a mask called the Brinks chemical respirator, which is effective in filtering fumes and other indoor pollutants. Try to stay away from anything that you know can cause an allergic reaction.

The conventional medical approach for treating chronic bronchitis can mitigate the symptoms to the extent that you adhere to the program. It is a chronic disease and requires daily treatment. If it is not strictly maintained, as is often the case, the bronchitis slowly progresses. The bronchial walls eventually thicken, and the number of mucous glands increases. The bronchitis sufferer becomes increasingly susceptible to lung infections—acute bronchitis and pneumonia—and the bronchial mucosa becomes more inflamed and secretes a higher volume of thicker mucus. Chronic bronchitis can be incapacitating, often leading to emphysema and eventually death. Chronic lung disease, including primarily bronchitis, emphysema, and asthma, is currently the fourth leading cause of death in the United States. Each year it is gradually gaining ground on the conditions that hold the top three positions: heart disease, cancer, and stroke.

Risk Factors and Causes

The most important risk factor for causing chronic bronchitis is *cigarette smoking*. All the physical and emotional causes for chronic sinusitis, especially air pollution, can also contribute to this condition.

ASTHMA

Symptoms and Diagnosis

Asthma is the most frightening and life-threatening of the common respiratory conditions. Its primary symptom is *difficult breathing*, with or without an audible wheeze, cough, a constricted chest, or painfully congested lungs. Affecting the small airways, called bronchioles, asthma causes swelling of the respiratory mucosa lining the airway, thicker and increased mucus secretion into the airway, and contraction of the smooth muscle lining the bronchiolar walls. These three obstructive changes occurring together leave little room for air to pass through. In addition to airway obstruction, asthma is also characterized by airway inflammation. This, in turn, causes airway hyperreactivity, resulting in a heightened sensitivity to airborne allergens, pollutants, and cold and dry air.

Asthma has always been difficult to diagnose in infants and preschool children because they have trouble following directions for *breathing-function tests*. These tests are easier to administer to older children and adults and they can provide the definitive medical diagnosis. However, most people with asthma relate a history of the onset of their symptoms that can also provide a dependable diagnosis. Shortness of breath, coughing, wheezing, chest congestion, constriction, or pain following the onset of a cold, sinus infection, hay fever symptoms, emotional stress, or exercise are all common descriptions of asthma. In fact, exercise can trigger wheezing and shortness of breath in up to 80 percent of individuals who have been diagnosed with asthma, and 70 percent require treatment for their symptoms.

Conventional Medical Treatment

According to the NIH "Guidelines for the Diagnosis and Management of Asthma," effective *management* of asthma relies on four integral components:

- Objective measures of lung function, not only to assess but also to monitor each patient's asthma
- Pharmacological therapy
- Environmental measures to control allergens and irritants
- Patient education

The general principles involved in managing (not *curing*) chronic asthma include:

- Treat the underlying pathology of asthma. First-line therapy should focus on preventing or reversing the airway inflammation that is a principal factor in the airway hyperresponsiveness that characterizes asthma and determines symptoms, disease severity, and possibly mortality.

- Tailor general therapy guidelines to individual needs. Specific asthma therapy, dictated by the severity of the disease, medication tolerance, and sensitivity to environmental allergens, must be selected to fit the needs of individual patients.

- Treat asthma triggers, associated conditions, and special problems. Exposure to known allergens and irritants must be reduced or eliminated; colds, sinus infections, middle ear infections (otitis media), and allergic rhinitis can set off or aggravate asthma. Treatment of a known trigger prior to exposure, such as exercise, is recommended. Influenza vaccinations and pneumococcal vaccines should be considered for patients with moderate or severe asthma.

- Seek consultation with an asthma specialist for pulmonary function studies, evaluation of the role of allergy and irritants, or evaluation of the medication plan if the goals of therapy are not achieved.

- Use step-care pharmacological therapy. An aim of this therapy is to use the optimum medication needed to maintain control with minimal risk for adverse effects. The step-care approach, in which the number of medications and frequency of administration are increased as necessary, is used to achieve this aim.

- Monitor continually. Continual monitoring, including pulmonary function tests and regular visits to your physician, are necessary to assure that therapeutic goals are met.

The *medications* include:

- *Anti-inflammatory agents:* oral corticosteroids such as prednisone, prednisolone, or medrol; or inhaled corticosteroids such as Azmacort, Beclovent, AeroBID, Vanceril, and Decadron Phosphate Respihaler.

- *Bronchodilators:* the most frequently prescribed beta-agonist inhalers are Alupent, Brethaire, Bronkometer, Isuprel Mistometer, Maxair, Metaprel, Proventil, and Ventolin. Theophylline is the principal methylxanthine (a type of bronchodilator) used in asthma therapy. It is found in the following frequently prescribed medications: Aerolate, Bronkodyl, Choledyl, Dilor, Elixophyllin, Lufyllin, Marax, Quibron, Respbid, Slo-bid, Slo-Phyllin, Tedral, Theo-Dur, Theo-24, Theolair, and Uniphyl. Primatene Mist and tablets and Sudafed are consistently available (OTC) bronchodilators. Sudafed, containing the drug ephedrine, is usually used as a nasal decongestant but also has a bronchodilating effect. Primatene tablets contain both theophylline and ephedrine. They should be used only as needed for asthmatic attacks and not on a regular basis.

- *Leukotriene antagonists:* Montelukast and Zafirlukast are examples of this new class of drugs used to oppose leukotriene inflammatory aggravation of chronic and recurring asthama.

- *Expectorants:* medications that thin the mucus and make it easier to cough up. Prescription expectorants containing either guaifenesin or iodinated glycerol include: Fenesin, Humibid, Organidin, Sinumist, and SSKI. There are also a number of OTC products that contain guaifenesin such as Guiatuss, Anti-Tuss, Genatuss, Glyate, Halotussin, Malotuss, Robitussin, Uni-tussin, Naldecon Senior EX, Breonesin, Hytuss 2X, and Glycotuss.

Risk Factors and Causes

The most commonly recognized causes of asthmatic attacks are:

- Common cold
- Sinus infection
- Allergen exposure—both airborne and food (especially milk)
- Exercise
- Cold air
- Emotional stress

Although asthma has been described by physicians for hundreds of years, no one within the medical community is willing to state conclusively the cause for the dramatic increase in both the prevalence and severity of this condition. Asthma is now considered an epidemic of its own, with the number of asthmatics in the United States more than doubling since 1980 to nearly 15 million. In spite of the fact that available treatment is better than it has ever been, the death rate has also doubled since 1980; about five thousand Americans (the majority are urban, male, and black children) now die each year.

Separate studies in New York, Connecticut, New Jersey, and Georgia from 1988 to 1990 all confirmed a strong association between the *ozone* levels in smog and the severity of asthma. Ozone inflames air passages, and swollen airways are one of the chief symptoms of asthma. A Canadian study in 1991 suggests that ozone can increase the lungs' responsiveness to allergens, such as ragweed or grass. Based on that research, it was recommended that during periods of high ozone, asthmatics should be inactive, stay inside, and use air conditioners. Asthmatics who exercise outdoors in highly polluted cities (especially with ozone and particulates), in cold temperatures, or on days with high pollen counts are at greater risk of inducing an asthma attack.

Although asthma was once regarded as a psychological malady, it is now seen by the medical community as a hereditary, immune system disorder that is sometimes linked to allergies. However, with any chronic disease there are multiple causes, and one of them is always *emotional*. Asthma is no exception.

For many children with asthma there is excessive *enmeshment*, a smothering love, between parent and child. This overpowering relationship can create a feeling of being stifled and a degree of dependence that nearly equates with the child's inability to breathe for himself. In many families with an asthmatic child, there is a lack of bonding between the parents. Asthma is also often associated with suppressed crying and a lack of nurturing, especially touch and affection.

The Holistic Medical Treatment and Prevention for Chronic Sinusitis, Allergic Rhinitis, Chronic Bronchitis, and Asthma

Because the holistic medical treatments for each of the chronic respiratory diseases are so similar, they are grouped together in this section. Recognizing how the nose, sinuses, and lungs are connected by one continuous mucous membrane, you can not only appreciate their intimate relationship but also understand how one affects another; why certain factors, especially colds, cigarette smoke and air pollution, and cold and dry air, can adversely affect all three parts simultaneously; and how an effective treatment program directed at one condition can benefit your entire respiratory tract. The primary goals of the holistic treatment for respiratory disease are: *(1) to heal the mucous membrane lining your nose, sinuses, and lungs; and (2) to strengthen your immune system.* If you suspect candida is involved with your condition, then its elmination will require a major commitment and will become your third goal. The *holistic treatment program is directed at loving and nurturing* your body, particularly the respiratory tract, and specifically *the irritated and inflamed mucous membrane*, to allow for maximum flow of oxygen to every cell in the body.

Physical and Environmental Health *Recommendations.* Unless otherwise stated, the following methods can be used to treat and prevent chronic sinusitis, allergic rhinitis, chronic bronchitis, and asthma.

Air. The simplest and most effective way to heal the damaged mucous membrane is to stop breathing unhealthy air. (For most urban Americans that would mean to stop breathing.) If you haven't already done so, the first step is *stop smoking*, followed by the prohibition of cigarette smoking in your home and workplace. Although it will be many years before we're able to see a substantial change in our outdoor air, technology has now made it possible for us to breathe optimal *indoor* air. Healthy air is clean (can't be seen or smelled), moist (35 to 60 percent relative humidity), warm (between 65 and 85 degrees), and rich in negative ions and oxygen (100 percent saturation). Negative air ions can create a profound difference in indoor air quality. Optimum levels for good health are between three thousand and six thousand ions per cubic centimeter, and the EPA reports that the average indoor environment in the United States contains only two hundred ions per cubic centimeter.

Negative ion generators are potentially the most efficient air cleaners—they attract dust, pollen, mold, animal dander, and even bacteria and then precipitate these particles out of the air; they have also been shown to help restore the damaged mucous membrane by stimulating the cilia (microscopic hairs that act as a filter) that line its surface. Negative ion generators, for use as room air cleaners, are becoming much easier to find. Look for one that puts out a minimum of one trillion ions per second and is self-regulating to avoid the excessive ion output that results in black residue on the walls. (This type of ionizer, along with most of the other products mentioned in this chapter, may be obtained by calling 1-888-434-0033 or ordered online at www.sinussurvival.com.)

If you're unable to locate an ion generator, the next best thing to use is an air cleaner with a *HEPA filter.* Some of these air cleaners also emit ions, but HEPA filters actually remove negative ions from the air, so it really isn't possible to benefit from both operating simultaneously in the same room. Place the ion generator or air cleaner in your bedroom and, if you spend a great deal of time there, in your office as well. There will soon be efficient ionizers for your car, too.

A *good furnace filter* on a forced air heating and air-conditioning system is also important. Look for a pleated filter in the $10 to $15 range. Remember, too, that while air-conditioning cools and dries the air, it also depletes it of negative ions.

Humidifiers are essential, even in humid climates. During the winter months, while the windows are closed and the heat is on, it's usually extremely dry. A warm mist room humidifier is best. Central humidifiers attached to the furnace can also be helpful. Be sure to install a flow-through type, one without a tray of standing water.

Plants can also add moisture to your home, as well as oxygen. Spider plants, aloe vera, pothos, philodendron, and chrysanthemums are all plants that function as effective air filters.

Don't forget the value of *good ventilation* as your primary source of more oxygen and fresh air. Adequate ventilation also helps to reduce indoor air pollution. Air duct cleaning and carpet cleaning (without using toxic chemicals) are both valuable steps to take in creating healthy indoor air. The outcome may be a condition of indoor air that could be described as Hawaii-like! This is air that not only does no harm but can actually help your mucous membranes to heal.

Water and moisture. In chapter 2, the value of *drinking good quality water* for optimal physical fitness was discussed. The mucous membrane of the respiratory tract also benefits from drinking an adequate amount of water. The wetter the membrane, the thinner the mucus, and the more easily it can flow and drain. When mucus dries, it tends to get thicker and plug things up, like a nose, sinus, or lung. One of the best ways to nurture your entire respiratory tract is to breathe *steam*, and especially from a device called a steam inhaler. It's not as hot and is more direct than holding your head over a pot of boiling water, and it is more efficient than a steam room. If you really want to treat your mucous membranes well, then add a couple of drops or spray *eucalyptus oil* to the hot water. Of the more than seven hundred species of eucalyptus oil, the most highly medicinal is a brand called V-VAX. It is very healing to the mucous membranes, and together with the steam it can act as an effective decongestant.

Nasal irrigation with salt water, using a rubber ear syringe, a porcelain Neti pot or a similar plastic device called SinuCleanse, or a Grossan nasal attachment to a Water Pik, is extremely helpful for flushing infected sinuses or cleansing the membranes of the nose and sinuses. For people with chronic sinusitis, this procedure should be performed at least once daily (two or three times is better), preferably in the evening. It's even more effective if you use the steam inhaler just before irrigating. Mix one-third teaspoon of noniodized salt into an eight-ounce glass of nonchlorinated or filtered water and add a pinch of baking soda to make your irrigating solution. This same salt water mixture can also be added to a nasal spray bottle to be used frequently throughout the day, especially when the air is very dirty and/or dry. The *saline nasal spray* acts as an irrigant, washing out the tiny particles of pollution, and as a humidifier, keeping the membranes moist. Be sure that the spray comes out of the bottle as a mist, not a stream. Dr. Ivker has recently formulated, with Dr. Steve Morris, his own saline spray called the Sinus Survival Spray, which also contains several medicinal herbs:

- Aloe vera—healing to mucous membranes
- *Berberis aquifolium*—antibacterial and antiviral properties
- Grapefruit seed extract—effective in killing candida
- Sodium selenite—has antiallergic properties

Diet

The recommended *diet* for treating and preventing respiratory disease is essentially the same healthy diet that was described in chapter 2. The foods to *avoid* if you have a respiratory condition are, first and foremost, *milk and dairy* products, in addition to sugar, caffeine, and alcohol. Milk can increase and thicken mucus and may be an unsuspected cause of food allergy; sugar can weaken immunity and is the primary fuel for bacterial infections and candida, as is alcohol; while caffeine has a multitude of potentially harmful side effects (see page 21). If you suspect you have candidiasis, it is recommended that you read the section on candida in chapter 9 and adhere to the candida-control diet.

There is a distinct possibility that *food allergy* may be one of the primary causes of your nasal allergies, chronic sinusitis, or asthma. There is a growing body of research to support this theory, and actual practice has demonstrated that the elimination of milk from the diet can provide dramatic relief for a significant number of allergy and sinus sufferers, as well as asthmatics. It often takes at least a month after stopping milk before the benefits are noticed. The other foods with a higher probability of triggering these respiratory conditions are wheat, eggs, corn, and soy. The best way to confirm this diagnosis is to eliminate from your diet for at least one month all of these foods that are most often responsible for food allergies (see the complete list earlier under Risk Factors and Causes of Allergies). Then begin to reintroduce each of these foods—in a pure form—into your diet at the rate of one every three days. Pay attention to your body and note any new symptoms such as headache, nasal congestion and itching, increased mucus secretion, nausea, diarrhea, gas, or mental fog. It should be obvious to you which food, if any, causes your body to react. Food allergy is often present with more severe cases of candidiasis and is discussed further in chapter 9.

If you find that your child is allergic to milk, then add a chewable calcium supplement to his or her diet. Avoid those with high sugar content. They are available in most health food stores, as are calcium-enriched orange juice, and either rice or soy milk to add to cereal.

Vitamins, Minerals, Herbs, and Nutritional Supplements

Most of the vitamins and minerals recommended for sinusitis, allergies, bronchitis, and asthma are discussed in chapter 2. They consist primarily of the *antioxidants*—Vitamins C and E, beta carotene, grape seed extract, zinc, and selenium. All of them are listed with their dosages for both treatment and prevention in the tables that follow.

There are also *herbs* that can strengthen the immune system and act as a natural antibiotic. They are usually recommended only for treating the acute respiratory conditions and whenever you feel as if you might be getting sick. Usually acute sinusitis and acute bronchitis, and often an asthmatic attack, will be triggered by a cold. Therefore, if you can prevent the cold, you can often prevent these infections and the asthma. The herbs and supplements to take to prevent the cold just as it begins are listed below under colds.

For *allergies*, the supplements that are most effective as a "natural antihistamine" are grape seed extract, quercetin (take with bromelain), and stinging nettles. The complete list of vitamins, minerals, and herbs for allergies and *asthma* are found in the relevant table that follows.

For *chronic bronchitis*, the amino acid N-acetylcysteine (NAC) has been usedful in reducing mucus viscosity. The dosage is one 500 milligram capsule three times per day. This is included on the table and should be taken along with everything else listed. The herbal bronchodilator ephedra can be used if wheezing accompanies the bronchitis. However, it is not advisable to use ephedra for more than a few days, and it should not be taken at all by anyone with heart disease, high blood pressure, thyroid disease, diabetes, or an enlarged prostate. Otherwise this condition can be treated in much the same way as chronic sinusitis.

Homeopathic drugs and nasal sprays and Chinese herbs and acupuncture can also be helpful for treating all four of the respiratory diseases. *Acupuncture* is particularly *effective for mild asthma*, with at least six sessions needed to demonstrate any positive effects and many more for long-lasting results. It is preferable to be evaluated by a homeopathic physician or a licensed practitioner of Chinese medicine (O.M.D.) rather than to self-administer any of these treatments. Acupressure and reflexology points can be another valuable addition to a holistic medical treatment plan. Apply direct pressure to these points for 20 to 30 seconds, two to three times a day. (See diagram on p. 30.)

Exercise

In treating respiratory diseases, exercise presents a unique challenge. In people with these conditions the mucous membrane is often the weakest part of the body, and diminished lung function is often present. Exercise can potentially harm both

NATURAL QUICK-FIX SYMPTOM TREATMENT

Cough

Gargle, then drink lemon juice and honey (1:1) with a tablespoon of vodka or a pinch of cayenne pepper

Ginger tea

Wild cherry bark syrup

Bronchial Drops (a homeopathic)

Sinus Survival cough syrup (with elderberry)

Fatigue

Ginseng

Antioxidants, especially vitamin C

Folic acid

Vitamin B-12, 500 mcg two times daily

Vitmin B-6, 75 to 100 mg daily

Pantothenic acid, 500 mg one or two times daily

Meditation

Exercise

Sleep

Fatigue (continued)

Pace yourself between activity and rest

Rule out anemia

Headache

Adequate water intake

Negative air ions

Steam

Eucalyptus oil

Acupressure/reflexology points

Hydrotherapy—alternate hot and cold shower

Garlic or horseradish (chew it)

Calcium/magnesium

quercetin, two caps three times daily

Fenu/Thyme (Nature's Way), two caps three times daily

Ginkgo biloba, 40 mg three times daily

Headache (continued)

Feverfew avena, 20 drops three times daily

Runny Nose

Adequate water intake

Saline spray every one to two hours

Nettles, one cap three times daily

Quercetin, 1000 mg, two tabs three times daily (on an empty stomach), take with bromelain

Vitamin C, 6,000 to 10,000 mg daily or higher—take as ascorbate or Ester C

Sneezing

Adequate water intake

Acupressure/reflexology points

Nettles two caps two to three times daily

Quercetin, 1000 mg, two tabs three times daily before meals (on an empty stomach) Take with bromelain

even more. Strenuous running or bike riding in polluted air can often precipitate a sinus infection, an allergy or asthmatic attack, or the flare-up of a bronchitic cough. Therefore, with respiratory conditions, there is an especially fine line between strengthening and further damaging the respiratory tract and immune system with aerobic exercise. When the proper precautions are taken, it can be the most beneficial of all forms of exercise. That's why it is recommended that respiratory patients gradually walk that fine line by beginning an aerobic exercise program with brisk walking. Even those who are already used to more demanding forms of exercise may need to decrease both the intensity and duration of their exercise in order to heal the mucous membrane and strengthen the immune system.

At a minimum, *aerobic exercise* (refer to this section in chapter 2) should consist of three 30-minute workouts weekly, maintaining your target heart rate for

NATURAL QUICK-FIX SYMPTOM TREATMENT *(continued)*

Sore Throat

Gargle with lemon juice and honey (1:1) and hot water

Gargle with a pinch of cayenne and one teaspoon salt in eight ounces water

Licorice-based tea (Long Life, Traditional Medicinals, or Throat Coat)

Lozenges (Zand Eucalyptus, Holistic brand Propolis)

Zinc picolinate, 30 mg three times daily—begin with zinc gluconate lozenges for three days, then switch to picolinate

Garlic, two caps three times daily

Zand Throat Spray

Stuffy Nose

Adequate water intake

Hot tea with lemon

Hot chicken soup

Steam

Stuffy Nose *(continued)*

Hydrotherapy (hot water from shower) or hot compresses

Eucalyptus oil

Horseradish

Acupressure/reflexology points

Massage

Orgasm

Exercise

Garlic

Onions

Cayenne pepper

Breathe Right—external nasal dilator

No ice-cold drinks

No dairy

No gluten: wheat, rye, oats, barley

Rule out allergies

Papaya enzyme, one or two tablets four times daily (dissolved in mouth)—use also for ear

Stuffy Nose *(continued)*

congestion, sinus congestion, and sinus pain

Anger release, especially punching

Wheezing

Lobelia, 25 drops in mint tea every half-hour to hour (may cause nausea)

No glutens or sulfites

No milk or dairy

Caffeine

Magnesium glycinate, citrate, or aspartate, 250 mg every three hours

Vitmin B-6, 200 mg two times daily

Vitamin B-12, 500 mcg (sublingual) two times daily

Vitamin C, 3,000 to 5,000 three times daily

Selenium, 200 mcg once a day

Onions, garlic, ginger

---

two-thirds of that time. For example, a 40-year-old's target heart rate is between 108 and 153 beats per minute. (It's easier to round it off to 110 and 150.) If you have an especially severe sinus or lung condition, keep it between 100 and 110 for no more than ten minutes for the first two weeks, and then very gradually increase time and rate. In the beginning check your pulse every five minutes. You can continue to walk for the full 30 minutes; just don't allow your heart rate to go beyond 110.

After starting your exercise program with brisk walking, you can vary it with hiking, jogging, swimming, and cycling. Treadmill, rowing, stair-climb, and cross-country ski machines are excellent indoor alternatives. Having an *indoor option* for aerobic exercise is especially important for respiratory disease sufferers. Given the highly polluted air of most cities, there might be days when you would

THE PHYSICAL AND ENVIRONMENTAL HEALTH COMPONENTS OF THE *SINUS SURVIVAL PROGRAM* FOR TREATING AND PREVENTING *SINUSITIS, BRONCHITIS,* AND *COLDS*

	Preventive Maintenance	Treating an Infection
Sleep	7–9 hours/day; no alarm clock	8–10+ hours/day
Negative ions or air cleaner	Continuous operation; use ions especially with air conditioning	continuous operation
Humidifier, warm mist	Use during dry conditions, especially in winter if heat is on and in summer if air conditioner is on	Continuous operation
Saline nasal spray (SS spray)	Use daily, especially with dirty and/or dry air	Use daily, every 2–3 hours
Steam	Use as needed with dirty and/or dry air	Use daily, 2–4 x/day
Nasal irrigation	Use as needed with dirty and/or dry air	Use daily, 2–4 x/day after steam
Water, bottled or filtered	Drink ½ oz./lb. of body weight; with exercise, drink ⅔ oz./lb.	½ to ⅔ oz./lb. of body weight
Diet	Increase fresh fruit, vegetables, whole grains, fiber Avoid sugar, dairy, caffeine, alcohol	No sugar, dairy
Exercise, preferably aerobic	Minimum 20–30 minutes, 3–5 x/week; avoid outdoors if high pollution	No aerobic; moderate walking only.
Postural Drainage[7]		

	Adults		Children (Over 3 years of Age)		Pregnancy	
	Preventive Maintenance[1]	For Sinusitis, Bronchitis, or a Cold	Prevention	For Sinusitis, Bronchitis, or a Cold	Prevention	For Sinusitis, Bronchitis, or a Cold
Vitamin C (polyascorbate or Ester C)	1,000–2,000 mg 3x/day	4,000–6,000 mg 3x/day	100–250 mg 3x/day	500–1,000 mg 3x/day	1,000 mg 2x/day	1,000 mg 4x/day
Beta carotene	25,000 I.U. 1 or 2x/day	50,000 I.U. 2x/day[8]	5,000 I.U. 1 or 2x/day	10,000 I.U. 2x/day	25,000 I.U. 1x/day	25,000 I.U. 2x/day
Vitamin E	400 I.U. 1 to 2x/day	400 I.U. 2x/day	50 I.U. 1 or 2x/day	200 I.U. 2x/day	200 I.U. 1x/day	200 I.U. 2x/day
Proanthocyanidin (grape seed extract or Pycnogenol)	100 mg 1 to 2x/day	100 mg 3x/day	—	100 mg 1x/day	—	100 mg 1x/day
Multivitamin[2]	1 to 3x/day	1 to 3x/day	Pediatric multivitamin		Prenatal multivitamin with 800 mg folic acid	
Selenium	100–200 mcg/day	200 mcg/day	—	100 mcg/day	25 mcg/day	100 mcg 2x/day

THE PHYSICAL AND ENVIRONMENTAL HEALTH COMPONENTS OF THE *SINUS SURVIVAL PROGRAM* FOR TREATING AND PREVENTING *SINUSITIS, BRONCHITIS,* AND *COLDS*

	Adults		Children (Over 3 years of Age)		Pregnancy	
	Preventative Maintenance[1]	For Sinusitis, Bronchitis, or a Cold	Prevention	For Sinusitis, Bronchitis, or a Cold	Prevention	For Sinusitis, Bronchitis, or a Cold
Zinc Picolinate	20–40 mg/day	40–60 mg/day	10 mg/day	10 mg 2x/day	25mg/day	40 mg/day
Magnesium citrate or aspartate or glycinate	500 mg/day	500 mg/day	150–250 mg/day	300 mg/day	500 mg/day	500 mg/day
Calcium (citrate or hydroxyapatite)	1,000 mg/day menopause: 1,500 mg/day	1,000 mg/day menopause: 1,500 mg/day	600–800 mg/day from diet		1,200 mg/day	1,200 mg/day
Chromium picolinate	200 mcg/day	200 mcg/day	—	—	in prenatal multivitamin	
Garlic	1,200 mg/day	1,200–2,000 mg 3x/day	—	1,000 mg 3x/day	—	1,200 mg 3x/day
Echinacea	—	200 mg 3x/day or 25 drops 4–5x/day	—	100 mg 3x/day or 7–10 drops 3x/day	—	200 mg 3x/day or 25 drops 4x/day
Goldenseal[9] or Berberis	—	200 mg 3x/day or 20 drops 4–5x/day	—	100 mg 3x/day or 7–10 drops 3x/day	—	—
Bee propolis	—	500 mg 3x/day	—	200 mg 3x/day or 500 mg 1x/day	—	500 mg 3x/day
Grapefruit (citrus) seed extract	—	100 mg 3x/day or 10 drops in water 3x/day	—	4 drops in water 2x/day	—	100 mg 3x/day or 10 drops 3x/day
Flaxseed oil (or omega 3 fatty acids in fish oil)	2 Tblsp/day	2 Tblsp/day	1 Tblsp/day	1 Tblsp/day	2 Tblsp/day	2 Tblsp/day

THE PHYSICAL AND ENVIRONMENTAL HEALTH COMPONENTS OF THE *SINUS SURVIVAL PROGRAM* FOR TREATING AND PREVENTING *SINUSITIS, BRONCHITIS,* AND *COLDS*

	Adults		Children (Over 3 years of Age)		Pregnancy	
	Preventative Maintenance[1]	For Sinusitis, Bronchitis, or a Cold	Prevention	For Sinusitis, Bronchitis, or a Cold	Prevention	For Sinusitis, Bronchitis, or a Cold
N-acetylcysteine (NAC)[3]	500 mg 3x/day	500 mg 3x/day	—	200 mg 3x/day	—	500 mg 3x/day
Yin Chiao (1 bottle = 8 tablets)[4]	—	1 bottle 3–5x/day for 2 days	—	½ bottle (4 tablets) 3x/day for 2 days	—	—
Acidophilus (lactobacillus acidophilus and bifidus)[5]	½ tsp. in ½ cup water 2x/day (AM & PM)[10]	½ tsp. 3x/day or 2 caps 3x/day	¼ tsp. 2x/day[10]	½ tsp. 3x/day	½ tsp. 2x/day[10]	½ tsp. 3x/day
Antibiotics[6]						

1. Use the higher dosages on days of higher stress, less sleep, more pollen, and increased air pollution.
2. Dosage depends on brand.
3. Use only for preventing and treating chronic bronchitis.
4. Use only at *onset* of a cold and influenza.
5. Use as part of the treatment program only if candiasis is suspected..
6. An option for sinusitis and bronchitis if taken infrequently, i.e., one or two times a year
7. Postural drainage for chronic bronchitis only.
8. Use this dosage for maximum of one month.
9. Use with caution if you have ragweed allergy.
10. Take this preventive acidophilus for only two weeks, three times per year, and when you're taking an antibiotic.

This table was created by Robert S. Ivker, D.O., Steve Morris, N.D., and Todd Nelson, N.D.

be doing yourself (and your mucous membranes) more harm than good by exercising outdoors. Since the 1970s, Boulder, Colorado has been a training center for many world-class runners and cyclists. During the early to mid-1990s, however, Boulder saw an exodus of many of these athletes due to their growing number of asthma, bronchitis, and sinus problems resulting from air pollution. Extremely dry and/or cold air are the other air quality factors to consider before exercising outdoors. Also try to avoid the main roads when you plan your walking, biking, or jogging route.

THE PHYSICAL AND ENVIRONMENTAL HEALTH COMPONENTS OF THE *SINUS SURVIVAL PROGRAM* FOR TREATING AND PREVENTING *ALLERGIES* AND *ASTHMA*

	Preventive Maintenance	Treating Allergies and Asthma
Sleep	7–9 hours/day; no alarm clock	8–10+ hours/day
Negative ions or air cleaner	Continuous operation (use negative ions, esp. if air conditioner is in use)	Continuous operation (esp. during allergy season)
Humidifier, warm mist	Use during dry conditions—in winter if heat is on; in summer if air conditioner is on	
Saline nasal spray (SS spray)	Use daily, several times/day, especially with dirty and/or dry air	
Steam	Use as needed with dirty and/or dry air	Use daily, 2–4 x/day
Nasal irrigation (allergies only)	Use as needed with dirty and/or dry air	Use daily, 2–4 x/day after steam
Water, bottled or filtered	Drink ½ oz./lb. of body weight; with exercise, drink ⅔ oz. lb.	
Diet	Increase fresh fruit, vegetables, whole grains, fiber; cayenne, ginger and garlic for asthma; decrease sugar, dairy, wheat, and alcohol; do food elimination diet to determine any food allergy	
Exercise, preferably aerobic	Minimum 20–30 min., 3–5 x/week. Avoid outdoors if high pollution and/or pollen	No aerobic; moderate walking okay. Avoid outdoors if high pollution and/or pollen

	Adults		Children (Over 3 years of Age)		Pregnancy	
	Preventive Maintenance[1]	Treating Allergies and Asthma	Prevention	Treating Allergies and Asthma	Prevention	Treating Allergies and Asthma
Vitamin C (polyascorbate or Ester C)	1,000–2,000 mg 3x/day	3,000–5,000 mg 3x/day	100–250 mg 3x/day	500–1,000 mg 3x/day	1,000 mg 2x/day	1,000 mg 4x/day
Beta carotene	25,000 I.U. 1 or 2x/day	25,000 I.U. 3x/day	5,000 I.U. 1 or 2x/day	10,000 I.U. 2x/day	25,000 I.U. 1x/day	25,000 I.U. 2x/day
Vitamin E	400 I.U. 1 or 2x/day	400 I.U. 2x/day	50 I.U. 1 or 2x/day	200 I.U. 2x/day	200 I.U. 1x/day	200 I.U. 2x/day
Proanthocyanidin (grape seed extract or Pycnogenol)	100 mg 1 or 2x/day	100 mg 3x/day	—	100 mg 1x/day	—	100 mg 1x/day
Multivitamin	1–3x/day	1–3x/day	Pediatric multivitamin		Prenatal multivitamin with 800 mcg folic acid	
Selenium	100–200 mcg/day	200 mcg/day	—	100 mcg/day	25 mcg/day	100 mcg/day
Zinc Picolinate	20–40 mg/day	40–60 mg/day	10 mg/day	10 mg 2x/day	25mg/day	40 mg/day

THE PHYSICAL AND ENVIRONMENTAL HEALTH COMPONENTS OF THE *SINUS SURVIVAL PROGRAM* FOR TREATING AND PREVENTING *ALLERGIES* AND *ASTHMA*

	Adults		Children (Over 3 years of Age)		Pregnancy	
	Preventive Maintenance[1]	Treating Allergies and Asthma	Prevention	Treating Allergies and Asthma	Prevention	Treating Allergies and Asthma
Magnesium citrate, aspartate or glycinate	500 mg/day	500 mg 2 or 3x/day	150–250 mg/day	300 mg/day	500 mg/day	500 mg/day
Calcium (citrate or hydroxyapatite)	1,000 mg/day menopause: 1,500 mg/day	1,000 mg/day menopause: 1,500 mg/day	600–800 mg/day from diet		1,200 mg/day	1,200 mg/day
Chromium picolinate	200 mcg/day	200 mcg/day	—	—	in prenatal multivitamin	
Vitamin B-6	50 mg 2x/day	200 mg 2x/day	10 mg 1x/day	25 mg 1x/day	25 mg 1x/day	25 mg 2x/day
Garlic	1,200 mg/day	1,200–2,000 mg 3x/day	—	1,000 mg 3x/day	—	1,200 mg 3x/day
Ephedra or Ma huang[2]	—	12.5–25 mg 2 or 3x/day	—	5 mg 2x/day	—	—
ALLERGIES ONLY[4] Licorice (*glycyrrhiza glabra*)[3]	—	10–20 drops 3x/day[7]	—	5–10 drops 2 to 3x/day	—	—
Nettles, freeze dried	—	300 mg 1 to 3x/day	—	—	—	—
Quercetin + bromelain	—	1,000–2,000 mg/day (into 3 to 6 doses/day)	—	250–500 mg 1 to 2x/day	—	—
Pantothenic acid	—	500 mg 3x/day (after meals)	—	50 mg 2 to 3x/day	—	—
Hydrochloric acid	—	1 or 2 after protein based meals	—	—	—	—
Antihistamines	—	OTC or Rx		OTC or Rx		OTC or Rx
Corticosteroid nasal spray	—	Rx	—	Rx	—	Rx
Allergy desensitization injections	Physician supervised					

THE PHYSICAL AND ENVIRONMENTAL HEALTH COMPONENTS OF THE *SINUS SURVIVAL PROGRAM* FOR TREATING AND PREVENTING *ALLERGIES* AND *ASTHMA*

	Adults		Children (Over 3 years of Age)		Pregnancy	
	Preventive Maintenance[1]	Treating Allergies and Asthma	Prevention	Treating Allergies and Asthma	Prevention	Treating Allergies and Asthma
Anti-inflammatory agents (corticosteroids or cromolyn sodium)	—	Rx	—	Rx	—	Rx
Bronchodilators (beta agonists and theophylline	—	Rx	—	Rx	—	Rx
Vitamin B-12[5]	500 mcg 1x/day sublingually (under tongue)	500 mcg 2x/day	—	—	—	500 mcg 1x/day
Ginkgo biloba	—	40 mg of 24% standardized extract 3x/day	—	20 mg of 24% standardized extract 3x/day	—	—
Coleus forskholi	—	3–4 mg/day	—	—	—	—
N-acetylcysteine (NAC)	—	500 mg 2x/day	—	250 mg 2x/day		
Lobelia	—	25 drops in mint tea every 3 to 4 hours	—	—	—	—
Ecomer (shark liver oil)	—	50 mg 3x/day	—	—	—	—
Flaxseed oil (or omega 3 fatty acids)	2 Tblsp/day	3 Tblsp/day	1 Tblsp/day	1 Tblsp/day	2 Tblsp/day	3 Tblsp/day

(Rows from Vitamin B-12 through Ecomer are bracketed as "ASTHMA ONLY 6")

1. Use the higher dosages on days of higher stress, less sleep, more pollen, and increased pollution.
2. Can be used for both allergies and asthma; do not use with high blood pressure.
3. Do not use with high blood pressure or an enlarged prostate.
4. Allergies only—take these only during your allergy *season*; natural products may be taken with or without Rx.
5. Magnesium, B-6, B-12, ginkgo, and coleus can be obtained in one product—Ventimax, made by CMC.
6. Asthma only—all of these can be taken together to control asthma, then *gradually* reduce Rx's while maintaining recommended dosages of natural products. This should be done under the supervision of a physician.
7. Watch for low potassium with long-term use.
8. Acidophilus can also be helpful for allergy and asthma treatment and prevention. Refer to the "Sinusitis" table for dosages.

This table was created by Robert S. Ivker, D.O., Steve Morris, N.D., and Todd Nelson, N.D.

Sinus Acupressure Points

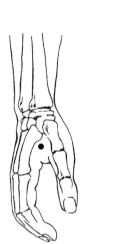
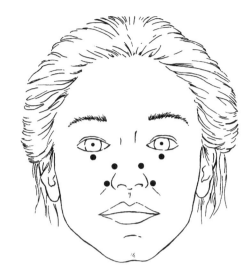

Reflex Points for Sinusitis, Allergies and Asthma

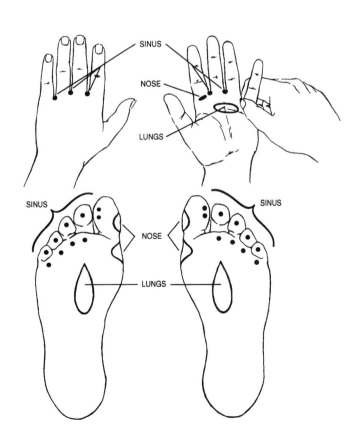

It is best to schedule exercise around the rise and fall of pollution levels. In the winter, cold night air can trap a layer of particulates, carbon monoxide, nitrogen dioxide, and sulfur dioxide that lingers into the early morning. In the summer, ozone builds up during the morning, reaches its maximum late in the afternoon, and then ebbs in the evening. A good general practice is to restrict outdoor exercise to afternoon and evenings during the winter and mornings during the summer.

Ultimately you must learn to listen to your body to determine whether you're doing too much or the air quality is hurting you. If you experience a wheeze, cough, tightness in your chest, or sinus pain during your workout, then it might be time to head indoors for aerobic exercise. Ozone levels in most homes, gyms, and pools are about half that of the outdoors—even less with a good air-conditioning system.

If you have a chronic respiratory condition and you exercise regularly, then try the following. After your heart rate has dropped to its pre-exercise level, get five to ten minutes of exposure to wet steam. This can be done in a steam room at a health club, in the bathroom of your home, or with the steam inhaler mentioned earlier. Breathe in slowly and deeply through your nose and exhale through your mouth. Do this as often as you can after exercise, whether it's indoor or outdoor.

Mental and Emotional Health Recommendations. Whether suffering from bad sinuses, allergies, bronchitis, or asthma, most people with chronic respiratory disease have repeatedly heard the message: "You're going to have to live with it," either from their physician or from themselves. This belief will often add to already existing feelings of anger, sadness, fear, and possibly hopelessness. Louise Hay recommends specific *affirmations* for a variety of ailments. Many of them have proven to be an effective component of Dr. Ivker's Sinus Survival Program. They are the following:

Allergies: *The world is safe and friendly. I am safe. I am at peace with life.*

Bronchitis and Sinusitis: *I declare peace and harmony are within me and surround me at all times. All is well.*

Asthma: *It is safe now for me to take charge of my own life. I choose to be free.*

Candidiasis: *I give myself permission to be all that I can be and I deserve the very best in life. I love and appreciate myself and others.*

There are many others that you can create on your own. For example:

I am always breathing freely and deeply.
The air that I breathe is strengthening and nurturing me.

I am comfortable in any environment.

My mucous membranes are healing with every breath I take.

My sinuses (lungs or allergies) are getting better every day.

My sinuses are now completely healed.

Remember to be as specific as possible with the affirmations and try to visualize what you want. In picturing healthy mucous membranes, it may help to look in the mirror and pull your lower lip down. The pink glistening tissue lining the inside of your lip resembles a healthy mucous membrane. This image will help in healing your nose, sinuses, or lungs.

Imagery can also be helpful in reducing allergic responses to sensitizing substances. The following visualization is an "allergy walk" taught by Dr. Jack Schwartz, an Oregon naturopathic physician.

Begin by placing yourself in a state of relaxation using abdominal breathing. Once relaxed, imagine yourself traveling to seven potentially allergy-producing sites.

1. An animal farm with a large variety of domesticated and wild animals and fearlessly petting and talking with them all

2. A family farm in springtime with everything covered with deep layers of tree, flower, and grass pollen

3. An old abandoned Victorian house in which you descend to the basement filled with dust, cobwebs, and mildew

4. An industrial park replete with strong odors of chemical solvents, polluted air, and heavy smog

5. A department store, walking up and down aisles filled with colognes and perfume, Naugahyde, new rugs, and potent detergents

6. A banquet hall with a large smorgasbord of a large variety of foods, sampling each

7. A large, well-appointed room in which you find every person you have ever disliked, greeting each briefly, wishing them well and moving to the next

In each of these scenes, imagine that you are breathing fully and deeply through your nose and bronchial passages without restriction, feeling energetic and confident.

Hypnosis has been effectively used in treating asthma, as has *psychotherapy*. It's best to find a psychotherapist who's been professionally trained in hypnotherapy. Suppressed anger, fear, and sadness seem to be a common theme causing respiratory diseases. Counseling could be a helpful adjunct in treating any of these conditions. However, if you choose to do the emotional work on your own, safely *releasing anger* on a regular basis can be far more effective treatment than years of antibiotics or multiple sinus surgeries. Punching, stamping, screaming, or any combination of sound (with the exhale) plus body movement for even a minute or two a day is sufficient. (Refer to the section "Anger Release" in chapter 3.) Giving yourself permission to cry allows the tears to flow while also helping your sinuses to drain. All of the recommendations for emotional fitness in chapter 3 are helpful in treating and preventing sinusitis, allergies, bronchitis, or asthma.

Bioenergy One recent study has documented the benefit of *journaling* in treating asthma (see pg. 57). Physical problems with the nose and sinuses are related to the sixth chakra (one of the seven primary energy centers described in Ayurvedic medicine—see the appendix). According to *Anatomy of the Spirit* by Caroline Myss, the mental and emotional issues associated with this chakra are self-evaluation, truth, intellectual abilities, feelings of adequacy, openness to the ideas of others, the ability to learn from experience, and emotional intelligence (the ability to identify, experience, and express feelings). The lungs are related to the fourth or heart chakra, and the concomitant issues are love and hatred, resentment and bitterness, grief and anger, self-centeredness, loneliness and commitment, forgiveness and compassion, and hope and trust.

Any *energy medicine modality*, such as therapeutic or healing touch, *Reiki*, or *qi gong*, can be beneficial in treating and preventing the respiratory diseases. These therapies can be directed at the specific chakra associated with your condition. It is also helpful to work on the specific mental and emotional issues that you feel apply to you. For instance, the perfectionism and strong need for control present in many people with chronic sinusitis would apply to the issues of self-evaluation, feelings of adequacy, openness to the ideas of others, and the ability to learn from experience. Just in becoming more aware of these possible factors that might be contributing to your dis-ease, you will begin the process of healing.

Colds, influenza and *otitis media* (middle ear infection) are *acute* respiratory conditions. All three are among the ten most common acute ailments in America. Although they are generally self-limiting (they'll usually resolve on their own), medication can sometimes be helpful in relieving discomfort and in shortening the duration of the symptoms. Each of the four *chronic* conditions discussed earlier—sinusitis, allergies, bronchitis, and asthma—can have acute flare-ups, which will usually resolve with treatment. However, with any chronic disease, the problem is never completely gone.

CONDITION

COLDS

Prevalence

In medical terminology, the common cold is called nasopharyngitis or upper respiratory infection (URI); it is an inflammation of the respiratory tract. There are an estimated one billion colds every year in the United States. The average adult develops two to four colds a year, usually between October and March. Children average six to ten colds, and people over sixty have less than one cold per year. The common cold is the nation's leading cause of absenteeism, accounting for seven lost workdays per person annually.

Symptoms and Diagnosis

Nasal congestion, a clear thin mucous discharge, and sore throat (early in the course) are the predominant symptoms of the common cold. For a complete list of primary and secondary symptoms, refer to the list on page 107. The duration of most colds is between four and ten days. If your cold is lasting longer than two weeks, be suspicious of a sinus infection.

Conventional Medical Treatment

There is very little that conventional medicine offers in the way of cold treatment, for the simple reason that there is no remedy that has been scientifically proven. The conclusion of the medical community is that the therapeutic benefits of vitamin C, chicken soup (it's just the steam above the bowl that helps—steaming water will have the same effect), rest and fluids, gargling, and most OTC cold tablets (especially those with a variety of ingredients) are overrated. *Zinc gluconate lozenges* did, however, test well in a study performed at the Cleveland Clinic. The zinc produced complete recovery in about four days, instead of a week in the untreated cold sufferers. The usual recommendations address the predominant symptoms:

- Decongestants—for a stuffy nose
- Antihistamines—for a runny nose
- Cough suppressants—to reduce cough
- Expectorants—to loosen mucus
- Aspirin or acetaminophen—to relieve muscle aches and/or fever

Risk Factors and Causes

Colds are caused by over two hundred different *viruses*. In the late fall and winter, colds are usually caused by either parainfluenza or respiratory syncytial viruses, while in spring, summer, and fall the predominant cold bug is one of the one hundred or more rhinoviruses. People become infected when exposed to the virus, either by inhaling it in airborne form or from contact with an infected surface, usually someone's hand. Rhinoviruses can survive for about three hours outside the nasal passages or on objects. The virus usually infects healthy cells by passing through the walls of the mucous membranes in the nose, eyes, or mouth.

Just as with any other illness, there are multiple factors impacting whether or not you get sick. Emotional *stress*, especially time pressure while attempting to accomplish too many things simultaneously, is perhaps the most prevalent risk factor in causing colds. This situation is often accompanied by a lack of, or not very restful, sleep. These factors combine to reduce immune responsiveness and weaken our resistance to the cold viruses to which we're frequently exposed during the winter months. Any of the previously mentioned environmental risks—cigarette smoke, heavy air pollution, or extremely dry or cold air—can irritate the mucous membrane of the nose or throat enough to allow the virus to enter the weakened cells.

Holistic Medical Treatment and Prevention

The common cold is often the trigger for causing acute sinusitis, acute bronchitis, and an asthmatic attack. Since recurrence of these acute problems often leads to chronic sinusitis and asthma, the most effective prevention for both the acute and chronic problems is to either prevent colds or greatly reduce their adverse effects. Your best line of defense against a cold is a strong immune system. Maintaining a healthy immune system not only is good prevention, but also will assist in a quicker and more complete recovery if you do get a cold.

The first physical symptoms of a cold are usually a sore throat, fatigue, feeling weak or achy, mucus drainage, and possibly some sneezing. If you respond quickly enough to the earliest signs of a cold, you can usually avoid the full force of the infection and not infrequently prevent the cold in its entirety. At the first hint of a sore throat or nasal symptoms, do the following:

- Rest and get more sleep
- Take vitamin C (in the form of Ester C), between 15,000 and 20,000 mg in the first 24 hours; either 5,000 mg three or four times daily, or 2,000 mg every two hours, or 1,000 mg every waking hour; very gradually taper this dose over the next three to five days
- Take vitamin A (kills viruses), 150,000 I.U. daily for two to three days; you can take 50,000 I.U. three times, then gradually taper over the next two to three days

- Take Yin chiao, a Chinese herb, five tablets four or five times daily in the first 48 hours

- Take garlic, eaten raw (one or two cloves a day) or in liquid or capsule form, 4,000 mcg (of allicin) per day

- Take echinacea, 1 dropperful in water three to five times daily for three to five days; or 900 mg four times daily. Do not take echinacea if you're pregnant or have an autoimmune disease like lupus, MS, or HIV

- Take zinc gluconate lozenges, containing at least 13 mg, every two hours

- Gargle with salt water

- Use a saline nasal spray hourly, preferably the Sinus Survival Spray containing antiviral herbs

- Take lots of warm or hot liquids; take ginger root or peppermint tea; you can include ginger, honey, lemon, cayenne, cinnamon, and a teaspoon of brandy

- Take a hot bath and inhale steam, adding a few drops of eucalyptus, peppermint, and/or tea tree oil

- Take the "homeopathic vitamin Cs," Aconitum (monkshood) and Ferrum phos (iron phosphate)

- Use acupuncture and acupressure

- Eliminate dairy products and sugar and eat lighter foods; eat less protein

The sooner you act, the more effectively this regimen will prevent the cold or lessen its severity and duration. The best treatment is obviously prevention, and that entails maintaining a strong immune system. A good preventive maintenance program is outlined in the preceding tables.

Keep in mind the basic objective of the physical aspect of holistic medical treatment—*love your body.* By creating the uncomfortable symptoms of a cold, your body is sending you a very strong message: there is a need for nurturing that isn't being met. You've been "doing" too much and not caring enough for yourself. Your actions and behavior, in conjunction with your genetic and emotional makeup, have combined to create an imbalance that manifests as physical discomfort. If balance is not restored and the body's warnings are not heeded, the problem can progress into a dis-ease of greater magnitude, for example, chronic sinusitis—a persistent state of imbalance and physical disharmony.

Louise Hay's affirmation for colds: *I allow my mind to relax and be at peace. Clarity and harmony are within me and around me.*

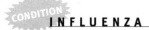

INFLUENZA

Prevalence

Many people are in the habit of describing almost every ailment as "the flu." In fact, influenza is a highly contagious and debilitating viral infection of the respiratory tract that can potentially be deadly. About 20,000 deaths occur each year in the United States from influenza. The infection occurs during the winter season, most commonly during the months of December, January, February, and March. A flu outbreak in a community typically begins abruptly, peaks after three weeks, then subsides in another three or four weeks after infecting 20 to 50 percent of the population. Children between the ages of 5 and 14 are the hardest hit. It takes about three to four days after flu symptoms appear before a person is no longer contagious.

The most common forms of influenza are types A and B. The former is more debilitating and lasts longer, sometimes ten days to two weeks. Type A flu is also highly unstable and constantly mutates, creating new strains that have been responsible for the deaths of hundreds of thousands of Americans during the twentieth century. The Swine flu in 1918, which killed between 20 and 40 million people worldwide, the Asian flu in 1957, and the Hong Kong flu in 1968 are all examples of type A pandemics (global epidemics). Approximately every ten years influenza pandemics have been caused by new strains of type A virus. Influenza A epidemics or regional outbreaks have appeared every two to three years, and influenza B outbreaks about every four to five years.

Symptoms and Diagnosis

The diagnosis of influenza is usually made on the basis of the symptoms. They most commonly include:

- Cough (usually dry) within 24 hours of onset
- Severe muscle aches
- Fever early on (approx. 103 in adults, higher in children)
- Extreme fatigue
- Sore throat
- Runny nose
- Headache
- Sudden onset with severe symptoms for first two days, gradually subsiding and resolving after five days

Secondary symptoms may include nausea, abdominal pain, diarrhea, light-headedness, and disorientation.

Conventional Medical Treatment

As in the case of medical treatment for the common cold, there is little to be offered for this potentially serious viral illness other than mitigating the symptoms. Bedrest and fluids, analgesics (but not aspirin for children, because of the risk of Reye's syndrome), cough suppressants, and decongestants can help flu sufferers to feel more comfortable.

The prescription drugs Symmetrel and Flumadine can be effective with influenza A if used very early in the course of the illness (preferably the first day). They can shorten both the intensity and duration of the symptoms. The latest drug, Relenza (available late 1999), will do the same thing and is effective for both type A *and* B viruses. Antibiotics are sometimes prescribed to prevent pneumonia in patients over 50.

Conventional medicine considers vaccination very important for people over age 65, those with heart or lung disease, and pregnant women. Since 1984, the Centers for Disease Control and Prevention (CDC) has added to this list the physicians, nurses, and other medical personnel who have extensive contact with high-risk patients.

Although an attack of influenza does confer immunity to that particular strain, the flu viruses alter themselves just enough so that you may still be vulnerable to the same type of flu in the future. This is especially true of type A. Flu vaccines have been developed that have been reported to be 60 to 90 percent effective for at least six months against either type A or B. A flu shot is definitely recommended if you have a chronic heart or lung ailment. But regardless of age, if you are healthy, then maintaining a strong immune system is your best defense against the flu, since vaccines are not always benign. Instances of healthy elderly people dying from influenza not long after receiving a flu shot are not uncommon.

Holistic Medical Treatment and Prevention

A good influenza prevention program incorporates the recommendations for sleep, air, water, exercise, food, and supplements listed in the preceding tables. However, if you do get sick, the sooner you begin the holistic treatment, the less severe the illness will be. The following regimen is highly effective in minimizing the symptoms and the duration of the infection. (Unless otherwise stated the directions are the same as for treating the common cold.

- Rest and lots of warm or hot liquids
- Vitamins C and A

- Yin Chiao and Yin Chiao Junior (for children)

- Garlic

- Echinacea

- Elderberry, taken as a tea or in extracts, 40 drops dissolved in a glass of warm water every four hours (especially for cough)

- N-acetylcysteine, 500 mg four times daily (for cough, bronchitis, or pneumonia)

- Quercetin with bromelain, 1000 mg three to five times daily (for congestion and aching)

- Oscillococcinum, a homeopathic remedy used primarily for aching, chills, and fever

- Ginger, taken as a tea or in capsules (for nausea)

- Diet: same as for a cold

CONDITION
OTITIS MEDIA
(Middle Ear Infection)

Prevalence/Anatomy and Physiology

Middle ear infection, medically known as acute otitis media, is the most common diagnosis in children treated by physicians and accounts for nearly one-third of all doctor's visits for children up to age five; half of all children have at least one episode. Acute otitis media typically results from the blockage of the eustachian tube (this tube allows for the equalization of pressure on the eardrum), which prevents the drainage of mucus from the middle ear space. Due to the anatomical positioning of the eustachian tube (see diagram), ear infections are very often seen in conjunction with the common cold and sinus infections. Just as these infections cause swelling and inflammation of the mucous membrane lining the nose and sinuses, they have the same effect upon the lining of the eustachian tube. The bacteria that most often cause this infection are the same as those responsible for sinus infections. But unlike a blocked and infected sinus, the infected middle ear space has the opportunity to drain through the rupture of the eardrum. This common occurrence relieves the pain and often resolves the infection. Occasionally, however, the eardrum does not heal and has to be surgically repaired. The other possible but uncommon complications of untreated otitis media include mastoiditis (an infection of the bone behind the ear) and meningitis (occurs in one out of four thousand ear infections). Chronic otitis media can also lead to scarring of the middle ear, causing hearing loss.

The ear is not typically thought of as being a part of the respiratory tract. But

Middle Ear Space and Eustachian Tube

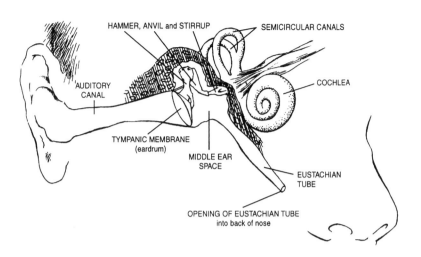

the fact that the middle ear space is lined by the same ciliated mucous membrane as the nose and sinuses and is connected through the eustachian tube (also lined by the same respiratory epithelium) to the back of the nose establishes the middle ear as an integral component of the respiratory tract. It is also impacted by the same factors that adversely affect the nose, sinuses, and lungs, although not as directly. One Canadian study found that children exposed to secondhand cigarette smoke at home before age three are twice as likely to get serious, persistent or recurrent middle ear infections. Another study showed that low humidity may be a contributing factor in otitis media.

Symptoms and Diagnosis

As a result of the build-up of pressure from the mucus trapped in the middle ear space, the primary symptom of otitis media is *pain*. This is often accompanied by fever, diminished hearing, and cold symptoms. The course of the illness is short, and very few children have more than two days of pain and fever, with or without antibiotics. In infants and younger children who aren't able to tell you if an ear hurts, the symptoms can be less specific, including runny nose, irritability, fever, and poor appetite (refusal to nurse or drink from a bottle because sucking aggravates the pain). The diagnosis is confirmed by a physician or health practitioner who can observe the inflamed and bulging eardrum through an otoscope, a hand-held instrument used to look into the ear canal.

Conventional Medical Treatment

Antibiotics are nearly always prescribed for otitis media. This is true in spite of the fact that many infections are viral and that several studies have shown little or no difference in the successful treatment of this condition with or without using antibiotics. In 1994, research performed at the National Academy of Sciences' Institute of Medicine concluded that antibiotics were no more effective than placebos in treating middle ear infections. *Analgesics* and *decongestants* are also usually prescribed. Most effective for this acute problem are the decongestant nose drops, but it's often a bit of a challenge to apply the drops. The use of antibiotics can reduce the risk of the potentially serious complications of otitis media, such as mastoiditis and meningitis.

Many European and Scandinavian physicians do not routinely use antibiotics. Instead, they have adopted an approach of watchful waiting (from 5 to 14 days), reserving antibiotics for the few children who do not resolve the infection on their own.

Many young children have repeated episodes of acute otitis media, as often as four or five times a year. After multiple courses of antibiotics, a significant number of these children are referred to an otolaryngologist (ENT physician) for *surgery*, called a tympanostomy. In this procedure a tube (called a tympanostomy tube) is inserted through the eardrum to facilitate drainage from the middle ear space. This is the most common operation for children that requires general anesthesia, numbering about one million procedures in the United States annually. Some studies have shown that this surgery results in a greater incidence of hearing loss than nonsurgical treatment. Another study, published in the April 1994 issue of the *Journal of the American Medical Association*, concluded that about one-quarter of middle ear surgeries to insert tympanostomy tubes in children are "inappropriate" and that another one-third are questionable. The Scandinavians have a much lower rate of ear tube placement and no increase in the rate of complications.

Holistic Medical Treatment

If your child does require an antibiotic, it is best to *follow* the antibiotic course with two to four weeks of *bifidus* bacteria (for children aged one to five) or *acidophilus bacteria* (for those six and older) to replace the good bacteria in the bowel. Buy only refrigerated brands of acidophilus and bifidus in the form of a liquid or powder that can be easily mixed with a glass of juice.

If your child is in pain, and the combination of acetaminophen and decongestant drops has not helped, and you'd rather not go the conventional route of antibiotics, there are several *homeopathic remedies* that are quite effective. Belladona, Chamomilla, and Pulsatilla can all be used for severe pain, while Ferrum phos, is recommended for milder pain and the early stages of a cold. If your child is prone to middle ear infections, and you'd like to try another method of treatment, a visit to a homeopathic practitioner would be valuable. You can be instructed on how to treat your child both preventively and therapeutically in the event of a recurrence of the infection.

A growing number of physicians are recognizing the role of *food allergy*, usually to milk and dairy products, in causing otitis media. Most holistic physicians agree that the elimination of milk from the diet of children with recurrent otitis will produce a significant improvement in at least one-half of the cases. In most hard cheeses, like cheddar, the milk protein has been broken down enough so that it will cause much less of an allergic response. Both cottage cheese and yogurt have a moderate milk allergy potential. Other potential food allergens for otitis media are wheat, eggs, corn, soy, chocolate, peanuts, and chicken. If your child has recurrent infections it would be wise to eliminate all these foods from his or her diet for several months (it sometimes takes that long to see a difference in the frequency of ear infections) and then gradually reintroduce them, one new food every three to four days. While treating an infection, milk and sugar should be avoided. Sugar has been shown to reduce immunity by diminishing the ability of the white blood cells to digest and destroy bacteria; this can last up to five hours following sugar ingestion. One study demonstrating this finding used full-strength fruit juice as the source of sugar. Either a holistic or, especially, a naturopathic physician is qualified to help you investigate your child's possible food allergies.

While treating a middle ear infection, it is helpful to boost your child's immune function with extra *vitamins C* (500 mg four times daily), E (200 I.U. per day), A, B-6, and the herbs *echinacea* and *astragalus*.

To help *relieve pain*, apply wet washcloths to your child's external ear, alternating three minutes of hot (to tolerance) with 30 seconds of a cold compress. If there are no ear drainage tubes, and you see no drainage coming from your child's ear (which means the eardrum is probably intact), you can instill drops into the ear to relieve both pain and inflammation, while also treating the infection. An effective combination is warm garlic oil with St. John's wort and mullein; then loosely plug the ear canal with cotton. This method works best if it is initiated at the first sign of an ear infection. The simplest way to do this is to buy the liquid form of each of the three herbs at a health food store, along with an empty dropper bottle. Mix the three in the empty bottle in the following proportions: garlic (2):St. John's wort (1):mullein (1)—the garlic is the most important ingredient. Place the bottle under warm tap water and test it by placing a drop on the back of your hand before instilling it in your child's ear.

If you can find skilled practitioners, *craniosacral therapy* and *Chinese herbs* can be very effective in treating otitis media, both acutely and in preventing recurrences. Research has also revealed that children who are breast-fed until age one or older have a lower incidence of otitis media.

7

Psychological Disease

Depression

Anxiety

Insomnia

Addictions and Alcoholism

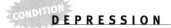 **DEPRESSION**

Prevalence

DEPRESSION IN ITS VARIOUS forms currently afflicts about 11 million people in the United States. This disorder does not distinguish among age, race, culture, or occupation—it is pervasive in all echelons of society. More than twice as many women are being treated for depression than men, but it is not known whether this is because women are more likely to be depressed or whether men tend to deny their depression. Suicide rates, especially for younger people, continue to rise. Some studies of high school children reveal that as many as 30 percent commonly think of suicide and feel hopeless. Depressed people are much more likely to develop cancer, die from a second heart attack, or die prematurely. The estimated yearly cost to this country of depression is $50 billion. According to the World Health Organization (WHO), depression is currently the fourth leading cause of disability in the world. Major depressions occur in 10 to 20 percent of the world's population in the course of a lifetime. By the year 2020, WHO estimates that depression will be second only to heart disease as the world's leading chronic disease.

Symptoms and Diagnosis

Depression is an all-inclusive term covering the spectrum from major depression and bipolar disorder, at one extreme, to adjustment problems, sadness, and the blues at the other. In the middle of the spectrum are the bulk of the depressed people, with chronic mild and intermittent depression. For the purposes of this book, the typical picture of a serious depression with its most common features is described. Before the diagnosis of depression is made, a complete physical examination by a primary care physician is recommended. It should include thyroid and adrenal function tests (including a salivary adrenal stress index test that measures both cortisol and dehydroepiandrosterone [DHEA]), a complete blood count (CBC), and a stool analysis for candida (a rapidly increasing cause of depression) and parasites. In general, the *diagnosis* of depression is made when there is a negative change in one's thought, mood, behavior, and physical responses, as indicated below.

According to the DSM-4 (the handbook of the American Psychiatric Association), one needs to display five of the following nine symptoms for at least two weeks to be diagnosed with depression:

- Depressed mood for most of the day
- Markedly diminished interest in usual activities
- Insomnia or excessive sleep nearly every day
- Significant loss of weight or appetite
- Agitated or markedly slowed movements
- Loss of energy or fatigue nearly every day
- Feelings of worthlessness or inappropriate guilt
- Diminished ability to think or concentrate
- Recurrent suicidal thoughts or plan

Typically, if you're depressed you have a significant loss of self-esteem, fatigue, and sexual drive. Other typical symptoms include crying spells, self-loathing, irritability and short temper, extreme pessimism, and thoughts of death. Everything seems hopelessly futile.

When the symptoms of the milder and more common forms of depression (the blues) increase in frequency, intensity and duration, they can become more disabling. Sufferers' relationships, work, and general functioning become more impaired. At that point, when one's symptoms and functioning are clearly perceived as distressing, one has a major depression, and treatment is required. About 40 percent of people with depression are neither medically diagnosed nor undergo professional treatment.

Conventional Medical Treatment

The most common treatment modalities for depression are *medications* and *psychotherapy*.

Medications. For treating depression, there are three basic groups of antidepressant medications. The first group is the *tricyclics*. Of these, the most common medications are: nortriptyline (Pamelor), desipramine, imipramine (Tofranil), and amitriptyline (Elavil). The *advantages* of this group are: helpfulness with sleep, improvement of depressive symptoms, a mild anti-anxiety effect, improved general functioning. The *disadvantages* of this group are: dryness of the mouth, constipation, drowsiness, longer time to become effective (up to four weeks), and possible heart rhythm problems.

The next group of antidepressants is the *SSRIs* (*selective serotonin reuptake inhibitors*). This "new generation" of antidepressants are currently more often prescribed than the tricyclics and include Prozac, Zoloft, Celexa, and Paxil. The *advantages* of this group include: less side effects than the tricyclics, more rapid onset of helpfulness (two to four weeks), more "friendliness" to the body. The *disadvantages* are: frequent sexual dysfunction, insomnia, headache, increased anxiety.

Two of the new antidepressants, Wellbutrin and Effexor, are in a class by themselves. They have fewer sexual side effects but seem to have a greater incidence of headache and insomnia.

None of the antidepressant medications are addicting, but they can become psychologically habituating. They generally have very few withdrawal effects. However, they can become a psychological crutch, and there is also some evidence that they may speed recurrence of depression. Since these drugs only treat symptoms of depression and do virtually nothing to address the multiple causes (see below) it is recommended that you undergo a thorough evaluation by a holistic physician or psychiatrist before starting on an antidepressant medication.

Psychotherapy. The term *psychotherapy* literally means *healing of the mind* and includes all forms of psychological therapy (see chapter 3). *Conventional psychotherapy* is generally limited to *talking* forms of treatment. In this era of managed care and HMOs, pharmacological treatment is increasingly being pushed because it is seen as more cost-effective in the short run. And most psychiatric care is given by primary care physicians, not psychiatrists. The combination of medication and conventional psychotherapy alone, without treatment of the body and spirit, is often not sufficient to effectively treat moderate to severe depression.

Risk Factors and Causes

Depression is not well understood. The following are believed to be the most significant risk factors contributing to its cause.

BODY: Physical (Medical) and Environmental

- Heredity—close to 50 percent of sufferers have a hereditary predisposition
- Candidiasis (yeast overgrowth)

- Inhalant and food allergies
- Childbirth—postpartum depression
- Female hormone dysfunction or insufficiency—PMS, perimenopause, menopause
- Hypothyroidism
- Hypoglycemia
- Obesity
- Folic acid deficiency
- Drugs and medications: Tagamet, Inderal, narcotics, benzodiazepines (see "anxiety" section), birth control pills, sleeping pills, prednisone, alcohol, marijuana
- Lack of exercise
- Biochemical—low levels of the neurotransmitters serotonin and norepinephrine
- Environmental toxicity—air pollution (decreased negative ions, increased positive ions, outgassing), heavy metal exposure (mercury, lead, cadmium)
- Decreased sunlight (seasonal depression)
- Overcrowding
- Lack of grounding in the earth

MIND: Mental and Emotional

- Distorted thinking
- Grief—feelings of loss following bereavement, divorce, or retirement
- Feelings of failure
- Lack of stimulation
- Addiction to work
- Sense of helplessness
- Lack of self-expression
- Sense of powerlessness
- Emotional traumas as a child: history of abuse or violence, abandonment or neglect

SPIRIT: Spiritual and Social

- Lack of purpose or meaning in life
- Feelings of isolation; lack of compassion or a committed loving relationship
- Lack of family or social connection

- Feeling disconnected from God/Spirit

- Spiritual issues are more prominent with severe or chronic depression

Holistic Medical Treatment and Prevention

The holistic treatment is most effective for mild to moderate depression. Severe depression will usually require antidepressant medication but can be combined with many of the following recommendations to enhance the therapeutic result.

Physical and Environmental Health Recommendations

Air and Exposure to Nature
These factors can benefit both depression and anxiety:

- Clean air

- Negative ion–filled air—studies have shown mood benefits with levels above 3,000 ions per cubic centimeter

- Sunlight

- Beautiful natural setting—provides a sense of both grounding and relaxation

Diet
The basic dietary recommendation for treating depression is a diet that is high in complex carbohydrates such as whole grains (brown rice, barley, corn, millet, oats, and whole wheat), vegetables, beans, and fruits. These foods will boost serotonin and promote feelings of well-being. The diet should be high in protein—no less than 60 grams daily divided into three or four servings. This will help to maintain a stable blood sugar level throughout the day. In addition to food, you may want to use protein powder in diluted fruit juice or soy milk, taken between meals as snacks, to meet your daily intake requirement. The diet should also include the spices of red pepper, garlic, and ginger. One or two servings of cold-water fish, such as salmon or sardines, per week is recommended, as they contain high amounts of essential fatty acids (see below). Caffeine, alcohol, sugar, and refined carbohydrates (products made from white flour—bread, pasta) should be eliminated. A food elimination diet (see chapter 19) to identify any food allergens can be very helpful.

Vitamins, Minerals, and Nutritional Supplements
In many cases, natural products can have an effect upon mood that is greater than or equal to that of antidepressants. Although you should start out slowly and carefully consider your unique biochemical individuality, the following amino acids,

vitamins, minerals, and essential fatty acids are usually effective in treating depression:

Amino acids. DLPA, or *phenylalanine*, is an amino acid found to be effective for treating depression. It is a precursor (directly on the formative pathway) to norepinephrine, one of the main neurotransmitters that govern mood. *Recommended dosage*: begin with 500 mg (one capsule) two times daily, on an *empty stomach with juice*. This can gradually be increased by 500 mg per day to two or three capsules, three times daily. For maximum effect, it is best to take 50 mg of vitamin B-6 at the same time, as well as niacin, 500 mg per day, and one gram of vitamin C. Vitamin B-6 is particularly important in regulating the absorption, metabolism, and utilization of amino acids.

L-tyrosine is an amino acid formed from phenylalanine and is one step closer to norepinephrine. *Recommended dosage:* exactly the same directions as for DLPA. *NOTE:* Glutamine is another "excitatory" amino acid that seems to combine quite well with L-tyrosine to improve its effectiveness. Some nutritional companies formulate both L-tyrosine and glutamine together. This combination capsule contains the correct ratio of both, and up to six capsules may be taken per day in divided doses, on an empty stomach.

With both DLPA and L-tyrosine, you need to be watchful for increased blood pressure, headaches, or insomnia. These side effects are indications that an excessive stimulation of the nervous system has occurred. *DO NOT take these amino acids if you are currently taking standard antidepressant medications* (the interaction between them is not well documented). *Also avoid taking these amino acids with the following conditions: phenylketonuria (PKU), hepatic cirrhosis, or melanoma.*

Like other essential amino acids, *L-tryptophan* cannot be manufactured by the body but must come directly from food or supplements. It is the building block for serotonin, the same neurotransmitter influenced by Prozac in the treatment of depression. When properly taken, tryptophan is extremely useful as a natural antidepressant as well as a sleep aid. Recently the FDA lifted its ban on tryptophan, although it must be prescribed. Decades of previous use have already proven this amino acid's broad therapeutic effectiveness. *Recommended dosage:* for depressive symptoms, take 2 grams (2,000 mg) of tryptophan two or three times daily. It should be taken between meals, with fruit or juice (simple sugars) to improve its utilization. It should not be taken with a protein meal, because tryptophan competes poorly with other amino acids for absorption. To convert tryptophan to serotonin, the body must have adequate levels of folic acid, vitamin B-6, magnesium, niacin, and glutamine.

The tryptophan metabolite *5-HTP*, which is much stronger than L-tryptophan, is a proven antidepressant and is available in some health food stores. *Dosage:* 100 to 200 mg twice daily between meals.

The amino acids DLPA, L-tyrosine, and L-tryptophan should be tried one at a time. If after six weeks at a high dosage there is no improvement, then you should take a different amino acid.

Other vitamins, minerals, and supplements include:

- *B-complex* (containing all of the B vitamins)—50 mg two times daily. (postpartum depression may result from a deficiency of B-6.)

- *B-12*—1,000 mcg daily, along with a weekly injection of B-12, 1,000 mcg combined with up to 5 mg of folic acid (especially for the elderly with cognitive dysfunction, or people with digestive disorders). Postpartum depression may result from a deficiency of B-12 and folic acid.

- *Folic acid*—5,000 mcg (5 mg) daily for one month, then reduce to 800 mcg daily

- *Niacinamide* (vitamin B-3)—500 mg two times daily

- *Vitamin C*—1,000 mg three times daily (as ascorbate or Ester C)

- *Vitamin E*—400 I.U. daily (as Natural d-alpha-tocopherol)

- *Magnesium*—1,000 mg daily; necessary for the production of neurotransmitters (as glycinate or aspartate)

- *Calcium*—1,000 mg daily (as citrate)

- *Zinc*—30–40 mg daily (as picolinate)

- *Essential fatty acids* (EFAs)—the best way to take the omega-3 EFAs is in capsules containing the combination EPA (300 mg) and DHA (200). Take one capsule two times daily. (The nervous system is composed of 60 percent DHA, and this EFA is essential for normal function.) For omega-6 EFAs, take evening primrose oil, 1,000 mg three times daily.

- *phosphatidylserine* (PS)—100 mg with breakfast and 200 mg with dinner (double-blind studies have proven its effectiveness with depression and insomnia)

Herbs
The therapeutic benefits of herbs often require more time than standard drugs. An advantage, however, is the safety in long-term use and absence of reported side effects.

1. *St. John's Wort (Hypericum perforatum)*. Several clinical studies have shown this herb to be as effective as standard antidepressants (amitriptyline and imipramine). The herb also has far fewer side effects. The active ingredient in St. John's wort is hypericin. The dosage is 900 mg daily of 0.3 percent concentration—600 mg with breakfast and 300 mg with lunch. A trial period of one month

is adequate to determine its potential benefits. Do not take St. John's wort along with the amino acids if you've just started the treatment program. After four to six weeks on DLPA or L-tyrosine, you can then begin St. John's wort. Likewise, do not take St. John's wort with the SSRI drugs (Prozac, Zoloft, Paxil).

2. *Ginkgo biloba* improves cerebral circulation, improving memory and often benefiting depression. Generally, ginkgo is not as effective as St. John's wort for depression, but it can be taken along with other herbs and nutrients to bolster one's overall mood. Ginkgo biloba should be in an extract that is standardized to contain 24 percent ginkgo flavone glycosides. The usual dose is 80–120 mg two times daily (breakfast and lunch).

3. *Yohimbine.* This herb, from tree bark in West Africa, has been used for decades in treating male impotence or diminished sexual interest. Recent research has indicated that yohimbine can also improve the overall effectiveness of standard antidepressant medications. In some cases, yohimbine can be used by itself to both stimulate sexual functioning in men and relieve mild depression. For mild depression and enhanced sexual functioning, take 5.4 mg of standardized yohimbine extract, three times daily. A suggested trial period for this yohimbine regimen would be two to three weeks. Yohimbine can then be taken periodically, as needed. *NOTE: For some individuals, yohimbine can cause increased anxiety or uncomfortable cardiac stimulation. It should be taken under the supervision of a health professional.*

4. *Siberian ginseng:* 400 mg of a standardized extract three times daily

5. Rosemary shampoo can be absorbed through the skin as well as providing aromatherapy for depression.

Professional Care Therapies

- *Hormonal Therapy.* Desiccated thyroid can often elicit a dramatic improvement, especially in middle-aged women. This can be true even with normal thyroid function. Lethargy, sense of cold, and fatigue are often symptoms of low thyroid function (see symptoms of hypothyroidism in chapter 20). One-half to one grain daily is a good starting dosage. DHEA can also be effective in treating depression, but the dosage should be based upon blood or saliva levels of DHEA sulfate. Your physician might also check your adrenal function via cortisol/DHEA testing. This can measure maladaptive responses to stress.

- *Traditional Chinese medicine* (acupuncture and Chinese herbs) and *homeopathy* can be helpful.

Exercise

The beneficial effects of regular aerobic exercise in the treatment of depression are well documented. Some psychotherapists believe that aerobic exercise, through its powerful release of endorphins, may be the most effective as well as the most economical antidepressant. (See to chapter 2 for more information on exercise.)

Mental and Emotional Health Recommendations

Psychotherapy

The *holistic psychotherapist* is concerned with the presenting psychological problems as well as the life force energy or spirit of each client. What are his or her purpose and unique talents, interests, dreams, and desires in life? This orientation can also be described as *spiritual psychotherapy*. Providing the encouragement and motivation to change are the hallmarks of a skilled therapist. This can only be done by evoking the assets and gifts in each person, as well as focusing on solutions to his or her current problems. Empowerment is the essence and goal of therapy—helping clients develop their own inner resources to be a catalyst for change. Being the source of your own choices and having the capability to reinterpret any painful experience as an opportunity for learning provides you with the energy to transform your life and cure depression.

Psychotherapy is most successful when the client establishes a comfortable therapeutic rapport with the therapist. Although this connection and trust is more important than the treatment model itself, there are several psychotherapeutic options in addition to conventional psychotherapy that are helpful in treating depression. They include:

- Cognitive/behavioral therapy—multiple studies have demonstrated its effectiveness in treating depression (see chapter 3). Affirmations and imagery are an integral part of this form of therapy.
- Psychosynthesis—a holistic type of spiritual psychotherapy
- Hakomi therapy—a body-centered form of psychotherapy
- Solution-focused/brief therapy—a goal-oriented form of psychotherapy
- Spiritual psychotherapy—just described above

Stress-Reduction Techniques

Each of the following can be helpful in treating both depression and anxiety.

Meditation is a technique for calming the mind. A sound or mantra can be used as an "object of meditation." Transcendental meditation uses a repetitive phrase to focus one's attention. Another method is to focus attention on the breath or other body sensations, a technique used in Vipassana and Zen meditation. Raja yoga is an integrative transpersonal approach that elicits responses of intuition and creativity. Whatever the specific method, the goal is to empty the mind of thoughts and to transcend feelings. Thus, the feedback loop—consisting of depressive thinking > anxiety > hopeless feelings > more depressive thinking— is diminished. This method of attaining inner peace and clarity has become increasingly popular in the West. It was discussed in chapter 3.

Relaxation training teaches you to relax the body by progressively tensing and then relaxing various muscle groups. Variations include tensing your fists while rolling your eyes upward and holding your breath. You then sequentially relax the eyes, exhale, and release the tension in your fists. This produces a "letting go" effect that can then be enhanced by focusing on counting down from five to one, picturing each number in a different color. Unlike meditation, this method emphasizes physical relaxation. Since you can't think depressing thoughts while relaxing, this method is effective for relaxing the mind as well.

Breath techniques include several breathing methods derived from yoga and various forms of meditation. More recently, these practices have been used with good effect by patients of psychotherapy to calm the mind and body. Sometimes called breath therapy, these breath techniques include quickly paced, connected (no pause between inhalation and exhalation) mouth breathing (to evoke emotions). Breath therapy (see Rebirthing in page 54) allows repressed emotions to surface and be released. Alternating mouth-nose breathing (for centering) and alternating nostril breathing can enhance creativity. Some of these breathing techniques can be enhanced with imagery and music. All breathing methods have their own intention and rationale and can be quite helpful in treating depression and anxiety. To get started, work with a qualified breath therapist. These methods are quite easy to learn and highly effective.

Biofeedback training is a systematized approach for learning relaxation that furnishes feedback evidence of reaching a calmer level of brainwave activity and physiological response. By allowing you to refocus energy in a self-empowering way, it gives you a greater feeling of control over your autonomic ("involuntary") nervous system reactions (heart rate, blood pressure), including those triggered by stress. With the help of a biofeedback technician, you are hooked up to an apparatus that measures your responses (heart rate, muscle tension, skin temperature, brain waves) while you focus on a sensory cue to help you relax. If you need technical confirmation that something is happening, this method is for you.

Discussed in chapter 3, *journaling* is a technique for recording your emotions and understanding patterns of action based on your feelings. To begin to focus on positive happenings, try keeping a *gratitude journal*. This consists of writing each day about something for which you can be grateful. By making a grati-tude entry each evening before bed, you neutralize the mindset that focuses on what's wrong in your life—the depression cycle—and you begin to appreciate what's right.

Hypnosis (hypnotherapy) is a form of treatment that can be quite effective with milder types of depression and anxiety. Hypnosis produces an *altered state of con-sciousness* (ASC) in which certain senses are heightened and others seem to fade into the background. It is not a state of sleep. While in a hypnotic trance, you be-come more aware of words and suggested images, and they grow more intense. Bodily sensations and time are often distorted. One does not require a deep trance for benefit to occur; a light trance is often adequate. Images of calm, relaxing scenes are often suggested for clients with anxiety. Although the visual imagery is quite effective, much of the benefit from hypnosis for anxiety is obtained by the simple act of learning to relax. It is often a revelation to learn that one *can* relax.

Progressive muscle relaxation is another form of hypnotherapy that is effective for anxiety. The client is instructed to start by tensing, then relaxing, the muscles of the feet, then repeating this process with each muscle group in succession, moving all the way up the body to the face and forehead (similar to relaxation training, described earlier.)

Depression is often a pattern of seeing yourself and your life with a bleak sense of entrapment. Hypnotherapy can be used to imagine, while in a heightened state of suggestibility, more hopeful options and better methods of dealing with painful issues. While in a hypnotic state, one can visually rehearse newer ways of perceiving oneself.

Self-hypnosis, which can easily be learned from a skilled therapist (and even from books), provides simple and effective methods for training yourself to enter hypnotic states. Audiotapes are also an excellent source of training in self-hypnosis and learning strategies to relax and reprogram habits of the mind.

Self-talk is rescripting self-dialogue from self-defeating to positive encour-agement. This is done through the use of affirmations or changing phrases from "if only" to "I will!" (See "Affirmations" in chapter 3.)

NLP (neurolinguistic programming) has proven extremely successful with in-tractable phobias and certain forms of anxiety. It utilizes transformational imagery to modify behavior and help reshape emotional patterns.

Spending consistent time immersed in *creative activities* such as painting or playing a musical instrument can help depression. The same holds true for daily and weekly scheduled time for *play* and/or *relaxation*, as well as periodic va-cations.

Energy Medicine

Therapies such as *Therapeutic Touch, healing touch,* and *Reiki* are all hands-on techniques that are helpful treating both depression and anxiety. You'll need to find a qualified practitioner.

Qi gong is a moving meditation practiced by over three hundred million Chinese on a daily basis that strengthens life force energy, or chi. It is relatively easy to learn and can be used to both treat and prevent depression and anxiety.

Regular exposure to *sunlight* and filtered sun (20 to 30 minutes daily) or full spectrum *lights* that simulate sunshine can help treat depression, especially with people suffering from seasonal affective disorder (SAD). This condition is most prevalent in locations with little sunshine during the winter months.

Soothing or stimulating *music,* or whatever sounds you resonate with, can also be helpful in treating depression.

Bodywork Therapies

A multitude of hands-on techniques can help to release deeply held or repressed emotions. Some of these methods are described as *body-centered psychotherapy* and often combine deep-tissue bodywork, such as *Rolfing,* with types of body movement, like *yoga* or *Feldenkrais.* (Some of these therapies are described in chapters 2 and 3.) Depression and anxiety are frequently more amenable to physical touch than verbal therapies. These therapies are particularly important for people with a history of physical and sexual abuse or poor body image.

Spiritual and Social Health Recommendations. Any of the recommendations made in chapter 4 are helpful in treating depression. However, of the *spiritual practices,* meditation, prayer, and altruism (volunteering) are probably the most beneficial.

Joining or maintaining a connection to a *support group* is especially helpful for depressed people in strengthening their degree of social health. Working on your committed relationship with a spouse or partner can often mitigate depression.

ANXIETY

Prevalence

Anxiety is a state of fear or worry in the face of perceived threat of danger. There is probably no one who has not experienced at least some degree of anxiety. Like depression, it covers a spectrum of emotional discomfort that ranges from mild appropriate concern to being overwhelmed by an excessive continuous state of worry. In fact, anxiety often accompanies depression, as well as obsessive compulsive disorders and post-traumatic stress disorder. When taken to the extreme, anxiety manifests as acute panic attacks and phobias. This section describes the chronic condition of fear known medically as anxiety neurosis. This mood disorder affects twice as many women as men.

Physiology

Anxiety and fear trigger the fight-or-flight response, which causes excess adrenaline to be produced by the adrenal glands along with other hormones called catecholamines, and the body prepares itself for action. When no action is taken and nervous energy is not discharged, there is physiological confusion. This could be described as an anxiety or panic attack, manifested by many of the symptoms in the following list.

Symptoms and Diagnosis

Anxiety neurosis, or generalized anxiety disorder, is characterized by *excessive* or unwarranted *worry* (usually over work, finances, relationships, and health), that occurs chronically for at least six months. The degree of fear is often unrelated to any obvious cause. The diagnosis can be made by the presence of several of the following symptoms (with some of them present for a majority of days in the past six months).

1. Restlessness, irritability, feeling keyed up or on edge/a sense of urgency
2. Heart palpitations (rapid or irregular heartbeat)
3. Muscle tension, especially in the neck, shoulders, and chest
4. Easily fatigued
5. Difficulty concentrating or mind going blank
6. Insomnia (difficulty falling or staying asleep, nightmares)
7. Rapid and shallow breathing, or feeling short of breath (hyperventilation)
8. Trembling or feeling shaky
9. Dry mouth
10. Generalized sweating, or sweaty palms
11. Headaches
12. Abdominal pain and/or diarrhea
13. Loss of appetite
14. Occasional panic attacks

Conventional Medical Treatment

Conventional medical treatment for anxiety consists of *medication* and *psychotherapy*. The class of anti-anxiety medications most often prescribed is the *benzodiazepines*. These include: Xanax (alprazolam), Klonopin (clonazepam), Ativan (lorazepam), and Valium (diazepam). Although these medications act rapidly and effectively and relieve panic attacks and general anxiety, they can be addictive, impair memory, and increase tiredness. When carefully used, however, these medications can be quite helpful for a short time.

Psychotherapy for anxiety includes those treatments described under depression.

Risk Factors and Causes

The causes of *anxiety* include:

- Fear—relationships and situations that contribute to insecurity
- Excess caffeine
- Excess sugar, chocolate, Nutrasweet
- Excess of highly acidic foods—tomatoes, eggplants, peppers
- Stimulants—decongestants, NoDoze, tobacco, asthma and cortcosteroid medications
- Hyperthyroidism
- Hyperadrenalism
- Hypoglycemia
- Nutritional deficiencies of B vitamins and magnesium
- History of trauma: physical, sexual, or emotional abuse

Holistic Medical Treatment and Prevention
Physical and Environmental Health Recommendations

Air
Same as for depression.

Diet
The recommended diet for treating anxiety includes complex carbohydrates (whole grains—especially brown rice, barley, millet, corn, and wheat), vegetables, seaweed, kasha, foods containing L-tryptophan (sunflower seeds, bananas, milk).

The diet is moderate in protein, fat (30 percent of calories), and strong spices. Caffeine, chocolate, alcohol, sugar, and highly acidic foods should be avoided.

Vitamins, Minerals, Nutritional Supplements

Gamma Amino Butyric Acid (GABA) is a nonessential amino acid in the brain that the body uses to calm anxiety naturally. Most tranquilizers (Xanax, Ativan, Valium, etc.) create a calming effect by stimulating the natural GABA receptors in the brain. But unlike Valium, GABA taken by mouth cannot pass the blood/brain barrier and is believed to be ineffective in calming the brain. However, it is very helpful in relieving anxiety symptoms originating in the digestive tract and adjacent organs, for example, diarrhea, "stomach butterflies," heart palpitations, and hyperventilation. This is due to its effect on what some scientists refer to as the second, or GI, brain (see page 251). It may take several weeks to appreciate the full benefit of GABA. *Recommended dosage:* for daytime relaxation, take 750 mg two times daily. For sleep, take 1,500 mg before bed.

As with depression, *tryptophan* is often quite effective in dealing with anxiety. This amino acid is readily converted into *serotonin*, which is a calming neurotransmitter as well as an antidepressant. It requires a carbohydrate such as fruit juice to facilitate its absorption and conversion, as well as vitamins B-3, B-6, and C. *Recommended dosage:* for anxiety, 500 mg twice a day between meals is often sufficient. As a sleep aid, tryptophan is also effective. One can take 2 or 3 grams before bedtime, with a carbohydrate.

Vitamin C, at least 1000 mg. three times daily; *vitamin B-complex*, 50 mg, two times daily, with extra *niacinamide* (up to 500 mg, three times daily), *vitamin B-1* (up to 1,000 mg three times daily), and *vitamin B-12* (an injection of 1,000 mcg per week with 2 mg of folic acid, or sublingual tablets at 2,000 mcg daily); and *vitamin E*, 1,200 mg daily, can all contribute to the easing of anxiety. *NOTE: a very small percentage of people will have increased anxiety with B-complex.*

Magnesium glycinate or aspartate, calcium citrate, and *essential fatty acids (EFAs)* are all essential in treating anxiety. Their daily requirements are the same as for depression.

Inositol is a unique B vitamin that research has found to reduce anxiety when taken in high doses. Its exact mode of action is unknown. Inositol may be an important nutrient, along with *choline*, for healthy brain cell metabolism. *Recommended dosage:* to reduce anxiety or promote a more calm state of sleep, one can take inositol at doses of 4 to 6 grams. The dose can be adjusted upward until relief is obtained. There is no known toxicity to inositol, even at doses as high as 50 grams.

Herbs

Kava kava (*Piper methysticum*) is a botanical herb has been successfully used by herbalists since the discovery of its use in Polynesia by Captain James Cook. It is used for treating anxiety and promoting sleep. Kava kava is one of the best-studied herbs with proven effectiveness, as well as being one of the best known and utilized. *Recommended dosage:* kava kava is available in both liquid and capsule form. The standardized extract potency of its active ingredient, kavalactone, should be 30 percent (15 mg per capsule). For daytime relief of anxiety, take 250 mg (one capsule or one-half dropperful), three times daily with meals. One can take four to six capsules for sleep (up to 1,500 mg). As with all other medications and nutrients, each individual has his or her own biochemical individuality and needs to take responsibility for finding his or her own unique level. Kava kava should not be taken continuously for a prolonged period of time (over four months).

The plant extract *valerian* has been the treatment of choice for over two hundred years throughout the world for anxiety and insomnia. Although it is quite safe to take for short periods of time, its long-term effects are not known. *Recommended dosage:* for daytime anxiety, take 150 mg (standardized extract of 0.8 percent valeric acid) three times daily. For difficulty with sleep, start with 150 mg, 45 minutes before bed. If that dose is insufficient, gradually increase to 600 mg.

Other herbs that can be used for treating anxiety include *chamomile*, *passion flower*, *lemon balm*, and *skullcap*. The latter two are best for acute anxiety.

Exercise

Longer, low intensity, aerobic exercise requiring greater endurance, such as jogging, swimming, and hiking, is best for relieving anxiety.

Professional Care Therapies

The following therapies can all be effective in treating anxiety: acupuncture and traditional Chinese medicine, Ayurvedic medicine, biofeedback training, bodywork (especially Rolfing), breathwork, chiropractic, environmental medicine (including detoxification therapy), homeopathy, mind/body medicine (guided imagery, meditation, hypnotherapy, NLP), naturopathic medicine, psychotherapy and professional counseling (especially cognitive therapy).

Mental and Emotional Health Recommendations

Almost every mental and emotional health technique recommended for depression is also effective for anxiety. These include:

- Psychotherapy

- *Stress-reduction techniques*—each of these can be even more effective for anxiety than for treating depression—meditation, relaxation training, breath therapy, and biofeedback training

- Journaling

- Energy medicine—healing and therapeutic touch, Reiki, qigong, along with working on the specific emotional issues associated with your condition

- Hypnosis

- Bodywork therapies

- Planned retreats and vacations—even long weekends away from home are helpful

- Creative activities—art, music

Spiritual and Social Health Recommendations

These are also the same as for depression; however, since fear is the primary cause of anxiety, prayer can be especially beneficial.

INSOMNIA

Prevalence

Insomnia, the most common type of sleep disorder, has become a rapidly increasing crisis of the 1990s. A 1995 Gallup poll found that 49 percent of adults reported some sleeping difficulty, up from 36 percent in 1991. Nearly 10 million people each year seek medical advice for insomnia. There is an epidemic of sleep deprivation in this country, yet most of the 70 million Americans who are afflicted are unaware to what extent their health is suffering from years of accumulated sleep debt. Most are aware, however, of its effect on their work, and estimates of lost productivity are as high as $70 billion. Poor sleep contributed at least in part to the *Exxon Valdez, Challenger,* and Three Mile Island disasters. An estimated 38,000 people die each year from sleep apnea (it can trigger heart attack and stroke), the most serious form of sleep disorder, and another 24,000 die in accidents caused by sleeplessness. The cost of sleep-related motor vehicle accidents is estimated at $50 billion annually. In 1910, Americans averaged nine hours of sleep per night, and today one-third of adults sleep little more than six hours on weeknights. Some sleep researchers believe that recent research on the serious consequences of our national sleep deficit will persuade society to change—psychologically, culturally, even legislatively. These investigators compare the sleeplessness problem to recognition of the risks of drinking and driving in the 1950s, or the documentation of the devastating health effects of cigarettes in the 1960s. Medical science is now helping us to recognize the magnitude of the health crisis resulting from sleep deprivation.

Physiology

Why do we need to sleep, and why does sleep have such a profound impact on our physical well-being? Although science has been seriously exploring the physiology of sleep since the early 1970s, it still remains largely a mystery. Although many prominent people (JFK, President Clinton, Martha Stewart, Jay Leno) have claimed they need only three to four hours of sleep, the evidence supports the fact that while sleep requirements are highly individualized, most people require seven to eight hours to function optimally. Although the quality of sleep diminishes with age, the need for sleep does not.

There are two distinct physiological states of sleep: nonrapid eye movement (NREM), with four stages defined by specific electroencephalogram (EEG) features; and REM sleep, characterized by episodic bursts of rapid eye movements, muscle relaxation, and dream activity. The two types of sleep alternate throughout the night in three to six 90-minute NREM-REM cycles. Recent research suggests that it is during REM sleep that the body is able to restore organs, bones, and tissue; replenish immune cells; and circulate a rejuvenating supply of growth hormone, making us less vulnerable to the diseases of aging. Studies also show that REM sleep is crucial for proper functioning of the brain and psyche.

Symptoms and Diagnosis

Insomnia is defined as *difficulty falling asleep or staying asleep*; it is the most common sleep disorder. It is medically classified as acute when it has been present for less than one month and chronic when it has persisted for more than six months. Primary insomnias are those having no apparent psychiatric, medical, or environmental cause. Secondary insomnias are caused by psychological and medical conditions and therapies. Sleep apnea is one of the less common but potentially most serious types of secondary insomnia. It is a sleep disorder in which there is intermittent cessation of breathing during sleep, which forces the individual to repeatedly wake up to take breaths. It affects predominantly men between 30 and 60. The three types of sleep apnea are:

1. Central sleep apnea—there is a defect in the central nervous system (brain and spinal cord) that affects the diaphragm.

2. Obstructive sleep apnea—occurs with blockage of the upper airway, usually resulting in snoring.

3. A combination of 1 and 2.

The most common *symptoms* accompanying insomnia are fatigue, immune deficiencies (increased susceptibility to illness), headaches, weight gain, irritability, depression, slowed reaction time, diminished short-term memory, decreased libido, poor job performance, and increased substance abuse.

If you would like a definitive diagnosis or a comprehensive medical evaluation of your sleep problem, there are more than 350 sleep-disorder clinics accredited by the American Sleep Disorders Association (telephone: 507-287-6006), plus almost 2600 others that are not accredited. They will usually perform an EEG to monitor brain waves and REM patterns and will evaluate heart rate and breathing while you sleep.

Conventional Medical Treatment

Conventional therapy addresses the treatment of the underlying cause if it can be identified, the improving of sleep habits, and the use of medications. A commonly used class of drugs are the benzodiazepine hypnotics (tranquilizers), such as Halcion (Triazolam) and Restoril (temazepam). They are most effective for the short-term management of insomnia, and they decrease the time to sleep onset while improving the quality of sleep. (Halcion is short-acting, and its sedative effect lasts for about three hours.) However, the sedative effects of the longer acting drugs can linger into the day, resulting in daytime sleepiness and impairment of cognitive function and performance. Habituation tends to develop, and when the short-acting benzodiazepines are stopped abruptly, they may cause rebound insomnia that is worse than the original problem. Tapering off of these drugs is recommended. Other benzodiazepines, antianxiety drugs like Valium, Xanax, and Ativan, are sometimes used for sleep.

In another class of drugs, Ambien (zolpidem) is the newest effective short-acting (lasts about four hours) medication for insomnia with fewer side effects and less potential for rebound than the benzodiazepines. If the insomnia is caused by depression, then an antidepressant such as Desyrel or Elavil is often prescribed. The antidepressants, in full doses (the sleep-inducing effect of low doses diminishes with repeated use), do not promote the dependence or the addiction often caused by the hypnotics. Most of the OTC sleeping pills contain antihistamines, which may cause lingering drowsiness.

Risk Factors and Causes
Physical and Environmental

- Age—sleep quality begins to diminish after age 40
- Menopause—estrogen deficiency

- Caffeine—in coffee, tea, soft drinks, chocolate, OTC drugs (analgesics and diet pills)
- Drugs—decongestants, thyroid medications, oral contraceptives, beta blockers, marijuana, and overuse of sleep-inducing drugs
- Stimulating herbs—ginseng, ephedra/ma huang, ginger, guarana, kola nut
- Sugar (in some sensitive individuals)
- Nocturnal hypoglycemia
- Allergies
- Pain—backache, headache
- Alcohol (initially sedating but lightens sleep as the night goes on)
- Environmental factors—noise, light, temperature, humidity, uncomfortable mattress
- Insufficient exercise
- Calcium, magnesium, and B vitamin deficiencies—less common
- Hypo- and hyperthyroidism; adrenal hyperactivity
- Chemical hypersensitivity

Mental/Emotional

- Anxiety, especially the fear of not sleeping
- Depression
- Grief
- Excitement/mania
- Anticipation of confrontational situations

Social/Spiritual

The underlying societal cause of this critical problem is that we are an overworked and overstimulated culture that is continually under pressure to accomplish more in less time. Insomnia is clearly a dis-ease of our modern age. But as technology helps us to achieve our material goals, we are sacrificing our relationships, our health, and our happiness.

Holistic Medical Treatment & Prevention of Insomnia

Physical and Environmental Health Recommendations:

Diet

Eliminate all caffeine in your diet, including coffee, tea, chocolate, and cola soft drinks. Also eliminate any other stimulants such as cigarettes, OTC drugs containing caffeine, some prescription drugs (discuss with your physician), some herbal supplements (see the preceding list), hot spicy foods (especially cayenne), sugar, refined carbohydrates (they deplete the B vitamins), alcohol (can lighten sleep), food additives, pork (bacon, ham, sausage), eggplant, spinach, and tomatoes. Some people with insomnia suffer from food sensitivities. The most common offending foods are dairy products, wheat, corn, and chocolate. Eliminate all of these foods for three to four weeks, then gradually reintroduce them, except chocolate. Avoid eating a heavy meal before bed. Establish a regular eating schedule to help promote circadian rhythm entrainment.

Foods that enhance sleep have high tryptophan to tyrosine (or phenylalanine) ratios: pumpkins, potatoes, bananas, onions, spinach, broccoli, cauliflower, eggs, fish, liver, milk, peanuts, cheddar cheese, whole grains (especially whole wheat, brown rice, and oats), cottage cheese, and beans. Eating tryptophan-rich foods for the evening meal or an evening snack may help induce sleep: milk products, turkey, chicken, beef, soy products, nuts and nut butters, bananas, papayas, and figs. If you are hypoglycemic, then follow a diet that stabilizes this condition. Foods that are high in carbohydrates raise the level of serotonin in the brain, which has a sedating effect. Without overeating you can try eating some pasta, half a baked potato, or a piece of toast half an hour before bed. Fruits, especially mulberries and lemons, can calm the mind. Chlorophyll-rich foods, such as leafy green vegetables, steamed or boiled, and microalgae—chlorella and spirulina (one-half gram at bedtime), are all sleep-inducing foods. The glutamine found in potatoes, red wine, and grape juice may enhance sleep. Drinking an adequate amount of water during the day will prevent waking up at night thirsty. But avoid drinking large amounts before going to sleep.

Vitamins, Minerals, and Supplements

- *Vitamin B-complex*, 50 to 100 mg daily with meals. *NOTE: a very small percentage of people have increased agitation and greater insomnia with B-complex.* The best food sources of the B vitamins are liver, whole grains, wheat germ, tuna, walnuts, peanuts, bananas, sunflower seeds, and blackstrap molasses.

- *Niacinamide (vitamin B-3)*, up to one gram (1,000 mg) at bedtime, for people who have trouble staying asleep, not falling asleep
- *Vitamin C*, 1,000 mg daily
- *Vitamin D*, 400 mg daily
- *Vitamin E*, 400 to 800 I.U. daily
- *Niacin*, 100 mg daily (reduce if flushing is a problem)
- *Pantothenic acid*, 250 mg daily
- *Calcium and magnesium*, 500 to 1,000 mg of each within 45 minutes of bedtime
- *Chromium*, 250 mg, twice daily, especially for people with hypoglycemia
- *Tryptophan*, three to five grams 45 minutes before retiring, and at least one and a half hours after eating protein; adding vitamin B-6 to the tryptophan along with fruit juice can improve results. Tryptophan is available by prescription only.
- *Hydroxytryptophan*, 100 to 200 mg before bed.
- *Phosphatidylserine*, up to 300 mg daily; an amino acid for those with insomnia due to elevated cortisone levels, usually induced by stress.

Hormones. Melatonin is a normally occurring hormone manufactured and released by the pineal gland in response to darkness. It is most effective for the type of insomnia that manifests primarily as difficulty falling asleep, and its recommended dosage ranges from 1 to 4 mg, one-half to one hour before bed. Melatonin can also be used for sleep maintenance with a sustained-release 1 mg preparation. There is also benefit with melatonin in treating jet lag. Natural *progesterone* has been used with good results for insomnia associated with menopause and PMS. Progesterone restores hormonal balance and has a calming effect. For additional information on natural progesterone, refer to "Osteoporosis," in chapter 8.

Herbs

- *Chamomile* tea has a mild sedative effect. It can be used for children. For adults, brew as strong as seven teaspoons of herb per cup of water.
- Sedative herbs include: *valerian, passionflower, lemon balm, hops,* and *skullcap*. You can use any alone or in combination as a strong tea. Of this group of herbs, *valerian* probably works best. Take one teaspoon of the tincture in warm water, or two to three grams of powdered valerian leaf (capsules) one hour before bed. However, as with the conventional sleeping pills, the effectiveness of valerian wears off with repeated use. Both capsules and tinctures (combination and single herbs) are available in most health food stores.

- *Kava kava* is useful for both anxiety and insomnia. Recommended dosage for sleep is two or three capsules (60 to 75 mg per capsule) an hour before bedtime.

- *St. John's wort* is best known as an antidepressant but can be used effectively for improving quality and length of sleep. Recommended dosage is 300 mg, three times daily of an extract standardized to contain 0.3 percent hypericin. Its full effects take about six weeks of continuous use to develop.

- *Chinese herbs* (and *acupuncture*) often produce dramatic and long-lasting relief from insomnia, but you'll need to find a qualified Chinese medicine practitioner, or O.M.D.—Doctor of Oriental Medicine.

Exercise

Exercising during the afternoon or early evening—five to six hours before bedtime is best—and avoiding strenuous exercise in the evening. *Outdoor exercise* is preferable, since studies show that people who get adequate natural sunlight tend to sleep better. Exercise for at least 20 to 30 minutes—brisk walking, jogging, bicycling, swimming, or yoga.

Hydrotherapy

Since sleep comes most easily when body temperature is falling, this process can be triggered by soaking in a *warm bath* or hot tub (below 105 degrees; if too hot, it can be stimulating) an hour to 90 minutes before getting into bed. Try keeping the bedroom temperature moderately cool (low 60s) to enhance the effect. To maximize the relaxation of tense muscles, you can add six to eight drops of *lavender oil* (used by aromatherapists for both anxiety and insomnia) to the bathwater. For maximum relaxation, a massage with lavender or chamomile oil following the bath is ideal.

Sleep Hygiene

- Make sure your bed is comfortable—most people do well with a medium-firm mattress that has a medium-soft top layer of padding.

- Restrict the bed to sleeping and sexual activity only—use other rooms for TV, reading, or conflict resolution.

- If you cannot fall sleep, or wake up and can't go back to sleep, then get up and go into another room and do something boring, including housework, until you're drowsy enough to go back to bed.

- Avoid taking naps.

- Go to sleep at the same time every night, at least eight hours before you have to get up, and set the alarm for the same time every morning; the best quality of sleep can be found between 10 P.M. and 6 A.M.

- Create optimum bedroom conditions—avoid bright lights after 9 P.M.; if it's noisy, buy a white noise generator or use foam earplugs; if it's dry, use a warm mist humidifier.

- Avoid obsessing about sleep, and turn the face of the clock away from you.

- Create a relaxing ritual before bed—read, listen to soothing music, do breathing exercises to quiet your mind.

- Love-making before sleep will usually induce good quality deep sleep.

Mental and Emotional Health Recommendations. The following options should be done just before bedtime:

- Meditation, with or without a mantra

- Visualization, with or without audiotapes

- Relaxing breathing exercises, with or without coordinating affirmations—repeat along with the breath: "I am sleeping soundly and peacefully"

- Journaling

- Attitudinal adjustment to reduce fear of insomnia (remember that even a couple of hours of sleep is adequate for basic survival); the less anxiety about insomnia, the better you'll sleep.

- For night awakening problems, affirm at bedtime that you will remember the thought of your unconscious mind as you awaken, and provide pen and paper on your bedside table. On awakening during the night, allow yourself to come to sufficiently full wakefulness to turn on the light and record a sentence or two about the first thoughts that come to mind. They will usually relate to the issue with which your unconscious mind has been struggling and stressing you into wakefulness. Several nights may be required to zero in on the topic. Once identified, the issue can be dealt with. Sleep is often dramatically better after using this technique.

CONDITION

ADDICTIONS AND ALCOHOLISM

Prevalence

An addiction is an overwhelming craving for or dependence on a mind-altering substance or activity, without regard for its health and social consequences. Addictions are either psychological or physiological, or both. In the United States, the most common forms of addiction are to drugs, alcohol, nicotine, caffeine, food, work, sex, and gambling. Drug usage in the United States has become an epidemic. The drug most studied is alcohol, which can serve as a model for the less studied drugs. Alcoholism among men is five times more common than among women; for illicit drugs the prevalence among men is three times greater than among women. The national cost of alcohol and other drug abuse in terms of health care, absenteeism, and lost productivity is approximately $166 billion per year. Over 15 million people are estimated to experience significant health problems as a direct result of their alcohol use, while one hundred thousand people will die every year as a result of alcoholism. The diseases most often associated with alcohol abuse are liver disease (cirrhosis), cancer, and heart disease. Among young alcoholics, the death rates from suicide, accidents, and cirrhosis are ten times higher than normal. Alcoholics shorten their life expectancy by about 20 years, and nearly half of the violent deaths from accidents, suicide, and homicide are alcohol related, as well as half of all automobile fatalities. One-third of all suicides and one-third of all mental health disorders are associated with serious alcohol abuse. At least 40 million spouses, children, and close relatives suffer from the destructive energy of alcohol abuse.

Drugs with the greatest addictive potential are: narcotics, including morphine, opium, heroin, and methadone; depressants such as alcohol, barbiturates, and sedatives; stimulants such as cocaine and amphetamines; hallucinogenic drugs; and marijuana.

These factors, combined with the effects of other drug abuse, add up to a significant social plague. Recent data show that 63 percent of all people arrested have illegal drugs in their urine. As for legal drugs, tobacco use kills about 420,000 Americans every year; the harmful effects of caffeine are discussed in chapter 2. Food addiction, especially to sugar, has been a significant contributor to the dramatic increase in obesity in this country. Although workaholism is surely one of our greatest addictions, there are few definitive studies on its prevalence. Sex addiction has only recently been recognized; the National Council of Sexual Addiction and Compulsivity estimates that 3 to 6 percent of Americans have this problem.

Symptoms and Diagnosis

- *Loss of control over the use of a drug or a behavior*
- Mood swings and irrational behavior
- The element of danger or risk (health, legal, social) is often present with an addiction
- Drug addiction: sore or red eyes, with dilated or constricted pupils, irregular breathing, trembling hands, itchy or runny nose, nausea

- Drug withdrawal: craving, depression, anxiety, restlessness, yawning, sweating, abdominal pain, vomiting, diarrhea, loss of appetite

If you are suffering ill effects or adverse consequences from the use of a drug or from a repeated behavior, then you are probably addicted.

Conventional Medical Treatment

Conventional alcohol and drug addiction rehabilitation programs usually involve detoxification, drug withdrawal, and counseling in both inpatient and outpatient settings. Through the 1980s many insurance companies were covering the costs of four-week stays at expensive (about $10,000 for one month of treatment) residential alcohol and rehabilitation centers. But with the growth of managed care and studies that show the inpatient programs to be no more effective than outpatient, the majority of the patients with addictions are now being treated as outpatients. In 1995, Kaiser Permanente of Colorado completed a study that revealed about 50 percent of the people who complete their out-patient addiction treatment programs remain clean and sober for at least one year.

Risk Factors and Causes

Physical/Environmental. Genetics are an important factor in determining your predisposition to addictions. In identical (same genetic makeup) twins, if one twin is alcoholic, the chance of the other twin being alcoholic is four times greater than if one fraternal (different genetic composition) twin is alcoholic. In researching genetic influences on cravings for addictive drugs such as nicotine, marijuana and alcohol, a UCLA study found that sons of alcoholics have a serious risk of developing a drug craving at an early age. This suggests that the genetically addictive brain is biochemically altered so that the individual is more susceptible to craving for a range of addictive drugs and even compulsive disorders such as sex, food, and gambling addiction. The conclusion from hundreds of studies is that *alcoholism, and to some extent drug abuse, is more of a disease than a personality disorder. The findings also confirm that irresistible cravings (alcohol, drug, and food addictions) and compulsive behavior disorders (sex and gambling addictions) are associated with a problem in the functioning of the reward-pleasure centers of the brain involving the neurotransmitters (serotonin, opioids, dopamine) and the enzymes that control them.* Researchers now believe that the root cause of addictive and compulsive diseases may be a defect in the gene that regulates the function of a specific receptor called dopamine D2, located in that part of the brain that is the center for feelings of reward and pleasure. The reason psychoactive drugs like morphine, cocaine, amphetamines, alcohol, and possibly sugar are so attractive to people with the genetically addictive brain is that these substances induce the brief release of abnormal amounts of dopamine which temporarily offset the diminished pleasure (low dopamine) experience created by these genetic defects. Although the malfunction begins with a gene, it can be altered by psychological, sociological and other environmental factors that can either trigger or mitigate the genetic predisposition.

Some scientists also believe that the alcohol and drug abuse itself may actually cause a relatively permanent disruption in the normal neurotransmitter pathways that mimics the defects that were thought to be purely genetic. For example, habitual use of cocaine can cause these neurotransmitter changes in just a few weeks or months, after which they become difficult to reverse.

Hypoglycemia is a significant risk factor in causing alcoholism—some studies have suggested it may be present in 90 percent of alcoholics. With a drop in blood sugar (hypoglycemia), a number of symptoms can occur—rapid heart rate, hunger, excessive sweating, craving for sweets, headaches, loss of concentration, and anxiety—all of which can be relieved by drinking alcohol, which works powerfully as a sugar. Since marijuana, amphetamines, cocaine, nicotine, and caffeine can all produce these hypoglycemic symptoms, it is not uncommon for users of these drugs to frequently drink alcohol as well. Hypoglycemia can be a significant cause of depression, anxiety, and mental confusion. Weak pancreatic and adrenal gland function, hypothyroidism, and a poorly functioning pituitary gland may all contribute to hypoglycemia. It is part of a vicious cycle that leads to a dependency on alcohol to alleviate its symptoms.

Another factor contributing to the altered neurochemistry of the addictive brain may be *poor nutrition*. Ironically, we live in one of the most affluent nations in the world, yet our diets often fail to provide minimum nutritional benefit and can even be harmful (see chapter 2). Our fast-food, high sugar diets—consisting of synthetic foods, heavily laced with pesticides, hormones, and herbicides—routinely deplete our vitality and contribute to a variety of diseases. There is certainly convincing evidence that our modern diet has created the growing problem of hyperactivity. Excessive sugar intake may also predispose children to developing the addictive brain neurochemistry that makes them susceptible to problems with alcohol, psychoactive drugs, and other compulsive disorders.

In addition to *contributing* to addictions, *nutritional deficiencies* can often *result* from alcohol and drug abuse. As deficiencies, in turn, create further cravings, the cycle of dependency can eventually alter brain biochemistry. The *secondary* loss of nutrients can include the minerals zinc, chromium, manganese, magnesium, calcium, copper, iron, and the B vitamins.

Food allergy is also a cause of alcoholism. Some people are allergic to the foods from which alcohol is made, such as wheat or potatoes in beer; grapes in wine; or corn in bourbon. Brewer's yeast, found in most alcoholic beverages, is another potential allergen. One of the ways the body reacts to foods to which it is allergic is to produce its own addictive opioid endorphins. These create feelings of euphoria, followed by subsequent withdrawal or hangover, which is then relieved with more alcohol.

By altering brain chemistry, *environmental toxins* such as gasoline, cleaning solvents, and formaldehyde (a common indoor air pollutant found in many building materials) can also contribute to causing alcoholism.

An excess of sugar and alcohol fuels an *overgrowth of yeast* (Candida albicans) organisms (see chapter 9). This condition can weaken the immune system, which even further stimulates the overgrowth of candida. *Candidiasis* mirrors many of the symptoms of hypoglycemia—especially fatigue and anxiety—the awareness of which can temporarily be relieved by drugs and alcohol.

Mental/Emotional

There are several reasons why men probably experience alcohol and drug abuse to a much greater extent than women. These primarily relate to men's repression of feelings.

- Men do not release their emotional pain as easily as women.
- Men are more "do-ers" and tend to act out their pain with alcohol and drugs.
- There is more societal permission for men to drink alcohol and take drugs.
- Men are more out of touch with their spirit than women and use drugs to try and "feel something."
- Men find the machismo of drugs more exciting than do women.

Regardless of your genetic predisposition, emotions and belief systems can have a profound effect on creating addictive behavior. The probable emotional causes contributing to alcohol abuse can include feelings of anger or rage, self-rejection, guilt, hopelessness, or inadequacy. Emotional factors with drug abuse may include fear of taking responsibility or an inability to accept and love oneself.

Holistic Medical Treatment and Prevention

Physical and Environmental Health Recommendations

Environment

As with the conventional approach, begin treating addictions in a somewhat secluded residential setting *away from home* in order to detach yourself from previous addictive behavior patterns. One of the most effective holistic retreat facilities for treatment of addictions is Dr. Gabriel Cousens's Tree of Life Rejuvenation Center in Patagonia, Arizona. His program focuses on specific *biochemical repair* and involves two steps: (1) avoiding alcohol, illegal drugs, sugar, nicotine, and caffeine; and (2) restoring the vitamin, mineral, and neurotransmitter deficiencies. The neurotransmitter pathways are maintained with a vegetarian diet and psychological and spiritual support.

Diet

Reaching optimal blood pH is critical for maximum mental and metabolic functioning. Measuring blood pH in response to diet is an important part of the Tree of Life program. In this way one is able to personalize the vegetarian diet to create optimal acid-base balance. Since hypoglycemia—low blood sugar—plays such a significant role in contributing to alcoholism, a *hypoglycemic diet* is recommended. This consists of a diet moderately low in protein and high in complex carbohydrates (beans, grains, vegetables). Healthy snacks (nuts, seeds, organic fruit or vegetables) between meals prevents a drop in blood sugar, which may trigger alcohol cravings. The first step in the process of biochemical repair is to *avoid all hypoglycemic activators such as sugar products, caffeine, and nicotine* (including chewing tobacco). The last two substances produce hypoglycemic symptoms, through an overstimulation of the adrenals, that can keep the addictive cycle going. The dietary emphasis for treating addictions is to eat whole and organic foods, free of additives, chemicals, and hormones. It is also important to identify and avoid any allergy-triggering foods or inhalants.

Vitamins, Minerals, and Nutritional Supplements

The following nutrients are an integral part of a holistic alcohol and drug addiction program, primarily because they help to relieve hypoglycemia, which contributes significantly to the cycle of addiction. Combined with an individualized neurotransmitter and endocrine rebuilding program, these nutrients are best administered by a highly skilled holistic practitioner. They include:

- *Chromium ubiquinone*—200 mcg two times daily—to rebalance sugar metabolism

- *Glutamine*—to reduce the craving for alcohol, other drugs, and sugar. It also stimulates GABA production (see holistic treatment for anxiety on page 143), which helps with sleep and relaxation. Dosage: 1,000 mg four to six times daily between meals on an empty stomach.

- *Calcium* and *magnesium*—to aid in detoxification, and to relax the system in a way that diminishes irritability, anxiety, unstable emotions, muscle spasm, and insomnia

- *Pantothenic acid*—to strengthen the adrenals for the normal production of all the adrenal hormones, and to diminish sugar cravings

- *Niacin*—150–350 mg daily in three divided doses—to stabilize blood sugar

- *5-HTP*—500 mg three times daily
- *Vitamin C* and *B-complex* (50 mg two times daily)—to help relieve adrenal stress
- *Vitamins B-6, B-3, copper, iron, zinc, folic acid, phenylalanine,* and *tyrosine* (see under depression for discussion and dosage of the latter two)—to aid in biochemical repair of the dopamine neurotransmitter system
- Evening primrose oil (Omega-6 fatty acid)—1,000 mg three times daily—alcoholics are often deficient in GLA (gamma linolenic acid)

Supplements needed to protect against the liver deterioration common in alcoholism are:

- *N-acetylcysteine* (NAC)—500 mg three times daily
- *Lipoic acid*—300 mg two times daily
- *L-carnitine*—300 mg three times daily
- *Choline* 1,000 mg three times daily and inositol (five–nine grams, two times daily)

Herbs

Herbs used to treat alcohol and drug addiction have two primary purposes—to support the liver and to support the nervous system. Those that detoxify the liver are:

- *Milk thistle extract (Silybum marianum)*—one or two 70 mg capsules, three times daily (standardized to 80 percent silymarin).
- *Dandelion (Taraxacum)*—200 mg three times daily

Herbs that help reduce nervousness associated with withdrawal symptoms include *valerian* (see under insomnia), *passionflower, oats,* and *chamomile. Kava kava* (300 mg three times daily) with 5-HTP can also be used. The withdrawal symptoms of *caffeine,* mainly headache, can be relieved with *feverfew, lime blossom,* and *chamomile. Lobelia* is especially helpful in reducing the craving for *nicotine,* since it has similar but gentler effects and a longer duration. Lobelia can be combined with *ephedra* or *Avena* (1:1, 20 drops four times daily) for even better results. Lobelia should be used no longer than one month. *Oatstraw* has been used in India for many years in treating *opium* addiction, but has also been shown to help reduce cigarette smoking. Oats help rebalance the endorphin levels in the brain.

Exercise

Regular aerobic exercise is useful in revitalizing a body debilitated by drug and alcohol addiction. It also improves the likelihood of maintaining abstinence by reducing anxiety and depression. Yoga is also an effective form of exercise in treating alcohol and drug addiction.

Professional Care Therapies

Ayurveda and *homeopathy* are both effective in treating most addictions. Nux vomica is a homeopathic remedy that works well for alcoholism and cigarette smoking. *Acupuncture* has been used successfully to treat addictions, especially heroin and cocaine, by Lincoln Hospital in New York City for over 20 years. Increasingly acupuncture has proven to be quite effective at both inpatient and outpatient treatment centers throughout the country for detoxification and withdrawal from drugs, alcohol, and nicotine.

Candida Treatment Program

This consists of a strict candida control diet. Antifungal prescription drugs, such as Diflucan, Nizoral, or Sporanox can be used with caution (they are potentially toxic to the liver). With alcohol addiction it is preferable to use a homeopathic remedy to kill the candida, along with an acidophilus/bifidus preparation (see under candidiasis, chapter 9).

Mental and Emotional Health Recommendations. Since addictions typically accompany depression, many of the following therapies are effective for both conditions. (See holistic treatment and prevention for depression above for an explanation of these therapies.)

- Psychotherapy
- Stress-reduction techniques—meditation works well in treating alcoholism
- Biofeedback—can be quite effective in overcoming the craving for cigarettes
- Journaling
- Energy medicine—qigong has helped with nicotine addiction
- Hypnosis
- Bodywork therapies

Spiritual and Social Health Recommendations. A number of twelve-step programs with a spiritual orientation are helpful in overcoming addictions. These support programs are particularly helpful in the first few weeks. The most popular perhaps, Alcoholics Anonymous (AA), is quite helpful in treating alcoholism by providing group support for abstinence and behavioral modification. Information on support groups or professional referrals for sex addiction may be obtained through the National Council on Sexual Addiction and Compulsivity at (770) 989-9754. The holistic spiritual and social recommendations are similar to those used in treating depression.

The effectiveness of the biochemical aspect of Dr. Cousens's holistic approach (outlined in this chapter in the "Diet" and "Vitamins/Supplements" sections) for treating *alcohol addiction* has been validated by an independent study done by Joan Matthews Larson, Ph.D., at the Health Recovery Center in Minneapolis, Minnesota, and a number of other studies. Dr. Larson's study was published in the *International Journal of Biosocial and Medical Research*. The study documented the following results:

- Alcohol cravings from the outset to discharge had dropped from 84 to 9 percent.
- Anxiety dropped from 64 to 11 percent.
- Poor memory dropped from 69 to 11 percent.
- Insomnia dropped from 44 to 6 percent.
- Tremors and shakiness dropped from 44 to 2 percent.
- Depression dropped from 61 to 5 percent.

Dr. Cousens's holistic treatment program has been found to be effective in treating *drug abuse* as well. With the biochemical approach alone, research at the Health Recovery Center showed that 92 percent of the clients were abstinent after six months, and 74 percent remained abstinent three and one-half years later. This compares to an average abstinence rate of 25 percent for clients using other drug treatment programs at one year. This is the same rate as for those who tried to break their drug addiction without using any program.

Dr. Cousens attributes the success of his holistic medical treatment program for alcohol and drug addiction to its emphasis on the repair of the body *as well* as the mind and spirit.

8

Musculoskeletal Disease:
Ailments Affecting the Bones, Joints, Muscles, and Connective Tissue

Osteoarthritis (Arthritis)

Rheumatoid Arthritis

Gout

Back Pain

Sciatica

Osteoporosis

CONDITION

OSTEOARTHRITIS

Prevalence

OSTEOARTHRITIS IS THE MOST common form of arthritis, afflicting about 27 million Americans of all ages. It rarely begins before the age of 40, but an estimated 40 to 80 percent of people over the age of 65 have some degree of arthritis. Under the age of 45, it affects men more than women. The majority of arthritis sufferers do not seek medical treatment. For some people with arthritis, the symptoms remain mild, while in others (about 16 million) symptoms grow progressively worse until they become disabling.

Anatomy and Physiology

Osteoarthritis, or arthritis, is an inflammation of the joints that causes a breakdown in the cartilage covering the bone inside the joint. Arthritis usually involves a synovial joint—one that is encased in a tough fibrous capsule lined with a membrane that secretes a thick clear synovial fluid. This type of joint connects one bone to another and, with the fluid lubricating the cartilaginous surfaces, allows for smooth motion. The cartilage, covering the ends of the bones, is made of a soft cushion-like material that acts as a shock absorber and prevents the bones from rubbing against one another. Arthritis is a progressive degeneration of the cartilage resulting from the wear and tear on the joint combined with the body's inability to regenerate the cartilage at the same pace. In an arthritic joint there may either be insufficient synovial fluid, causing stiffness, or an excess, causing swelling. If the cartilage has broken down enough to allow the bones to rub against one another, there is significant pain. The body often attempts to repair the joint damage by producing bony outgrowths at the margins of the affected joints. These spurs can also cause pain and stiffness.

Symptoms and Diagnosis

There are no definitive laboratory tests for arthritis. The diagnosis is usually made from a physical examination, an X-ray, fluid withdrawn from a joint, and especially from the medical history. The primary symptoms of arthritis are:

- Intermittent pain with motion of affected joints
- Stiffness and limitation of movement, with audible cracking in the joints
- Swelling and deformity of the joint
- Pattern of gradual onset

Although arthritis can occur in any joint in the body, the most common sites are the fingers (particularly the two joints closest to the fingertips), the knees, hips, neck, and lower spine. The degenerative changes of osteoarthritis can often be seen in the spine on X-rays, but the majority of people with these changes do not have back pain.

There are two types of osteoarthritis:

1. Primary—results from normal wear and tear
2. Secondary—results from an injury to a joint; from disease; or chronic trauma, such as obesity, postural problems, or occupational overuse

Conventional Medical Treatment

Conventional treatment of osteoarthritis includes:

- *Reduction of stresses* (or *rest*) on joints is usually advised, using a splint, brace, neck collar, crutches, or a cane.
- *Physical therapy* is often recommended, including exercises—swimming, water aerobics, walking, bicycling, and cross-country skiing, in addition to strengthening and stretching; hot and cold packs; diathermy and paraffin baths.
- *Drugs.* Treatment usually begins with acetaminophen and progresses to non-steroidal anti-inflammatory drugs (NSAIDs), which may either be prescription or

OTC. Those most commonly used are: ibuprofen (Advil, Nuprin), Alleve, Orudis, Naprosyn, Tolectin, Indocin, and Feldene. Aspirin is not recommended for osteoarthritis because the high doses needed to reduce pain may damage the stomach lining. The NSAIDs do not stop joint deterioration. In some instances they may even *accelerate* it, by reducing a critical ingredient (glycosamino glycans) in cartilage. Long-term use can also lead to a significant incidence of kidney and liver damage, capillary fragility, stomach ulceration and small bowel irritation.

- *Corticosteroids* such as prednisone are used as a second step drug to suppress the inflammation of arthritis. Long-term use tends to suppress immunity and diminishes production of the patient's own cortisone from the adrenal gland, accelerating degenerative changes such as osteoporosis.

- *Surgery*, which may be used as a late-stage intervention, might include reconstruction or replacement of knees, hips, knuckles and other joints.

Risk Factors and Causes

- Heredity

- Severe or recurrent joint injury from heavy physical activity

- Skeletal postural defects and congenital joint instability

- Excess overweight—excessive body weight and high body mass index are significant predictors of osteoarthritis of the knee. The risk for arthritis of the knee in men is 50 to 350 percent *greater* in men who are the heaviest compared to those of normal weight. This principle probably relates to other weight-bearing joints as well.

- Exercise—there is some evidence that only the most violent joint-pounding activities (long-distance running, basketball, etc.) performed over many years will predispose to the development of arthritis.

- Cold climate and barometric pressure changes

- Food allergy, especially nightshades (potatoes, tomatoes, peppers, and eggplants), wheat, and dairy

- A diet high in animal products

- Nutrient deficiency: calcium, magnesium, manganese, protein, D-glucaronic acid, essential fatty acids

- Low-grade infections (e.g., dental infections) and autoimmune disease

- Dehydration

- Excessive acid in the body causing increased amounts of calcium, minerals, and acid toxins to be deposited in the joint, resulting in inflammation and pain

- Other systemic disorders often associated with arthritis include nutritional deficiencies, digestive disorders, constipation, fatigue, emotional stress, and endocrine disorders

Holistic Medical Treatment and Prevention

Physical Health Recommendations. Arthritis, like any other chronic condition, is a systemic (whole body) dis-ease. It is not usually just a local dysfunction of a particular joint. If there is no major joint degeneration, it is curable using a holistic approach.

Diet

The first step in treating arthritis is to *remove* all inflammatory causes. Many people with arthritis have food allergies that cause joint inflammation. Dairy products, wheat, and *nightshade plants*, including potatoes, peppers, eggplant, tomatoes, and tobacco, are most often responsible for these food allergies due to the acid they contain, called solanine. Eliminating all of them from your diet for at least one month will help to determine if food allergy is contributing to your arthritis; gradually reintroducing them (one new food every three to four days), will show which specific foods are involved.

The next step is to *remove* or decrease consumption of *all animal products* other than fish, which will help to eliminate excess calcium, mineral deposits, and acid from the joints. The most effective way to do this is to *eat a raw food vegetarian diet*. This is also called a vegan diet (vegetarian plus elimination of all animal products, especially dairy). Periodic supervised fasting also has a very high success rate. This is not a new idea. For more than 50 years, fasting clinics throughout Europe have had outstanding results with periodic juice fasting. Gabriel Cousens, M.D., at his Tree of Life Rejuvenation Center in Patagonia, Arizona, has administered a juice fasting program for treating arthritis to a number of people and has been consistently successful. Fasting enhances the eliminative and cleansing capacity of the lungs, skin, liver, and kidneys. It also rests and restores the digestive system and helps to relax the nervous system and mind. If you're considering fasting as a therapeutic option, it is best to do it under the supervision of a well-trained physician.

Besides green vegetables, your diet should *include:* carrots, avocado, seaweeds, spirulina, barley and wheat grass products, sprouts, pecans, soy products, whole grains (such as brown rice, millet, oats, wheat, and barley), seeds (sesame, flax, and pumpkin), and cold-water fish (such as salmon, sardines, herring, and tuna).

In addition to the preceding, the following foods should be *avoided:* alcohol, coffee, sugar, saturated fat, hydrogenated fat (margarine), excess salt, spinach, cranberries, plums, buckwheat, nuts.

Weight reduction, through diet and exercise, is also recommended in treating arthritis.

Vitamins, Minerals, and Supplements

The *antioxidants,* vitamin C, 1,000 to 6,000 mg daily, in an ascorbate or ester C form (essential for collagen synthesis and connective tissue repair); vitamin A, 10,000 to 25,000 I.U. daily; and vitamin E, 400 to 1,200 I.U. daily (inhibits enzymes that break down cartilage) have all demonstrated benefits in treating arthritis. A vitamin B-complex (especially B-6), 50 mg daily is recommended. Proanthocyanidin (*grape seed extract* or *pycnogenol*), in a dosage of 100 to 300 mg daily, can act as a strong anti-inflammatory. The *minerals* zinc picolinate, 30 to 50 mg daily; selenium, 200 mcg; copper aspirinate, 2 mg; calcium, 1,000 mg; magnesium, 400 to 800 mg; and manganese, 10 to 20 mg, should also be taken daily.

Glucosamine sulfate is a building block of cartilage and can be used to repair damaged cartilage or to grow new cartilage. Although it is not an anti-inflammatory, a multitude of studies (nearly three hundred, including 20 double-blind studies) have shown that glucosamine can relieve the pain of osteoarthritis. This supplement is considered safe, but it can occasionally produce heartburn and diarrhea. It usually takes four to eight weeks to get significant benefit from glucosamine. It is available in most health food stores. The recommended therapeutic dosage is 1,000 mg three times daily for 12 weeks, followed by a maintenance dosage of 500 mg three times daily. It can often be found in combination with the mineral *boron*, which can also improve the symptoms of arthritis. The daily dosage of boron is 6 to 9 mg.

Niacinamide is a B vitamin (*B-3*), similar to niacin, which has been beneficial in treating arthritis. The dosage is 500 mg four times daily, but some people will benefit with as little as 250 mg three times daily. The only reported harmful side effect is that on rare occasions it can be harmful to the liver. A periodic liver profile (blood test) can monitor your liver function.

Methionine, an amino acid needed for cartilage formation, has been shown in some studies to be more effective than ibuprofen in treating osteoarthritis.

Essential fatty acids in the form of omega-6 oils, such as evening primrose oil, black currant seed oil, and borage oil; and omega-3 oils from cold-water fish (salmon, sardines, and tuna) and *flaxseed oil* have been effective in treating arthritis. Flaxseed oil should be taken in a dosage of two tablespoons daily, and is better absorbed if taken with a small amount of cottage cheese. The best omega 3 and 6 combination is EPA (1,000 mg)/DHA (500 mg) or any 2:1 combination of EPA:DHA.

Bovine cartilage and supplements containing chondroitin sulfate may also be helpful, although there is some evidence that chondroitin may not be effective if taken orally.

The supplement *S-adenosylmethionine (SAM)*, has only recently become available in the United States, but has been successful for the past twenty years in treating arthritis in Europe.

Herbs

- *Ginger* (zingiber officinale)—acts as an anti-inflammatory; 0.5 to 1 mg of powdered ginger daily or as a tea—one grated teaspoon of fresh ginger in a cup of hot water two times daily; more simply, you can take a standardized extract of ginger combined with 500–1,000 mg of mixed bioflavonoids or include it in your diet

- *Curcumin* (Curcuma longa)—an extract of the common spice *turmeric;* an effective anti-inflammatory, 400 mg three times daily; take on an empty stomach and combine with 1,000 mg of bromelain

- *Devil's claw* (Harpagphytum procumbens)—an analgesic and anti-inflammatory; one to two grams, three times daily

- *Cayenne* (Capsaicin)—available as a capsule, 500 mg three times daily, and as an OTC cream for analgesia (blocks substance P, present in arthritic joints); apply three or four times daily for at least a week

- *Licorice root* (Glycyrrhiza glabra)—an anti-inflammatory. Long-term use can elevate blood pressure and increase potassium loss; effective doses are one-eighth to one-quarter teaspoon of a 5:1 solid extract up to three times daily

- *Yucca*—has long been used to reduce arthritic pain

- *Celery seed extract*—acts as an anti-inflammatory

- *Castor oil hot packs*—apply to affected joint

Exercise

Yoga can be especially beneficial as part of the treatment program for arthritis. Whatever form of exercise you choose, it should not cause direct pounding or contribute to the deterioration of the affected joints. Swimming is a good choice for arthritis sufferers.

Professional Care Therapies

Traditional Chinese medicine, both acupuncture and Chinese herbs; Ayurvedic medicine, especially Boswellin cream, camphor, and eucalyptus oil; bodywork (Rolfing and Hellerwork); body movement therapies, such as Feldenkrais, Trager, and Pilates (can improve mobility of the affected joints); chiropractic and osteopathic manipulation (can increase circulation to the joint); homeopathy; and craniosacral therapy can all be helpful in treating arthritis.

Mental/Emotional Health Recommendations

Louise Hay, in *You Can Heal Your Life*, lists as the probable emotional cause of arthritis: "Feeling unloved. Criticism, resentment." The affirmation that she recommends is: "I am love. I now choose to love and approve of myself. I see others with love."

Caroline Myss, in, *Anatomy of the Spirit*, writes that she believes the mental/emotional issues related to arthritis are:

- *Sensitivity to criticism*—this is probably the most significant emotional factor
- Trust
- Fear and intimidation
- Self-esteem, self-confidence, and self-respect
- Care of oneself and others
- Responsibility for making decisions
- Personal honor

There are a number of *affirmations* that you could create, directly related to the joints affected by arthritis or to the activity the arthritis prevents you from doing . For example, "My fingers move freely and easily." "My hands are filled with energy and vitality as I (write, type, work at my computer, paint, sculpt, play the piano)." Remember that you cannot use negative words. So you can't say, "I am (writing, painting, etc.) without pain. You could say, "My hands are free of pain," but that still focuses your attention to some extent on the pain. Try to make the affirmations as positive as possible.

In addition to writing and reciting the affirmations, don't forget to visualize and feel them. In addition to seeing your own affirmations, another effective *visualization* for arthritis would be to picture the surface of your arthritic joint as if it were healed. To do so, you could imagine the most perfectly smooth grayish-white glistening cartilaginous surface of a chicken or turkey drumstick that you've ever seen. Every day you could take a few minutes to picture in your mind's eye an irregular inflamed discolored cartilaginous surface being transformed into a perfectly healthy joint surface.

One recent study has documented the benefit of *journaling* feelings in treating arthritis (see pg. 57).

RHEUMATOID ARTHRITIS (RA)

Prevalence

Less common and often more disabling than osteoarthritis, rheumatoid arthritis affects between 2 and 3 percent of the American population. Women are affected three times more than men. Although it most commonly occurs between the ages of 30 and 40, it can begin at any age. In childhood it is called juvenile onset rheumatoid arthritis and afflicts 71,000 children every year—six times as many girls as boys.

Anatomy and Physiology

Rheumatoid arthritis is chronic and progressive and is thought to be an autoimmune disease. These conditions occur when the body fails to recognize its own tissues or cells and initiates an immunological response in which antibodies attack parts of the joint tissue, as well as skin and muscles.

The joint damage caused by RA begins with an inflammation of the synovial membrane. This then leads to thickening of the membrane resulting from the overgrowth of synovial cells and an accumulation of white blood cells. The release of enzymes and other substances by these cells can erode the cartilage that lines the joints, as well as the bones, tendons, and ligaments within the joint capsule. As the disease progresses, the production of excess fibrous tissue limits joint motion.

Symptoms and Diagnosis

Since RA is a systemic disease, symptoms can affect the entire body. Early in the course of the illness, even before the joints are involved, there can be fatigue and weakness; general feeling of malaise (feeling ill); low-grade fever; inflammation of the eyes; loss of appetite and weight loss.

Joint symptoms include:

- Pain, swelling, and red/purple color of joints of the fingers (but not usually the joints closest to the fingertips), wrists, ankles, and toes—occurs symmetrically on both sides of the body (osteoarthritis does not present symmetrically)

- Warm and tender joints

- Stiffness, usually early morning, improves during the day

- Red, painless skin lumps called rheumatoid nodules, over the affected joints
- Bent and gnarled deformities (usually in fingers and hands) in long-term RA

The disease can occur in many forms, from a mild short-term illness with little damage in only a few joints to a severe progressive condition with significant destruction of many joints. Most people are somewhere between these two extremes.

There is no specific diagnostic test for RA, but from the medical history, physical examination, joint X-ray, blood tests, and joint fluid analysis, a definitive diagnosis can usually be made. The diagnosis, as defined by the Arthritis Foundation, requires seven of the following diagnostic criteria, with the symptoms of the first five lasting over six weeks:

- Morning stiffness for longer than one hour
- Pain on motion in at least one joint
- Swelling (soft tissue: not just bony overgrowth) in at least one joint
- Swelling of at least one other joint
- Symmetrical joint swelling, not including terminal phalangeal joint (joint closest to fingertip) involvement
- Subcutaneous (beneath the skin) nodules usually on the forearm below the elbow
- X-ray changes typical of RA
- Positive agglutination test: +RF

Conventional Medical Treatment

The degree of pain determines the potency of the anti-inflammatories prescribed for RA. They range from aspirin and the OTC NSAIDs such as ibuprofen (Advil, Nuprin), to corticosteroids, gold compounds, D-penicillamine, antimalarials, and methotrexate (an immune suppressant used for treating cancer). The latter group of drugs can slow the destructive progression of the disease but can also cause serious, even life-threatening, side effects. A new drug, Arava, is an immune suppressant that diminishes the body's attack on the joints without compromising its ability to fight infection (as methotrexate does). It is also the first drug that has been clearly shown to inhibit the progression of RA. Preliminary information about the new COX-2 drugs (cycloxygenase inhibitor nonsteroidals, e.g., Celebrex) that have been newly approved by the FDA indicate that risks of gastrointestinal irritation and bleeding should be less common. A synthetic compound mimicking joint fluid, called Synvise, has also recently been approved for injection into affected joints. In more severe cases, physical therapy is often an option, and surgery may be recommended for the most disabling joint symptoms.

Risk Factors and Causes

As with all chronic conditions, there are multiple factors that predispose to the development of RA. Although the exact cause is unknown, there is strong evidence of a *genetic* component and an *immunological* problem. Evidence for the latter etiology places RA in the category of an autoimmune disease (the body reacting against itself). Some researchers believe RA is triggered by either a *viral infection* or a *hormonal imbalance*. There is some evidence that the disorder is related to distorted permeability of the small intestine. Others have identified *food allergies* and *psychosocial* factors as possible prime contributors to this condition.

Certain personality traits tend to be associated with the disease; those at risk tend to be more compulsive, perfectionistic, over-conscientious and helpful, excessively moralistic, and more frequently depressed. Many people suffering with this disease are rigid and stubborn, inflexible and immobile. In a survey of 88 children with juvenile RA, the most striking findings were the psychosocial factors: children whose parents were unmarried comprised 29 percent, while adoption occurred three times more often in this population. The onset of the disease, in 51 percent of the cases, occurred very close to the traumatic event—divorce, separation, death, or adoption. RA sufferers of any age may be more vulnerable to any instance of separation, either real or imagined.

Holistic Medical Treatment and Prevention

Although we know some physicians who have observed significant improvement in patients using food elimination, there are very few well-documented cases of RA being successfully treated with holistic medicine. This may be a result of the advances made by conventional medicine in slowing the progression of the disease, coupled with the likelihood that many people with RA consult a holistic practitioner only during the later, more disabling stages of their disease. The holistic treatment is most effective for milder cases of RA and is very similar to the approach used to treat osteoarthritis (see the preceding section), with the following exceptions and suggestions.

Physical Health Recommendations. Early intervention is essential, before there is significant joint destruction.

Diet

A *vegan* diet—vegetarian diet with all animal products, especially dairy and eggs, eliminated. The exceptions to this diet are fish and high-DHA eggs (found in some health food stores). This diet can also serve as a food elimination diet to identify possible food allergens. The most highly allergenic foods associated with

RA are dairy products, wheat, and corn. Some authorities find *food sensitivities* significantly related to RA in up to *50 percent* of cases.

See the osteoarthritis section for the remainder of the dietary suggestions.

Vitamins, Minerals, and Supplements

The antioxidants, minerals, and supplements are essentially the same as for osteoarthritis, with the following *prioritized items:*

1. *Glucosamine sulfate*—not to the same extent as for osteoarthritis, but also considered moderately effective in treating RA; 500 mg three times daily.

2. *Vitamin C,* as ascorbate or Ester C—1,000 mg three times daily.

3. *Essential fatty acids* (especially EPA, an omega-3)—flaxseed oil is the most effective and economical means of taking it; daily dose is one to two tablespoons per day.

4. *Copper,* 2 mg daily

5. *Quercetin* or *curcumin* (with bromelain)—250 mg between meals three times daily

6. *Manganese*—30 mg daily

7. *Selenium*—200 mcg daily

Digestive enzymes such as *pancreatin* have been helpful in treating RA, possibly by mitigating the effects of food allergies. The dosage is 500 to 1,000 mg with each meal. *Probiotics,* such as acidophilus- and bifidus-containing products, can help relieve the symptoms of RA by reducing bowel toxicity.

Herbs

- *Curcumin (turmeric)*—the best-documented herb for treating RA; a potent anti-inflammatory; 400 to 600 mg three times daily, usually given with the following:

- *Bromelain*—a pineapple extract and enzyme that also acts as an anti-inflammatory

- *Ginger, devil's claw*, and *licorice root*—same dosages as with osteoarthritis

- *Bupleuri falcatum*—a Chinese herb that seems to be as effective an anti-inflammatory as steroids and without the harmful side effects; two to four grams daily.

- *Siberian ginseng (eleuthrococcus)*—a Korean herb that strengthens the adrenal glands; 500 mg two times daily

- *Hawthorn berries*—a rich source of flavonoids that helps to heal collagen and joint membranes; one-half teaspoon or two capsules three to four times daily.

Professional Care Therapies

The same therapies used for treating osteoarthritis can be used for RA. Some holistic practitioners have had success in treating RA with bee venom therapy.

Mental and Emotional Health Recommendations. In addition to the recommendations made for osteoarthritis, *psychotherapy* can be quite helpful for people suffering with RA. There are usually painful deep-seated emotional issues related to RA that need to be addressed and released before significant healing can occur. *Affirmations* and *visualizations* can also be of great value with this condition.

Social Health Recommendations Enhancement of family support and family counseling are strongly recommended with RA.

GOUT

Prevalence, Symptoms, and Causes

Gout is a form of arthritis that affects more than one million Americans, mostly men between the ages of 40 and 50. It is caused by the deposit of chalky urate crystals in joints, tendons, kidneys, and other tissues, when the *uric acid* level in the body is *elevated.* Symptoms include: acute joint pain, swelling, tenderness, redness, and heat of sudden onset followed by pain-free intervals. Initially the attacks are short-lived and usually occur at night with throbbing and excruciating pain. But usually there are recurrences, and eventually these flare-ups can last for days or weeks. When allowed to persist, gout can cause severe inflammation and destruction of joints, as well as kidney damage and stone formation. In addition, soft nodules may form in the earlobes, tendons, and cartilage. Gout usually attacks a single joint, most often the innermost joint of the *big toe.* Other joints commonly affected are those of the knee, ankle, wrist, elbow, and hands.

The high blood levels of uric acid are caused by foods rich in proteins called purines, such as liver, organ meats, and poultry. There also appears to be a hereditary factor that can contribute to the elevation of uric acid. Alcohol can often precipitate an acute attack of gout. People with gout are typically obese, prone to diabetes and hypertension, and have a high risk for heart disease. Low-dose aspirin therapy and some diuretic high blood pressure medications can also elevate uric acid and cause secondary gout.

Gout is considered a disease of affluence—the "rich man's disease"—affecting mostly people who eat a diet rich in *animal protein, fat,* and *alcohol.*

Conventional Medical Treatment

The pain and inflammation of acute gout is usually controlled with OTC NSAIDS. An older drug, colchicine, works well, but inadvertent excess dosages cause nausea and diarrhea. As the inflammation subsides, usually within two or three days, the drug dosage is gradually reduced and then stopped. In some severe cases, a corticosteroid drug may be injected into the joint. To prevent recurrences, uric acid–lowering drugs are taken on a daily basis. Allopurinol is the drug most often prescribed for prevention. Although it is effective, the drug can be toxic to the liver. Blood tests at regular intervals are advised.

Holistic Medical Treatment and Prevention

Physical Health Recommendations

Diet

A low purine diet is the essence of the holistic treatment. Prior to the availability of allopurinol, this diet was the primary recommendation of conventional treatment. But the effectiveness of the drug in preventing recurrences of gout has made dietary compliance more difficult. However, with strict adherence to this diet you can usually eliminate medication. *Foods to avoid* include: all meats, especially organ meats, milk and dairy products, refined carbohydrates, saturated fats, herring, sardines, mackerel, anchovies, brewer's yeast, baker's yeast, spices, alcohol, and shellfish. *Foods to eat:* a *vegetarian* diet is highly therapeutic, especially celery, kale, cabbage, parsley, green leafy vegetables, seaweed, tomatoes, strawberries, bananas, and cherries (up to one pound daily). Drinking lots of vegetable and fruit *juices*, especially carrot, apple and cucumber, celery and parsley, red cherry, and red grape juice is helpful. You should stay well hydrated with a high intake of purified *water*. Although drinking an adequate amount of water is always a key component of optimal health, gout is one clear instance where it can be therapeutic (flushing the kidneys of urate crystals and preventing kidney stones) in prevention.

Weight reduction is also helpful in treating gout.

Vitamins, Minerals, and Supplements

The full complement of antioxidants, minerals, and supplements recommended for osteoarthritis and rheumatoid arthritis should also be taken for treating and preventing gout. Those that are most beneficial are vitamins C and E, *essential fatty acids, quercetin,* and *bromelain.* Vitamin C triggers the excretion of uric acid by the kidneys; combined with adequate liquid intake to prevent urate crystal formation, a dose of three to four grams daily can slowly lower uric acid blood levels. To this list add *folic acid*, which is very effective for gout because it inhibits the enzyme that produces uric acid. The dosage is 10 to 40 mg daily. Be aware that folic acid can mask the signs of B-12 deficiency, so *B-12* should also be taken, two to ten mg daily. High doses of folic acid can also cause gastrointestinal upset and interfere with epilepsy drugs.

Herbs

- *Celery:* tincture of seeds, 10–30 drops two or three times daily; you can also eat celery stalks in large amounts every day.

- *Devil's claw:* one to two grams of powder three times daily; or 10 drops of the tincture three times daily; this herb reduces uric acid levels and helps relieve pain.

- *Colchicum:* tincture, 5–15 drops three times daily during an acute attack; this can be toxic in high doses.

- *Cherry extract*, sufficient to provide the equivalent of one half to one pound of cherries a day

Professional Care Therapies

Acupuncture is often helpful in easing the pain of an acute attack but is usually unsuccessful for long-term relief. Homeopathic remedies, such as arnica and pulsatilla, can also relieve acute pain, and homeopathy can also be beneficial in preventing recurrences.

Exercise

Exercise is recommended with gout to not only improve circulation but help with the elimination of uric acid. Aerobic exercise (brisk walking, bicycling, jogging), yoga, t'ai chi, or dancing can all be helpful if practiced regularly.

Mental and Emotional Health Recommendations

See osteoarthritis and rheumatoid arthritis.

BACKACHE

(Low-Back Pain)

Prevalence

About 80 percent of all Americans will suffer from low back pain at some point in their lives. Backache becomes more common between the ages of 30 and 50 as the intervertebral disks lose some of their ability to absorb shock and backs become more unstable from inactivity. According to the National Center for Health Statistics, back pain is the fourth most common chronic ailment, the sixth most common reason for visiting an emergency room, and accounts for 13 million visits to primary care physicians' offices each year. Back pain is responsible for 60 million lost working days each year, which in turn costs the economy $5.2 billion.

Anatomy and Physiology

Although we often think of the back as a single entity, it is actually a complex connection of *many parts*. These include:

- *Bones*, including: the vertebrae at each level of the spine; the sacrum or last five bones of the spine above the tailbone, which rests between the bones of the pelvis and the back; and the pelvic bones themselves
- *Nerves* of the low back, which includes a pair of nerves that leave the spinal cord at each level, one on each side below each vertebra. These then join together to form the nerves of the low back, the pelvis, and the legs. Several nerves come together in the buttock and run down the back of the leg as the sciatic nerve. This nerve then divides and innervates the entire leg all the way to the tips of the toes
- *Muscles*, which connect the spine and pelvis to the lower back, upper back, ribs, hips, legs, and abdomen; and muscles that connect the pelvis to the low back
- *Ligaments*, which form static supports between the vertebrae, sacrum and pelvic bones

The *functions* of these different structures are as follows:

- *Bones* provide support and form for the body and protect the internal organs.
- *Nerves* carry signals from the brain and spinal cord to the muscles to allow for movement, sensations of pain and pleasure, heat and cold, pressure, and sharpness; they also send information back to the nervous system regarding the position of the body, how far it is bent, how fast it is moving, and where it is in space.
- *Muscles* perform various movements, including bending, squatting, rotating, walking, standing, sitting, and rising up.
- *Ligaments* hold the vertebrae together in their linear alignment.

Together, all these parts of the back allow us to do a variety of activities, to comfortably remain in one position, to balance ourselves, and perform very complex movements. The nervous system also helps coordinate various motions so that the different muscles and joints in a particular area work together to allow for coordinated movements and actions.

Symptoms and Diagnosis

Backache is the term used to describe a variety of conditions. Since X-rays usually reveal no abnormality, your symptoms and a physical exam are the major components in establishing a diagnosis. However, in the majority of cases the exact diagnosis is still not known. The most common types of backache are:

1. *Sprain and strain:* often used interchangeably, these are the most prevalent forms of low-back pain. A strain is usually an overstretched muscle, and a sprain a partially torn ligament, but in most cases of backache it isn't clear which one it is.

2. *Muscle spasm* is a painful, sustained, and involuntary contraction of muscles in the back.

3. *Disc problem* (A slipped disc): this accounts for only 2 to 4 percent of backaches. In actuality, the disc *herniates* or bulges from between two vertebrae and may eventually rupture. This bulging disc may push against a spinal nerve causing shooting pains, tingling, or numbness to extend into the leg. Most often the affected spinal nerve is the sciatic, the largest one, and when that occurs the condition is called *sciatica*. (Sciatica is discussed separately in the following section.)

4. *Structural problems* and *underlying medical conditions* account for a small percentage of backache.

The *symptoms* of muscle strain and muscle spasm include:

- Persistent pain in the lower back ranging from mild to excruciating
- Muscle spasms often follow muscle strain
- Stiffness, especially after sitting for extended periods
- Changes in posture, limitation of mobility and activity

The normal healing process can take from two to four weeks in 90 percent of people with backache, but the pain usually starts to decrease after a few days or a week.

The following types of back pain need the urgent attention of a physician. If you have any of these symptoms, have them evaluated as soon as possible.

1. Sudden severe back pain associated with pain in the abdominal area and shortness of breath, especially when there is no injury, could be an aneurysm in the aorta (large blood vessel in the back).

2. Weakness or inability to move your leg or legs, with or without back pain, could be a stroke or a severe ruptured disk.

3. Persistent back pain in one place could be a sign of bone disease or cancer. X-rays or other tests may be helpful in making the diagnosis.

Conventional Medical Treatment

1. *Bedrest*, usually for no more than two days; and *limited activity*.

2. *Sleeping on the back* with a big pillow under the knees or on the side with a big pillow between the knees.

3. *Ice* to the affected area for the first two days. It can be applied hourly for 20 minutes at a time to help decrease swelling and pain.

4. After two days, change to *moist heat* (heating pad, hot bath or shower) to help loosen the muscles and decrease spasm. Begin gentle *stretching* to the point of tolerance (no pain). It is very important to listen to your body and not over-stretch it. The intensity of the stretches may be very gradually increased daily until a return to full motion (or even better motion than originally) is attained. If you're not patient with this healing process, you may reinjure the muscle and have to start over. An excellent guide for stretching is a book entitled *Stretching*, by Bob Anderson (not the coauthor of this book).

5. *Pain medications* might include: Tylenol, one or two extra-strength 500 mg tablets, four times a day (maximum eight per day); aspirin, one to two tablets every four hours; ibuprofen (Advil, Nuprin, Motrin), 200 mg tablets, two tablets three or four times a day; or naproxen sodium (Aleve), 220 mg, one tablet two or three times a day. Tylenol has fewer potential side effects than the other medications but may not provide as much pain relief. For short periods of time, all these medications are relatively safe. The exceptions are for persons with stomach ulcers or kidney and liver problems. None of these should be taken with alcohol, including the Tylenol. These medications can be purchased OTC, or similar stronger versions can be prescribed by a physician.

6. *Muscle relaxants* may be prescribed if muscle spasm is a significant component of the back pain. These medications are often effective but are not meant for long-term use. Most of them can cause drowsiness.

7. Addressing *posture*, the *ergonomics* of the work station, and proper instruction in lifting and carrying. Lifting should be done by bending the hips and knees, while keeping the back straight and the spine and shoulders over the hips. It is best to grab the object, pull it as close to your body as possible, and then stand up by straightening the knees and hips while keeping the spine straight. Follow this same procedure when putting a heavy object down—all the bending should be

done with the hips and knees and not with the back. It is also very important when moving heavy objects to turn the entire body by turning the feet and legs, to avoid twisting the back. If the back is twisted while lifting, it is much more prone to injury.

8. *Injections* into muscle trigger points. This procedure often gives temporary and sometimes long-lasting relief.

Causes and Risk Factors of Backache from Muscle Strain, Sprain, or Spasm

Physical

1. Lifting heavy objects improperly, for example, moving too quickly or awkwardly

2. Poorly conditioned muscles (both back and abdominal) due to lack of exercise and flexibility; and excessive exercise

3. Posture problems and leg length discrepancy

4. Prolonged standing, insufficient arch support, and inappropriate footwear, such as high heels

5. Obesity and pregnancy

6. Inadequate support from a soft mattress

7. Uncomfortable work stations, such as chairs with improper support or working under an automobile or with heavy equipment.

8. Nutritional deficiencies, especially low protein, manganese, and magnesium intake (diuretics used to treat high blood pressure can lower magnesium); and constipation

Mental/Emotional

Fear is the underlying emotion contributing to backache. Louise Hay believes it is a fear of money and lack of financial support. Carolyn Myss believes the mental/emotional issues that may be associated with low back pain are:

- Family relationships and group safety and security

- Ability to provide for life's necessities

- Ability to stand up for self

- Comfortably occupying one's home

- Social and familial law and order

- Blame and guilt

- Money and sex

- Power and control
- Creativity
- Ethics and honor in relationships

Holistic Medical Treatment and Prevention
Physical Health Recommendations for Acute Back Pain

1. Osteopathic or chiropractic adjustment—a brief course of structural treatments; the Jones counterstrain technique (osteopathy) is particularly helpful.

2. Acupuncture, acupressure, and therapeutic massage

3. Calcium citrate or lactate, 1,200–1,500 mg; and magnesium citrate or glycinate, 500–750 mg—divide this total daily dosage into three or four doses

4. Herbs:

   - *Valerian* and *passionflower*—help relieve muscle spasm
   - *Bromelain*—a pineapple extract, 500 units, three times daily
   - *Cayenne (capsaicin)*—500 mg three times daily, or apply cream three or four times daily
   - *Ginger*—100 mg, two times daily; can also be massaged into the back
   - *White willow bark* (a natural aspirin-like compound)—one-half to one teaspoon, three to four times daily
   - *Cramp bark*—relieves muscle tension and spasms—one-half to one teaspoon, three to four times daily; can also be massaged into the back
   - Soft tissue injections of *Sarapin* (from the North American pitcher plant); 2–15 cc injected into several large and tender muscle sites or trigger points. This agent has a local anesthetic effect that lasts up to three weeks and gives superb relief from acute pain of muscular origin. Your physician can find it in the PDR under high chemical.

   The advantage of the herbs is that they are safe to take even if one has ulcers or has an allergy to the standard pain medications. The disadvantage is that they may not be as effective in relieving this type of pain.

5. Homeopathic remedies:

   - Arnica as a topical oil or gel or taken internally
   - Aconite can be taken when the pain comes on suddenly or in cold or dry weather
   - Magnesium phosphate—acts as a muscle relaxant

Physical Health Recommendations for Chronic Low Back Pain.

Holistic treatment follows a comprehensive medical history including the mental, emotional, and social status of the patient. It would also include the same thorough physical examination and diagnostic tests that would be performed conventionally. Less testing might be done if the practitioner is more comfortable with a structural examination.

Bodywork and Body Movement

Maintaining the *structural alignment* of the muscles, tendons, joints, bones, and fascia (the lining of muscle) is an essential component of the holistic treatment for chronic back pain. Several treatments by an osteopathic physician, chiropractor, or other trained or certified practitioner may be needed. Lasting benefit is most likely to be obtained with the more indirect types of treatments, such as *myofascial release* or *craniosacral osteopathy*. The more direct or high-velocity thrusting techniques, which force areas that are out of alignment back into alignment, are usually more helpful with acute injuries than with chronic back pain. However, other forms of *osteopathic* or *chiropractic* treatments, which usually consist of gentler techniques, can be helpful in some cases of chronic pain. But if these modalities or any other form of therapy do not offer noticeable improvement after three to six treatments, it is important to evaluate whether to continue.

Physical therapy performed by a highly skilled therapist using a variety of modalities, such as heat, ice, ultrasound, and electrical stimulation, is often helpful. However, these are adjunct therapies and are not substitutes for structural treatment. They are unlikely to provide lasting relief with chronic pain when used alone. Standard physical therapy often utilizes strengthening exercises to overcome areas of weakness or malalignment. A holistic treatment program is designed to help the body to realign itself, thus healing the weakness and directly treating the cause of the problem.

There are several other forms of *bodywork* or *body movement therapies* that may be helpful in treating chronic low back pain. These therapies utilize methods to retrain the nervous system to improve posture, alignment, balance, coordination, and self-awareness. They can help you to move more efficiently and to be more aware of your body and how it works. Some of the more common body-based therapies include *Trager psychophysical integration, Feldenkrais awareness through movement, the Alexander technique, Rolfing structural integration,* and *Pilates.* The *Loren Berry Method* of bodywork is not as well known but is also highly effective. These approaches often involve both hands-on treatments and instruction from the practitioner for exercises to be done by the patient at home. These exercises can directly address the cause of the back pain by helping the body to integrate its functions and resolve areas of dysfunction. These practitioners are becoming much easier to find. You can either evaluate them on your own (see the appendix) or you can obtain a referral from a holistic physician.

Exercise

Yoga has demonstrated remarkable success in both treating and preventing chronic low back pain. Find a teacher, a class, or a videotape, and start out *very* gradually. Remember—DON'T PUSH YOURSELF. If you keep it slow and steady, practicing every day, you might very well end up with a healthier back than you had prior to the onset of your back pain.

If you do not practice yoga, you should at least do several *stretching exercises* every day. A physical therapist can teach you, or you can refer to the book *Stretching* by Bob Anderson.

Brisk walking, swimming, or any other gentle form of *aerobic exercise* is recommended for treatment and prevention of chronic backache.

Acupuncture

Acupuncture may be helpful both for both acute and chronic back pain. It may offer substantial and long-lasting relief, and it often works wells in combination with structural approaches. The sooner the problem is addressed with acupuncture, the better the chance that it will work.

Hydrotherapy

Hot baths with mineral salts (Epsom salt) and/or the following essential oils: chamomile, marjoram, lavender, or a combination of wintergreen, camphor, and eucalyptus. These same oils can also be applied as a *hot compress* or *massaged* into the back. There are also exercises that can be performed in a hot shower or bath. A good book on the subject is *Hot Water Therapy* by Patrick Horay, D.C.

Sleep support

Be sure your bed provides good support. Waterbeds and soft mattresses should be avoided.

Diet

- Lose weight if overweight
- *Eat* whole grains, especially barley, brown rice, millet, corn, and oats; fish; fiber-rich foods, especially beans; fresh vegetables, especially leafy greens; fruits
- *Avoid* animal products, coffee, alcohol, tobacco, soy, and hot spices such as cinnamon, cloves, and garlic

With any of these therapies for treating chronic back pain, you need to continually evaluate their benefit. If you are receiving the same treatment repeatedly without lasting results, the therapy is probably not addressing the underlying cause. Not only can continuing this course of treatment become expensive, but it can also create a dependence on the practitioner. Holistic medicine attempts to address causes while empowering patients to learn to heal themselves.

Mental/Emotional Health Recommendations. The affirmations recommended by Louise Hay for low back pain are as follows: "I trust the process of life. All I need is always taken care of." "I am safe."

She believes that backs represent the support of life and suggests an affirmation for backs (a preventive measure)—"I know that life always supports me." Just as with any other malfunctioning part of the body, there are a wide variety of affirmations that you can create that will represent a healthy back to you. Some examples might be; "My back is strong and flexible." "I am sitting, standing, bending, and lifting normally." "My back is now completely healed." "I am stretching every day and my back continues to heal."

Relaxation techniques and biofeedback work well for backache related to muscle spasm and muscle tightness—the variety of backache often related to chronic stress.

Visualizations that represent healing are very powerful. Whatever your understanding of the cause of your back pain, it can be used to create a healing image. If the cause of your pain is unknown, then just ask for a healing image to come to you and use it every day while doing a breathing exercise. You could imagine each abdominal breath filling your abdomen and low back with light and energy, or a laser beam of light zeroing in on any abnormal tissue or contracted muscle. The light could either heal the tissue or relax the muscle enough to allow for a realignment of the spine to take place. Since the regular practice of visualization has been known to successfully dissolve cancerous tumors, it can certainly help to relax tight muscles and move bones.

Counseling or any of the other emotional health recommendations in chapter 3 are helpful in treating chronic low back pain. The focus of your emotional work will be on one or more of the emotional issues associated with backache that were listed earlier under "Risk Factors and Causes."

Bioenergy recommendations

Energy medicine, using healing or Therapeutic Touch, Reiki, or more advanced techniques (see the appendix) can be helpful in treating chronic low back pain. They work similarly to acupuncture, but instead of the specific meridians used by acupuncturists, these modalities should be applied directly to the low back. Using imagery while being treated by a practitioner of energy medicine seems to enhance the effectiveness of both treatments.

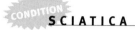

SCIATICA

Prevalence, Anatomy, and Physiology

Sciatica refers to aching or pain along the route of the sciatic nerve, the largest and longest nerve in the body. It is actually a group of nerves encased in a sheath. The right and left branches of the sciatic nerve extend from the base of the spinal cord through the buttock and the back of each thigh to the knee, where it branches and extends down into the feet. Sciatica most often affects people in their forties and fifties.

Symptoms and Diagnosis

The irritation of the sciatic nerve causes:

- Pain in the low back, lower buttock, or back of the leg, which may radiate down to the foot; can be either mild and intermittent, or severe and persistent. Pain is usually worse with movement, laughing, sneezing, coughing, straining with a bowel movement, and at night

- Muscle spasms, weakness, numbness, or tingling (pins and needles) in buttock or leg

- As a result of the chronic pain, other symptoms might include severe fatigue, inability to sleep, irritability and increased anger, and loss of ability to perform typical activities of daily living. Sometimes, severe depression can also be present, including feelings of extreme sadness and hopelessness, crying spells, insomnia, and loss of appetite. These symptoms can occur even without a prior history of depression and should be treated by a physician

In about half of all cases of sciatica, the pain resolves spontaneously within four weeks.

A definitive *diagnosis* should be made by a well-trained physician. A thorough history will include a careful accounting of all of your symptoms: the type of pain and its location, body positions that relieve or aggravate the pain, activities you were engaged in just before the onset of the pain, and the current stressors affecting your life. This evaluation, coupled with a careful, well-focused physical examination, are often all that's necessary to make a diagnosis. Many primary care physicians are capable of evaluating back pain, especially more recently trained family physicians or osteopathic physicians (D.O.) who have maintained their skills in osteopathic manipulation.

If a severe nerve injury is suspected following the physical exam (symptoms may include the loss of reflexes and true muscle weakness), then tests, such as an MRI, may be warranted. Otherwise, these tests often reveal many "incidental" or common minor abnormalities that are not significant and are probably not related to the pain. These findings may create unnecessary anxiety for the patient and could lead to further testing and procedures, including surgery. Bulging intervertebral disks, minor "degenerative joint changes," and flattened, narrowed disks, especially at the L5-S1 level, are all common on MRI scans, especially in older people.

Conventional Treatment

1. Chronic use of *pain medications*, including Tylenol, ibuprofen (Advil, Nuprin, Motrin), naproxen sodium (Aleve), and other similar products in OTC or prescription strength

2. *Narcotic medications*, such as codeine, hydrocodone, or oxycodone

3. *Bedrest* for one or two days, using a firm mattress. Lie on your unaffected side with your affected leg straight and supported by several pillows under the knee

4. Try alternating *heat* and *cold* as described earlier for backache

5. *Physical therapy*, traction devices, and home exercise programs, often including walking

6. *Nerve blocks*—injections into the joints of the spine or near the spinal cord—can sometimes offer dramatic relief in more extreme cases. However, it is a high-risk procedure because the injections are given in close proximity to the spinal cord and other vital structures. Therefore, it must be performed by a trained anesthesiologist, orthopedist, or neurosurgeon.

7. *Surgery* on the spine or disks between the bones of the spine, called laminectomies and discectomies, in some instances can be very helpful and afford immediate relief of pain. Surgery should only be done if the abnormalities seen on tests and scans correspond well to the exact location of the symptoms. For some back problems arthroscopic surgery can be performed through a small instrument inserted into the back by either an orthopedic surgeon or neurosurgeon. Some of the potential problems with surgery include a long recovery period even if the surgery is successful, scarring near the spinal cord, and, rarely, infections of the spine. It is essential to consider the potential benefits before choosing surgery, since many procedures are performed that result in no relief of pain. When performed in the right circumstances, surgery can work quite well.

8. *Pain clinics* may do further testing and are often helpful in combining a program of physical therapy and learning to cope with the psychological effects of chronic pain.

9. A *support group* can be helpful, but only if it is based on a positive attitude and works to improve the situation. If the support group becomes a complaining session, then it could be detrimental.

Risk Factors and Causes

Physical.

1. Ruptured ("slipped" or "herniated") intervertebral disks in the low back that can push against the sciatic nerve

2. Accumulation of injuries that have not completely healed due to repetitive lifting or constant exposure to mechanical vibrations (e.g., long hours of driving a truck or car)

3. Chronic muscle tension from poor posture or stress

4. Loss of motion at the joints of the lower spine, particularly the sacroiliac joint or the spine joints of the pelvis, and tight muscles in the hip area that can press on the sciatic nerve, especially the piriformis muscle

5. Severe degenerative osteoarthritis of the spine (mild and even moderate osteoarthritis usually do not cause pain)

6. Inflammatory types of arthritis, such as spondylitis and rheumatoid arthritis

7. Other types of bone disease, including cancer of the bone or cancer that has spread to the bone

Mental/Emotional. For sciatica, Louise Hay believes the probable emotional cause to be: "Fear of money and of the future. Being hypocritical." All the mental/emotional issues associated with low back pain listed earlier would apply to sciatica and any other cause of chronic low back pain.

Holistic Medical Treatment and Prevention

Physical Health Recommendations. Most of the recommendations for treating and preventing recurrences of *low back pain* and *osteoarthritis* can also benefit sciatica. In addition, the following suggestions are especially helpful for sciatica.

Diet

Both *thiamine* (B-1) and *magnesium* are natural muscle relaxants, so the diet should include foods high in both, such as: dark green leafy vegetables, yellow vegetables, whole grains, and raw nuts and seeds. Avoid those foods that deplete the body of both nutrients, such as caffeine, chocolate, and refined sugars.

Vitamins, Minerals, and Supplements

Vitamins C, D, and E; the minerals calcium, magnesium, and manganese; and the supplement glucosamine sulfate can all be beneficial for treating and preventing sciatica. Some health food stores now carry products that combine most or all of these ingredients. Proper dosage for all of these can be found in the arthritis and backache sections.

Intramuscular injections of vitamin B-12 (1,000 mcg daily for one to two weeks), with folic acid (2 or 3 mg) added in the syringe at least three times per week, has proven to be highly effective in relieving the pain of sciatica in about one-half of cases. If after the first ten injections there's no improvement, then stop. If there has been a good response, then after the initial two weeks decrease the frequency of the injections to two or three injections a week for a month, then one to four injections for a month if needed. Another variation of this technique is to use Sarapin with B-12 in a 1:1 ratio (0.5 cc of each) in four injections given two times per week.

Herbs and Homeopathy

The herbs and homeopathic remedies used to relieve the pain of sciatica are the same as those used for acute low back pain. Additional recommendations include:

1. A mixture of equal parts *willow bark* and *St. John's wort* one half teaspoon of each herb three times daily

2. *St. John's wort oil* (warm) can be massaged into the low back to alleviate pain

3. *Bromelain* and *turmeric*—200 to 600 mg of both four times daily (between meals and at bedtime), to relieve inflammation

4. *Juniper berries*—apply as a massage oil

5. *Homeopathic Hypericum*—for acute pain use 30x, four pellets every half-hour to hour during the first two days

6. *Colocynth* and *Rhus tox.* are both effective homeopathics

Professional Care Therapies

Acupuncture, bodywork (osteopathic and chiropractic manipulative therapy), *bioenergy* (including treatment with a Transcutaneous Electrical Nerve Stimulation [TENS] unit), and *physical therapy* (stretching and strengthening exercises) applied by skilled practitioners can all be helpful in treating and preventing sciatica.

Acupressure. To relieve sciatica lie down on your back with your legs bent, and feet flat on the floor. Place your hands underneath your buttocks (palms down) beside the base of your spine. Close your eyes and take long, deep breaths and rock your knees from side to side for two minutes. Reposition your hands for comfort and to enable different parts of the buttocks muscles to be pressed. Also try swaying your legs from side to side with your knees pulled into your abdomen and your feet off the floor.

Simply touching one of the acupressure points for 15 to 30 minutes can give prompt and prolonged relief. Place the pad of the tip of the middle finger over the sciatic nerve about one-half inch above the buttock-thigh crease, midway between the inside and outside margins of the thigh.

Mental and Emotional Health Recommendations

Louise Hay's affirmation for sciatica: "I move into my greater good. My good is everywhere, and I am secure and safe." *Visualization* is especially helpful in treating sciatica. If there is irritation and inflammation of your sciatic nerve as it emerges from the spinal cord, you can picture red, inflamed, swollen tissue that gradually becomes pink as it shrinks down to normal size. Any visualization that represents to you diminished pain and inflammation will work.

The mental and emotional issues contributing to sciatica are the same as those associated with backache.

CONDITION

OSTEOPOROSIS

Prevalence

Potentially a disabling disease, osteoporosis affects approximately 25 million Americans. It can affect men, but it is eight times more common in women. Although about one-half of all women between the ages of 45 and 75 have some degree of osteoporosis, nearly one-third of all postmenopausal women suffer from serious bone deterioration. Caucasians and Asians are more often afflicted. Osteoporosis affects more women than heart disease, stroke, diabetes, breast cancer, and arthritis. The United States has the highest rate of osteoporotic fractures in the world, and interestingly, the hip fracture rates begin to rise abruptly between the ages of 40 and 44—much earlier than menopause begins in most women. Treatment of this condition costs about $3.8 billion each year.

Anatomy and Physiology

Osteoporosis literally means *porous bones*. The bones lose their density, becoming fragile and brittle due to progressive loss of calcium and protein. Bone mass reaches a peak in women between the ages of 30 and 35; but between 55 and 70, the average woman will have lost 30 to 40 percent of her bone mass. The most rapid rate of bone loss occurs in the first five years after menopause: at least 5 to

10 percent. It then levels off to about 1 percent per year. Most men don't experience bone loss until after age 70.

Two types of bone cells function in bone maintenance. Osteoclasts remove damaged or weak bone tissue, and osteoblasts replace it with new bone. As long as these cells maintain an equilibrium, bone mass remains stable. Estrogen slows the activity of the osteoclasts, while progesterone has the opposite effect on osteoblasts. In males, testosterone has the same functions. A thyroid hormone, calcitonin, helps to maintain proper levels of calcium, thus enhancing bone formation. In addition to calcium, bones also require adequate amounts of the minerals magnesium, phosphorus, manganese, zinc, copper, and silicon, plus vitamins A, C, and K. Physical stresses on a bone, caused by gravitational pull and muscle contraction (walking and other forms of exercise), are also necessary. A balance and interaction of all these essential factors is required to maintain normal bone mass.

Symptoms and Diagnosis

A gradual loss of height is the most common symptom, due to compression of the vertebrae. This can lead to a stooped posture, the classic "dowager's hump," and low back pain. Often there are no obvious symptoms until a relatively minor fall results in a fracture, usually of the hip, arm, or wrist.

The initial test to diagnose osteoporosis is to measure for a loss in height. Your doctor should check your height routinely at each office visit, or you can do it yourself at regular intervals. A loss of one-half inch from your usual height is significant, and should then be followed by a bone density test. This is best measured by DXA—dual X-ray absorptiometry—since it has only a 1 percent rate of error. Other commonly performed tests, DEXA and DPA, have error rates of 2 and 8 percent. Regular X-rays can only detect osteoporosis after 25 percent of the bone mass has been lost. The bones most recommended for testing are the vertebrae of the lumbar spine.

Conventional Medical Treatment

- Estrogen or a combination of estrogen and progesterone—called HRT (hormone replacement therapy) is usually continued until age 70, when the rate of bone loss subsides. The longer estrogen is taken, the greater the risk of adverse side effects, including water retention, increased fat synthesis, uterine fibroids, heart disease, gall bladder and liver disease, stroke, and breast cancer. The risk of endometrial cancer can be offset by taking progesterone along with the estrogen.

- Fosamax—a prescription drug—increases bone mass. It must be taken with a full glass of water in the morning on an empty stomach at least 30 minutes before eating. The usual dose is 10 mg once a day.

- A recently approved salmon-based calcitonin nasal spray, called Miacalcin, may provide benefit.

- A calcium-rich diet and calcium supplements are usually recommended.

- A weight-bearing exercise program, including walking, jogging, dance, or weight training, should be followed.

Risk Factors and Causes

- Gender—being female

- Age—postmenopausal, fifties and sixties

- Race—Caucasian or Asian

- Family history of osteoporosis

- Sedentary lifestyle, or insufficient weight-bearing and resistance exercise; one of the most important risk factors

- Cigarette smoking—poisons the ovaries, which decreases both estrogen and progesterone

- Dietary factors—high sodium (salt), fat, protein (especially meat and milk), processed food, sugar, alcohol (two or more alcoholic drinks per day significantly increases risk), soft drinks (high in phosphate, which depletes magnesium from bone), and caffeine can all increase calcium loss. Inadequate intake of calcium, vitamin K, silicon, boron, folic acid, magnesium, and manganese can contribute to osteoporosis

- Hormonal deficiency—low progesterone is even more significant than low estrogen

- Environmental factors—heavy metals (lead, cadmium, tin from tin cans, aluminum), and acid rain derivatives cause the body to extract calcium from bone for use as a buffer to balance the acidity

- Insufficient calcium absorption—both vitamin D and adequate hydrochloric acid (HCl) are needed for adequate absorption.

- Low body fat, chronically underweight—causes reduced progesterone

- Hyperthyroidism or excessive thyroid medication—may cause excess bone depletion

- Women who have never had a child

- Fluoride—toxic to bone cells

- Broad spectrum antibiotics—destroy intestinal flora, which can cause malabsorption of nutrients and diminish production of vitamin K; take acidophilus supplements following course of antibiotic

- Corticosteroid medications (prednisone)—impairs calcium absorption, and inhibits osteoblasts

Holistic Medical Treatment and Prevention

Since osteoporosis is a gradual, invisible, and insidious disease, it isn't easy to determine whether or not your holistic treatment program is working. Therefore, you might want to monitor your progress with periodic (annual) DXA or DEXA tests to see if your therapeutic regimen is improving or at least maintaining your bone status. If it is not, you might then consider starting Fosamax and HRT.

Physical Health Recommendations

Diet

A *vegan* diet (no animal products—meat or dairy) is recommended, one that is rich in the foods high in calcium: whole grains; fresh vegetables, especially dark greens, such as collard, kale, mustard greens, broccoli, cabbage, and dark lettuce; legumes; nuts; sprouted seeds and beans; microalgae; and seaweed. If you're unwilling to make that level of commitment, then eat a *high complex carbohydrate, low fat*, and *moderate protein* diet, while *avoiding* the dietary excesses listed on page 203—red meat (eat lean cuts, no more than three times per week), alcohol, cigarettes, soft drinks, salt, coffee, and hot spices. Also avoid the following foods: spinach, chard, beet greens, chocolate, cranberries, and plums. They contain calcium oxalate, which binds with calcium, making it nutritionally unavailable. It is interesting to note that countries with the highest consumption of milk products have the highest incidence of osteoporosis. Although milk is a good source of calcium, it is often the cause of food allergy and contributes to heart disease, diabetes, and other health problems. Use only cultured dairy products, such as yogurt. Research has also shown soy to be effective in promoting bone health.

To eliminate the risk of both lead and aluminum, drink bottled water. If you avoid foods packaged in tin cans, you will greatly reduce your exposure to tin.

Vitamins, Minerals, and Supplements

For osteoporosis, these are all bone nutrients. They should include:

- *Calcium*—500 to 1,000 mg daily (1,500 mg is usually recommended, but too much calcium can interfere with the uptake of other bone nutrients such as magnesium, manganese, and zinc). If your diet is relatively low in protein, much less calcium is necessary. If you take the following minerals and supplements and avoid the foods listed earlier, this lower daily dose of calcium should be adequate. Take calcium (and magnesium) in the more efficiently absorbed forms. The most effective and well-studied form of calcium is microcrystalline hydroxyapetite. It may be absorbed into bone up to two hundred times more directly than any other form, because it is a complete bone matrix containing all the essential minerals in the appropriate ratios. Other well-absorbed types of calcium are citrate, malate, or fumarate

- *Magnesium*—500 to 800 mg daily
- *Zinc*—30 mg daily
- *Copper*—2 to 3 mg daily
- *Manganese*—20 mg daily
- *Silicon*—1mg daily
- *Boron*—2 to 3 mg daily
- *Vitamin K*—300 mcg daily
- *Vitamin D*—200 to 600 I.U. daily (highest dose is for postmenopausal women)
- *Folic acid*—1 mg daily
- *B-complex*—25 to 50 mg daily
- *Vitamin B-6*—100 mg daily
- *Beta carotene*—15 mg daily or 25,000 I.U. daily
- *Vitamin C*—1,000 to 3,000 mg daily as ascorbate
- *Vitamin E*—400 I.U. daily as d-alpha-tocopherol
- *Hydrochloric acid* (HCl)—if needed (especially over 70); take only after protein meals

Many health food stores have excellent "bone nutrient" combination products that contain many of the above ingredients.

Natural Hormonal Therapy

Conventional medicine relies chiefly upon HRT therapy (estrogen and progesterone) to treat osteoporosis. The synthetic progesterone used is progestin, and it is frequently prescribed along with estrogen to minimize estrogen's uterine cancer risk. Extensive testing at the Department of Obstetrics and Gynecology at Vanderbilt University has shown that *natural progesterone*, found in wild yams, is both safe and effective in treating osteoporosis, premenstrual syndrome (PMS), and menopause (without being accompanied by estrogen). Other studies have demonstrated the significant benefit of natural progesterone, usually applied as a cream, in increasing bone mass in postmenopausal women.

For postmenopausal women, the recommended dosage of natural progesterone cream is one-eighth to one-fourth teaspoon twice a day for the first 21 days of the month, then none for the last 7 days. Alternate among different smooth skin sites, such as the face, neck, inner arms, abdomen, inner thighs, or soles of the feet. Occasional vaginal spotting may occur with the use of this cream but is usually only temporary. If it persists, or if you feel estrogen supplementation is necessary for hot flashes or vaginal dryness, consult your physician. (See page 428.) Progesterone cream comes in several different brands, and is available in most health food stores. Progesterone also mitigates the detrimental effects of cortisone on bone density.

If this regimen does not relieve other menopausal symptoms such as vaginal dryness or hot flashes, then *estrogen* can be used in addition. When progesterone levels are adequate, however, a much lower dose of estrogen will be needed. Estrogen replacement therapy for osteoporosis does reduce the incidence of fractures by 50 percent, but it may also increase the risk of some cancers and other health problems, as noted earlier. However, estriol, one of the three naturally occurring forms of estrogen in the body, may actually prevent breast cancer. (See page 428.) Some physicians are now prescribing a combination, called triple estrogen, which contains 80 percent estriol, 10 percent estrone, and 10 percent estradiol. It is usually effective in treating menopausal symptoms and is probably safer than pharmaceutical estrogen preparations. Another advantage is that while it can be used along with natural progesterone cream, this cream may not be strong enough to prevent the uterine-cancer-promoting effect of pharmaceutical estrogens. Triple estrogen is available by prescription through pharmacists. A holistic physician can usually prescribe a safe and balanced natural hormone regimen for you.

Although both are considered male hormones, the ovaries also produce testosterone and DHEA. Both of these hormones are bone builders and may be deficient in postmenopausal women, especially DHEA. Your physician should test your blood or salivary (more sensitive and accurate) levels and, if low, begin supplementation with the appropriate hormone.

Herbs

Wild yam, from which natural progesterone is derived, has been the primary herb used in treating osteoporosis. However, when taken orally it is not well absorbed. *Black cohosh* is the herb most studied that contains estrogen-like substances that can protect against bone loss. *Dong quai* is a Chinese herb that is helpful in maintaining hormonal balance. Herbs that contain calcium are: *nettles, parsley, alfalfa, dandelion leaves, kelp,* and *horsetail.*

Exercise

Weight-bearing exercise is a highly essential component of the treatment program. The form of exercise should involve the parts of the body most susceptible to fractures, such as the legs, hips, upper spine, wrists, and arms. Walking, jogging, stair-climbing, bicycling, skiing, dancing, and weight-training are all beneficial. Christiane Northrup, M.D., reports that her patients who do yoga regularly seem to have the lowest incidence of osteoporosis. Exercise for 30 to 45 minutes three times a week or 25 minutes five times a week. If you're lifting weights do three sets, with eight to ten repetitions per set.

Mental and Emotional Health Recommendations

It is not clear what specific mental and emotional issues are associated with osteoporosis. However, Carolyn Myss does mention that "bone" problems may be related to: physical family and group safety and security; ability to stand up for oneself; ability to provide for life's necessities; feeling at home; and social and familial law and order. Todd Nelson, N.D., a contributing author of this book, believes that the primary emotional issues associated with osteoporosis are "being upright and focused in purpose" and "having clarity with your fundamental beliefs."

A consistent practice of affirmations, such as "My bones are getting stronger every day," along with a visualization that represents increased bone mass to you, would be most beneficial. This imagery might include breathing in white light that you see whitening and filling in your bones with each breath. After 10 to 15 minutes, your entire skeleton, but especially your hips, arms, and spine, are radiating this bright white light.

Peri- and postmenopause is a time of great transformation, and there are many powerful emotions that need to be expressed. This can be done in counseling, with your spouse or partner, with journaling, or with any other method that feels comfortable to you. Acceptance and appreciation for this normal life transition requires your commitment and understanding. Remember to be compassionate to yourself, and perhaps your bones will respond by being more supportive.

9

Systemic Conditions

Chronic Fatigue Syndrome

Fibromyalgia

Candidiasis

THE CONDITIONS DISCUSSED in this chapter are called systemic because they affect the entire body. All three are debilitating and at times can even be incapacitating. Although it is possible for the holistic treatment program to help you experience a dramatic improvement with self-care therapies, to realize the full potential of this approach it is recommended that you consult with a holistic practitioner and establish a personalized approach to treating these conditions.

CHRONIC FATIGUE SYNDROME (CFS)

Prevalence

Fatigue is probably the most common complaint among Americans today. It is no doubt a result of a combination of factors related to our modern way of life with its many stressors, lack of sleep and exercise, and unhealthy diets and environments. But the condition medically known as chronic fatigue syndrome (CFS) involves severe, at times incapacitating, fatigue. At one time referred to as "yuppie flu," CFS was first identified in the early 1980s. About 80 percent of the sufferers are women between the ages of 25 and 45, and the majority of them had allergies prior to the onset of CFS. Not until recent years have most physicians recognized it as a true illness. It was assumed that patients complaining of this syndrome were either depressed or hypochondriacs. However, in 1988 the CDC officially recognized the existence of CFS as an actual disease. It is still not clear whether CFS is a specific condition, several related conditions, or a group of symptoms that can't be attributed to any particular cause. It's so often misdiagnosed that there are no accurate estimates of its prevalence.

Symptoms and Diagnosis

The diagnosis is made on the basis of the typical symptoms and the exclusion of other ailments that might be causing these symptoms. Some of the other illnesses that can cause excessive fatigue are: hypothyroidism, anemia, Lyme disease, and chronic hepatitis.

Symptoms include:

- Debilitating fatigue, so severe that activities such as taking a shower or brushing your teeth may be too strenuous; the fatigue is not relieved by rest or sleep, and is made worse with exercise
- Recurrent flu-like symptoms, including low-grade fever, sore throat, enlargement of lymph glands, headache, muscle and joint aches
- Sleep disorder
- Depression, anxiety, mood swings
- Weight loss
- Exercise intolerance
- Maladaptive immune response with increased allergy and chemical sensitivity
- Cognitive dysfunction—including memory loss, mental fog, difficulty concentrating, poor analytical thinking, and spatial disorientation

Conventional Medical Treatment

The role of conventional medicine in treating CFS is primarily to rule out treatable conditions, with a detailed medical history and laboratory tests. Once that evaluation is completed and the diagnosis of CFS is made, conventional medicine can sometimes offer symptomatic relief with analgesics and antidepressants to improve sleep and decrease mood swings. Some doctors prescribe a six to eight-week trial of Zovirax, an antiviral drug commonly used for treating herpes and shingles.

Risk Factors and Causes

A definitive cause for CFS has never been determined, although it was first (in the early 1980s) thought to be caused by the Epstein-Barr virus, which causes mononucleosis, or other viruses such as herpes and polio. Scientists have discarded that theory and now believe that it may be an autoimmune disorder in which the immune system reacts (or overreacts) to a perceived threat (such as a virus) by attacking otherwise healthy tissues. That has led to CFS sometimes being referred to as chronic fatigue and immune dysfunction syndrome, or CFIDS. It is not contagious. The actual cause is probably a combination of a weakened immune system plus the presence of a virus. The majority of people who develop CFS have led *exceedingly busy, productive, and often stressful lives.* The other common risk factors that are most often associated with this condition are:

- A history of recurrent courses of antibiotics, NSAIDS, or other medications
- Inhalant and food allergies and sensitivities
- Adrenal exhaustion and low DHEA from chronic stress or following a serious illness
- Significant emotional stress and/or excessive work
- Insufficient sleep and relaxation
- Chronic candidiasis
- Hypoglycemia
- Chronic infection—sinusitis, prostatitis, or dental abscesses
- Clinical hypothyroidism (with normal thyroid lab tests—see hypothyroidism in chapter 20)
- Chemical exposure or sensitivity (can be triggered by paints, refinishing oils, or other chemicals)
- Intestinal parasites
- Poor diet, especially excessive sugar, caffeine, alcohol, or chronic nutrient deficiency
- Mercury toxicity from amalgam dental fillings (they contain over 50 percent mercury)
- Dysbiosis/leaky gut syndrome

Holistic Medical Treatment and Prevention
Physical Health Recommendations

Diet
A balanced, whole foods diet, focused on high nutrient, high protein complex carbohydrate foods—organic vegetables (parsley, cabbage, kale, carrots, beets, yams, lots of greens), whole grains, beans, fish, eggs, and poultry (avoid mercury toxins in fish and antibiotics in poultry). Try to identify and eliminate all foods to which you may be allergic (see chapter 19). A rotation diet is recommended in order to minimize low-grade food sensitivities that may have an ongoing trigger effect on the immune system. Sugar, caffeine, milk products, alcohol, aspartame, and refined carbohydrates (white flour, white rice) should all be avoided.

Vitamins, Minerals, and Supplements

- *Beta carotene*—100,000 I.U. daily
- *Vitamin C* (Ester C)—2,000 mg, three times daily
- *Vitamin E*—400 to 800 I.U. daily
- *Vitamin B-complex*—50 to 100 mg of all B vitamins daily (take in evening)
- High-potency multivitamin/mineral daily—Natrol's My Favorite Multiple—Take One is recommended
- *Zinc picolinate*—30 mg daily
- *Magnesium glycinate*—1,000 mg daily
- *Calcium citrate or lactate*—1,000 mg daily with vitamin D, 400 units
- *Manganese*—15 mg daily
- *Omega 3 EFAs* (EPA/DHA)—300 mg/300 mg three times daily
- *Pantothenic acid*—250 mg two times daily
- *Acetyl-L-carnitine*—1,000 mg two times daily for three months, then 250 to 500 mg daily
- *Coenzyme Q10*—100 to 200 mg daily for three months (an oil/resin-bound form for maximum absorption)
- *L-Lysine*—1,000 mg, three times daily for three months, then 1,000 mg daily
- *Malic acid*—600 to 1,000 mg daily
- *Alpha lipoic acid*—100 mg three to four times daily
- *L-glutathione*—50 mg two times daily
- *Adrenal extract*—one or two tablets three times daily
- *Thymus gland extract*—one or two tablets three times daily
- *Probiotics:* one-half teaspoon of mixed acidophilus/bifidus in pure water, first thing in the morning and at bedtime
- *Vitamin B-12* injections, 2,000 mcg with folic acid, 5 mg one or two times per week
- *Gamma globulin* injections weekly for several months

In addition to this list, some holistic physicians will treat CFS with an intravenous "nutrient cocktail" consisting of vitamins and minerals—especially vitamin C and magnesium.

Herbs

The herbs used to treat CFS have antiviral and immune-boosting properties. The first four herbs should be taken during the early acute phase of CFS (the herbs are best taken on an empty stomach):

- *Echinacea*—300 to 325 mg three times daily (use for weeks weeks, stop for one week, then resume)
- *Licorice*—300 mg three times daily (20–28 percent glycyrrhizic acid)—do not take with high blood pressure
- *Lomatium*—25 to 35 drops three to four times daily

During the convalescent or chronic phase you can use:

- *Astragalus*—150 mg three times daily
- *Licorice*—250 mg three times daily
- *Siberian ginseng*—250 mg three times daily
- *Oats* (avena)—500 mg three times daily
- *Ashwaganda root*—25 mg three times daily (1.7 percent with anolides, 1.5 percent alkaloids)
- *Ginkgo biloba*—60 to 100 mg three times daily (24 percent ginkgoflavon glycosides)

Hormones

- *DHEA*—dosage dependent on results of saliva or blood tests
- *Hydrocortisone*—dosage dependent on lab tests, but not exceeding 20 mg daily

Candida treatment program

If candidiasis is suspected, and it is often present with CFS, use the recommended treatment program on pg. 222. If you're not sure if you have candidiasis or not, then adhering to the candida diet and taking acidophilus supplements would still be helpful. Stool testing can be helpful in detecting both yeast overgrowth and parasites. If parasites are identified, appropriate treatment is necessary (see chapter 11).

Treat insomnia

See the holistic treatment for insomnia in chapter 7.

Professional care therapies

Acupuncture alone and in combination with *Chinese herbs* has been successful in treating CFS. The treatment is directed toward strengthening the immune system and relieving soreness in the musculoskeletal system. Periodic *detoxification, liver function enhancement,* and *leaky gut repair* have been well-documented and are highly effective treatments for CFS.

Exercise

Walking and mild aerobic exercise is recommended, but avoid any activity that increases fatigue or any of the other symptoms associated with CFS. You can begin with as little as five minutes of exercise and gradually increase it. Stretching exercises, yoga, qigong, and breathing exercises are especially helpful since they stimulate lymph flow. Be very gentle with yourself, listen to your body, and increase the intensity of your exercise very gradually.

Mental and Emotional Health Recommendations. Almost all the mental and emotional treatment techniques used to treat depression (see chapter 7) are also effective in treating CFS. The same holds true of the emotional issues associated with CFS. There is usually such a strong emotional factor contributing to CFS that some form of psychotherapy is recommended as a part of the treatment program. Most CFS patients report that their illness has made them stop, slow down, reassess their values and priorities, and refocus their lives in a more balanced direction.

Social and Spiritual Health Recommendations. CFS is a condition in which life force energy has been depleted and in this sense can be thought of as a spiritual disease. This is usually associated with a deprivation of love. Any and all of the therapeutic recommendations described in chapter 4 would be an effective complement to the holistic treatment of CFS. Practicing these techniques, such as intimacy-enhancing exercises, meditation, prayer, gratitude, and especially forgiveness, can help to strengthen the immune system while giving your body, mind, and spirit an infusion of the healing energy of love. If you would like to find a support group in your area, call the CFS Association (in Kansas City) at (913) 321-2278, or the CFS Society (in Portland, OR) at (503) 684-5261.

CONDITION FIBROMYALGIA (FM)

Prevalence

Fibromyalgia, or fibrositis, as it is sometimes called, is a mysteriously debilitating syndrome that afflicts between 6 and 12 million people in the United States. The condition bears a striking resemblance to chronic fatigue syndrome and affects mostly women (female to male ratio is about 10:1) between the ages of 25 and 50. It is estimated that 15 to 20 percent of patients seen by rheumatologists have FM. Health care costs for people afflicted with this condition average about $10,000 per year, and FM patients are almost six times more likely than the general public to apply for disability payments. More than 25 percent of FM patients who remain employed report missing more than 120 days of work per year due to their disease.

Symptoms and Diagnosis

The primary symptoms of fibromyalgia are generalized *muscle pain*, MUSCLE TENDERNESS, *stiffness*, and *aching*, along with significant *fatigue*. Other symptoms include: sleep disorder, depression, poor memory and concentration, headache (tension or migraine), dizziness, tingling of the extremities, irritable bowel syndrome, irritable bladder (urgency and frequency of urination), temporomandibular joint syndrome (TMJ), cold intolerance, and allergic reactions to drugs, chemicals, and environmental toxins. Blood tests and X-rays normally do not reveal any specific abnormality. Ruling out rheumatoid arthritis, lupus, and other conditions with similar symptoms (especially pain and fatigue) to FM is an important part of the diagnostic evaluation. Some physicians believe FM to be a variant of chronic fatigue syndrome, since 90 percent of patients with FM report significant fatigue. In 1990, the American College of Rheumatology, established the following criteria for *diagnosing* FM:

1. History of widespread pain of at least three months' duration. Pain must be present in all four quadrants of the body, that is, on both the left and right side of the body and above and below the waist. Axial skeletal pain (cervical spine, anterior chest, thoracic spine, or low back) must also be present.

2. Pain, and not just tenderness on physical examination (digital palpation with an approximate force of four kg), in at least 11 of 18 tender points in muscles, tendons, or bones.

Conventional Medical Treatment

After many years of research, there is still no effective conventional treatment for fibromyalgia. Antidepressants have been used to provide short-term relief for sleep disorders and depression, while anti-inflammatory medications have been used for treating the pain with poor to fair results.

Risk Factors and Causes

Although the cause of FM is unknown, most of the risk factors associated with chronic fatigue syndrome—especially food allergy (dairy products, wheat, fermented foods, and nightshades—potatoes, eggplant—are most common), emotional stress, intestinal candida overgrowth, nutritional deficiencies, and adrenal exhaustion—are also present with fibromyalgia. Recent research suggests that *damage to the cells' energy production in the mitochondria* (the energy production center of the cells), as a result of an excess of free radicals, is the primary cause of FM. Reduced circulation to muscle cells and low levels of the neurotransmitter serotonin may also contribute to causing FM. The metabolic shutdown in the muscle cells might possibly be due to the accumulation of phosphate and uric acid. Some of the standard medications (Zyloprim) used to treat gout (elevated uric acid) and other drugs that increase output of uric acid and phosphate (Probenecid, Sulfinpyrazone, and Robinul) have significantly improved some FM patients. Guaifenesin, a common expectorant used to thin mucus, has recently been shown to help FM patients by increasing uric acid excretion. In people who have FM, it is now known that the body breaks down muscle protein at an unusually high rate and converts it to glucose for energy. It has been theorized that this increased level of muscle tissue breakdown is one of the primary causes of the pain, aching, and fatigue. Aluminum toxicity may also play a role in causing FM.

Almost all FM patients have a history of chronic *overdoing*. Not knowing one's boundaries and limits is the hallmark of a person suffering with FM. They often lack the ability to balance activity and rest.

Holistic Medical Treatment and Prevention

The holistic treatment for FM is nearly identical to that of chronic fatigue syndrome; the following are especially helpful:

1. *Malic acid*—1,200 to 2,400 mg daily, in combination with magnesium—300 to 600 mg daily, vitamin B-1, and other synergistic factors. This product is available as Fibroplex from Metagenics in San Clemente, California, or Mitochondrial *Resuscitate* from Healthcomm in Gig Harbor, Washington (must be obtained through a physician). These supplements help restore normal energy production in the muscle cells as well as aid in aluminum detoxification.

2. Especially important to take for FM from the list of vitamins and supplements for CFS are those that help to stimulate mitochondrial function—*Acetyl-L-carnitine, Coenzyme Q10, L-Lysine, magnesium, lipoic acid, L-glutathione, EFAs, vitamin E*, and *B-complex*, as well as *vitamin B-1* (thiamin) and *manganese*.

3. *5-HTP*—50 to 100 mg morning and night—can reduce muscle pain and insomnia.

4. Intravenous vitamin and mineral injections often produce significant improvement but will usually have to be administered more frequently (three or four injections over a two-week period) than for CFS.

5. Trigger point injections, massage therapy, biofeedback, acupuncture, hydrotherapy, and electrostimulation have all been reported to be effective for some people with FM.

6. Periodic use of UltraClear or UltraInflam (both are available through physicians from Metagenics) detox programs have been of great benefit to FM patients as a result of their effect on leaky gut, enhancement of liver function, and reduction of free radical activity.

Exercise

Exercise is an essential part of the treatment program for FM, but impact-loading exercises such as jogging, basketball, or any other activity that involves jumping up and down should be avoided. Ideal exercises include walking, using a stationary bike or a treadmill, swimming, Qigong, t'ai chi, and yogic breathing. Another excellent type of exercise is the use of an Aquajogger. This is a buoyancy belt that fits around the chest and allows the person to stand up in a swimming pool and either walk or run against the resistance of the water. Try to gradually work up to 40 minutes of exercise, three times a week. You may have to begin with only five to ten minutes per exercise session. Learn to listen to your body, and do not push yourself to meet unrealistic goals. This is especially hard to do if you have been used to leading a very active, busy life. You must slow down and give your immune system a chance to heal.

Mental and Emotional Recommendations. Counseling is strongly advised with FM patients. They need to learn to strike a healthier balance between work and relaxation along with establishing a slower pace, a healthier rhythm, in all of their activities. Learning to say no is vital to this process of healing.

Support Groups You can find a local FM support group through the *Fibromyalgia Network*, an organization based in Tucson, Arizona. Their phone number is (602) 290–5508. The *Arthritis Foundation* in Atlanta, Georgia (800-283-7800) also helps organize support groups and educational classes.

CANDIDIASIS
(Yeast Overgrowth)

Prevalence

Candida albicans is the scientific name for the yeast organism. Physicians are quite familiar with its physical manifestations as skin rashes, oral thrush, and vaginal infections. But still largely unrecognized, in individuals whose immune systems have been compromised, is the potentially devastating systemic ailment known as candidiasis, candida-related complex, or candida toxicity syndrome. It affects many millions of Americans, most of whom unknowingly suffer from this condition of yeast overgrowth. Along with food allergy, with which it is often interrelated, candidiasis is one of the most commonly overlooked or misdiagnosed chronic disease conditions in America.

Physiology

Yeast is an integral part of life. It is a hardy fungus found in air, in food, and on exposed surfaces of most objects. There are more than 250 species of yeast organisms, and more than 150 of them can be found as harmless parasites in the human body. The most prevalent type of yeast found in and on the human body is Candida albicans. It is an innocuous single-cell fungus and a normal inhabitant of the intestines, mouth and vagina. Although not well documented, it is believed that its only function is to help absorb the B vitamins.

Candida is kept under control by the good bacteria that also make their home in the gastrointestinal and genital tracts. Lactobacillus and bifidus make up the largest percentage of the billions of these friendly bacteria. Similar to the bacteria in yogurt or in raw fermented foods, the lactobacilli make enzymes and vitamins, help fight undesirable bacteria, and lower cholesterol levels. While assisting us in keeping our bowel function and digestion normal, these friendly organisms, also referred to as acidophilus bacteria, regard candida as their food. Since they are the chief "predator" of candida, they are critical to maintaining a "balance of nature" in our intestines. As long as this homeostatic relationship is maintained, candida poses no problem. Unfortunately, this balance is delicate and can be easily disrupted.

Once an overgrowth of yeast occurs (usually in the small intestine), the organisms invade the tissues lining the gastrointestinal tract. If it persists long enough they can bore holes in the intestinal wall, allowing candida, bacteria, undigested food particles, pollen, environmental pollutants, and other material to enter the bloodstream, creating a condition known as "leaky gut syndrome." Candida are then carried throughout the body and take up residence in those parts of the body with the most favorable environment for their growth—moist mucous membranes, especially those of the sinuses and lungs. In whatever tissue the candida have colonized, they cause inflammation and subsequent discomfort such as sinus pain, muscle aches, joint pain, and itchy anus or vagina. Deliberate exposure to a large innoculum of candida organisms has been unequivocally shown to lead to invasion of the bloodstream in healthy volunteers. There is still great controversy on this point. In most clinical situations, are the symptoms being caused by the presence of candida organisms in the bloodstream or by absorption of the candida toxins from the intestine?

Symptoms and Diagnosis

As a direct result of widespread inflammation in the small bowel from the direct toxicity of candida, *symptoms of the gastrointestinal tract* are usually noticed first. Due to incomplete digestion and poor absorption of nutrients, these symptoms might include bloating, a feeling of fullness, diarrhea, constipation, alternating diarrhea and constipation, rectal itching, gas, and cramping. If the inflammation is severe and/or longstanding, it may be a contributing factor in leaky gut syndrome. As a result of this condition, particles of incompletely digested food, especially proteins, pass into the bloodstream and trigger multiple food allergies and sensitivities.

There are 79 identified toxins that are released by candida. These toxins can damage tissues directly, cause problems in distant organs, and weaken the immune system by inhibiting the function of suppressor T-cells. These white blood cells are responsible for modulating antibody production. When they are not working properly there is a resulting excess of antibodies. The combination of this overabundance of antibodies and absorption of incompletely digested protein helps to explain the exaggerated, multiple adult-onset allergies and sensitivities, both airborne and in food, experienced by people suffering from candidiasis.

A yeast impaired immune system also has less than the normal tolerance for ordinarily safe levels of common chemical odors such as gas and oil fumes, cleaning fluids, chlorine, perfume, and so on. An increasing number of people with candidiasis have become so allergic that almost every odor, all clothing except cotton, almost all foods, or anything in their immediate environment has become a major health problem. This condition has several names: *multiple chemical sensitivity*, environmental or ecological illness, or the universal reactor phenomenon. An immune system weakened by candida can also produce antibodies to the body's own tissues, especially the ovaries and thyroid, resulting in PMS and hypothyroid symptoms. These symptoms often include: *FATIGUE*, irritability, *sugar craving*, *headache, depression*, and constipation.

One of the major toxins produced by yeast is acetaldehyde. Its multiple effects can be devastating. It is converted by the liver into alcohol, depleting the body of magnesium and potassium, reducing cell energy, and causing symptoms of intoxication—disorientation, dizziness, or mental confusion. The *spaciness* or *mental fog*, as it's often described by patients, is one of the most frequent symptoms of candidiasis. Patients report a detached state of mind, poor concentration, faulty memory, and difficulty making decisions. The longer this condition persists, the more likely it is that *depression* will be added to the list of symptoms.

Energy is depleted because acetaldehyde interferes with glucose metabolism—a key component of energy production. Along with other yeast toxins, acetaldehyde reduces the absorption of protein and minerals, which in turn diminishes the production of enzymes and hormones needed for energy. The state of fatigue also leaves little energy for exercise, and the decrease in physical activity supplies less oxygen to the body, aggravating all the symptoms just mentioned. The combination of these multiple factors explains why *excessive fatigue* is the chief complaint of people with candidiasis. It usually comes on gradually but is most noticeable after a night's rest, after eating, and in mid- to late afternoon.

In addition to those already mentioned, other *frequent symptoms* include: insomnia, muscle aches and pains, joint pain, recurrent sinusitis, chronic runny or stuffy nose, vaginal itching or burning, irregular and painful periods, decreased libido, recurrent prostatitis, scaly skin, generalized itching, tinnitus (ringing in the ear), intolerance to heat and cold, and excess weight. It is precisely because of this wide range of symptoms that candidiasis so often goes undetected.

Since there is still no consistently reliable laboratory test to *diagnose* candidiasis, a thorough history and a review of symptoms will usually work well. William Crook, M.D., author of *The Yeast Connection*, has developed a candida questionnaire and score sheet that has proven to be an extremely reliable diagnostic tool in managing candidiasis. It can be ordered from Professional Books, P.O. Box 3494, Jackson, TN 38301. The questionnaire can also be found in Dr. Crook's books, as well as in Dr. Ivker's *Sinus Survival*.

Currently, the laboratory tests most often used to diagnose candida are *stool cultures*. The problem is that these cultures are often false negatives (about 20 percent of the time), which means they show no yeast when in fact yeast is present. The greatest value of the stool test may be that it can accurately determine the amount of good bacteria. If the lactobacilli are missing, then candida have an excellent chance of overgrowing.

A blood test for *candida antibodies* and immune complexes is also frequently performed. This measures the level of antibodies your immune system cells have made to fight candida. But it too is often unreliable since the body normally has candida antibodies, and high counts don't always mean a current yeast over-growth. To increase the odds of making a correct laboratory diagnosis of candidi-asis, the antibody test should be done in conjunction with a stool culture.

Conventional Medical Treatment

Due to the unreliability of the currently available diagnostic tests, the vast major-ity of physicians *do not believe the problem of candidiasis even exists.* But interestingly enough, during the past decade the pharmaceutical industry has developed a num-ber of powerful and quite expensive antifungal drugs to treat the problem of can-didiasis—such as Diflucan, Sporanox, and Nizoral. Although the statistics are not available, one can assume that an increasing number of physicians are prescribing them.

Risk Factors and Causes

In many respects, candidiasis is a twentieth-century disease, since many of its causes are directly due to modern-day factors such as antibiotics, birth control pills, environmental pollutants, and today's typical devitalized American diet. The most frequent cause of candidiasis is *recurrent or extended use of antibiotics,* which kill not only the harmful bacteria implicated in the condition for which the antibiotic is prescribed, but also the good bacteria needed to keep candida in check. Broad-spectrum antibiotics are particularly suspect, because the broader their scope, the greater the likelihood that they will destroy the body's reserves of lactobacilli and bifidus. Vaginal candida infections often occur soon after women use antibiotics, for example. The majority of people with chronic sinusitis who have taken three or more courses of antibiotics (10 to 14 days per course) within a six-month period also tend to suffer from some degree of candidiasis. Since most antibiotics are admin-istered orally, the friendly bacteria in the intestines are particularly susceptible to these medications. Antibiotics are also commonly found in commercially grown meats and poultry from non-range-fed animals, making these foods potential sources for yeast overgrowth.

Hormones, especially progesterone, and birth control pills can also contribute to causing candidiasis, which is why the condition is more prevalent in women than in men, children, or nonmenstruating women. Progesterone, found in most birth control pills and also secreted at high levels prior to menstruation, has been shown to stimulate the growth of candida. The combination of high progesterone levels just prior to menstruation and an existing excess of candida can contribute to particularly severe symptoms of PMS (premenstrual syndrome). Pregnancy is also favorable for candida, since it is accompanied by continuous high levels of progesterone.

Anything that weakens the immune system can contribute to yeast over-growth. *Cortisone medications*, such as prednisone and prednisolone, often used to treat chronic diseases such as asthma, arthritis, lupus, and colitis, are well-known immune suppressants. They too have the potential for stimulating yeast over-growth and can actually aggravate the disease the cortisone was treating. *Chemo-therapy* and *radiation treatments* given to cancer patients can also weaken immunity and open the door to candida.

Any medication that can potentially cause gastrointestinal ulcerations or in-flammation and weaken the lining of the gut can allow candida to gain a stronger and deeper foothold. These drugs might include *aspirin, cortisone,* and *NSAIDs* such as Feldene, Alleve, Motrin, Advil, and Nuprin. *Ulcer medications,* such as Tagamet and Zantac, can reduce acidity and increase pH levels in the stomach, creating an ideal environment for yeast to proliferate. Candida thrive in a pH of 4 to 5, and normal stomach acidity is 2 to 3.

Environmental toxins and chemicals such as pesticides, herbicides, solvents, paints, formaldehyde, combustion products of natural gas and coal (sulfur and ni-trous oxide), and heavy metals such as lead, cadmium, arsenic, mercury, alu-minum, and nickel can also weaken the immune system. People with occupational exposure to these substances are at highest risk for candidiasis. However, most of us in urban America are living in an unhealthy environment and are exposed to many of these toxins.

Poor diet is usually a major contributor to candida, especially one that is high in sugar. Other risk factors for candidiasis include *alcohol, food and environmental allergies, chronic viral infection, parasites* (especially giardia and amoeba), *emotional stress, physical trauma, adrenal dysfunction, hypothyroidism,* and *deficiencies in hy-drochloric acid, pancreatic enzymes, and bile.*

Once the scale has been tipped and yeast overgrowth begins, it is fueled by the staple of the typical American diet—sugar. Like most of us, yeast consider sugar to be their favorite food. While candida thrive on it, sugar weakens our im-mune system and diminishes the ability of white blood cells to attack and destroy unwanted organisms. It is therefore not surprising that *diabetes,* a chronic condi-tion of high blood sugar, is also a predisposing factor to candidiasis.

Like other chronic diseases, candidiasis usually results from a number of fac-tors occurring simultaneously. But the three *primary causes* seem to be:

1. Recurrent use of broad-spectrum antibiotics

2. A sugar-filled diet

3. Significant emotional stress

Holistic Medical Treatment and Prevention

Candidiasis usually results from a variety of factors, each of which needs to be addressed directly. Because candidiasis overgrowth slowly develops when these conditions occur over a prolonged period of time, patients must realize that there is no quick-fix cure. In order to achieve success, both time and personal commitment to dietary and lifestyle changes are required. Treatment also depends on the degree of yeast overgrowth and how severely immune function has been compromised. When yeast overgrowth is confined only to the GI tract or vagina, the treatment tends to be shorter and less involved. In systemic cases, however, where yeast toxins have spread throughout the body, treatment protocols can last as long as six months to a year. And in severe cases of leaky gut syndrome, successful treatment (requiring the healing of the bowel lining) takes at least a year or more. The comprehensive holistic approach consists of four components, and for best results you should start with stages 1 and 2 before progressing to 3 and 4.

1. Kill the overgrowth of candida.

2. Eliminate the fuel for the growth of candida through diet.

3. Restore normal bacterial flora in the bowel.

4. Strengthen the immune system.

Stage 1. The holistic treatment of candidiasis can be effective if used entirely as a self-care approach. However, if you're convinced you suffer from candidiasis and would like the the most effective method for *killing candida*, then it would be helpful to seek medical consultation with a physician willing to prescribe one of the *antifungal medications*, such as Nizoral, Diflucan, and Sporanox. Although each of these drugs has some minimal risk of liver toxicity, periodic liver function tests and taking the herb milk thistle (silymarin), which protects the liver, will usually mitigate this risk. A far more common side effect of these drugs is the "Herxheimer reaction," or die-off effect. These medications are often so effective in killing yeast that as the organisms die they release a "flood" of toxins into the bloodstream that can cause fatigue, headaches, nausea, loose stools, flu-like aches and pains, and any other symptom that yeast are known to produce. Increasing intake of distilled or filtered water, using water enemas, and taking vitamin C and ibuprofen all help to relieve these die-off symptoms. Although it's possible that for a short time you might feel worse than you did before, you might also choose to look at a relapse resulting from die-off as a confirmation of your diagnosis of candida, as well as a hopeful sign that you are eliminating yeast and will be feeling much better very soon. Another prescription drug that's been used for many years (prior to the new antifungals already mentioned) is Nystatin. It's available in tablets and powder and is much more effective for killing candida in the bowel, but not elsewhere in the body.

In spite of the potential side effects and expense (these drugs range in price from $3 to $13 a tablet), there is nothing that works as well in eliminating yeast overgrowth. Typically, the prescription will be 200 mg per day for at least one month, and depending upon the severity of the condition and the response to the drug, another two weeks or one month will be suggested. The second month might be every other day, or a similar strategy will be used for tapering off the medication rather than stopping abruptly.

For patients who are unable to obtain these drugs or who cannot take them due to their potential side effects, a number of other options are available, although none of them usually works as quickly or effectively. Among these are a variety of *homeopathic remedies* (many are available in health food stores). Other products are also available at most health food stores to combat candida, including Yeast Fighters, Candida Cleanse, Cand-Ex, Caprystatin Yeast Defense, and Cantrol. Caprylic acid, garlic, pau d'arco, and other herbs that either act directly on candida or indirectly by strengthening the immune system can be helpful as well. In addition, there are a number of new herbal/supplement combinations. Flora Balance, a unique strain of bacteria called Bacillus laterosporus B.O.D., can also be effectively used in killing candida (take two capsules 20 minutes before breakfast for two months, then reduce to one capsule for one to two more months). The herbal formula Intestinalis (available through physicians from BioNutritional Formulas, 800-950-8484) can treat both candida as well as certain types of parasites. Two other effective products available through physicians are Candicin (from Metagenics) and SF 722 (from Thorne).

Bowel cleansing during this stage of your program is also important. If you suffer from candidiasis, chances are you also have mucus and impacted food residue built up as a thick coat along the walls of your large intestine. This encrusted matter diminishes colon function, contributes to disease by preventing the absorption of vital nutrients, and creates an ideal environment for yeast to thrive. One rapid method of cleansing the bowel and removing excess candida is colonic therapy. These treatments are best done on a weekly basis during stage 1 and need to be administered by trained practitioners. (To find one, you might inquire at the office of a holistic physician, chiropractor, or naturopath.) Enemas, although not as effective, can also be performed. It is possible to clean the colon by following a yeast-free diet, drinking plenty of water, getting regular exercise, taking caprylic acid, and drinking 8 to 10 ounces of water or diluted juice mixed with one heaping teaspoon of psyllium and two tablespoons of liquid bentonite twice a day. Both psyllium and bentonite eliminate colon toxicity. You may experience some bloating if you try this combination. If so, take half doses of these amounts, but still take it twice a day.

Stage 2. In addition to killing off candida, *eliminating their fuel through diet and strengthening immune function* are also essential. Dietary considerations comprise the second part of candidiasis treatment and should be adopted at the same time that you begin stage 1. Although there is no single anticandida diet that perfectly meets everyone's unique biochemical needs, the following principles can help most people. Eat primarily protein and fresh vegetables, with a limited amount of complex carbohydrates and foods rich in healthy fats, along with a small amount of fresh fruit (avoid fruit and juices for the first two to three weeks of the diet). Avoid sugar and all concentrated sweets. For best results, rotate all acceptable foods, eating particular foods (especially grains) no more than once every three to four days. Usually three to six months is the minimum time required for maintaining the diet, although it can become less restrictive the longer you follow it. The more involved you become in shopping, planning your meals, and cooking, the easier and more rewarding you will find the diet to be.

Acceptable foods include raw or lightly steamed, fresh, organic *vegetables*, especially those high in water content and low in starch. These include all green and leafy vegetables, such as lettuce, spinach, cabbage, kale, sprouts, greens, and parsley; and low starch vegetables such as celery, zucchini, squash, green beans, broccoli, cauliflower, bell peppers, asparagus, tomato, onion, cucumber, garlic, radish, and Brussels sprouts. Carrot, beet, turnip, eggplant, artichoke, avocado, and peas can also be eaten, although they contain moderately higher levels of starch. *Proteins* can be eaten freely. Meats that are free of antibiotics and hormones (free-range, organic meats) and deep-water ocean fish are recommended. (Beef and pork should be avoided, however.) Organic seeds and nuts are also permissible. *Complex carbohydrates* can also be used, but try to limit yourself to no more than one serving a day. These include potatoes, sweet potatoes, yams, legumes, and whole grains (eat only nongluten grains—brown rice, millet, quinoa, amaranth, buckwheat), either sprouted or cooked. For best results, wait until you are in the third week of your program before introducing legumes, and be sure to rule out any food allergies (see chapter 19) you might have. *Flaxseed oil* (one to two tablespoons daily) used on grains or vegetables, or as a salad dressing, should also be consumed (do *not* heat it or cook with it). Other acceptable oils are cold pressed olive, linseed, walnut, and soy. Certain *fruits* are also permitted after the first two weeks, although you should limit yourself to one serving per day until you are sure they are not aggravating your symptoms. For the first 21 days, start with melons and berries. Then add grapefruit, apple, pear, peach, orange, nectarine, apricot, cherry, and pineapple. Fruit juices in general are best avoided unless they are freshly squeezed or are diluted 1:1 with water. Candida cookbooks are relatively easy to find in most book and health food stores.

Foods to avoid include all foods containing *sugar* (cakes, cookies, donuts, ice cream, soft drinks, etc.), *sucrose, fructose, maltose, lactose, glucose, dextrose, corn sweetener, corn syrup, sorbitol,* and *manitol; honey; molasses; maple syrup; date sugar; barley malt; rice syrup; NutraSweet;* and *saccharine.* Use sea salt instead of table salt. *Milk* and *dairy products (including cheese)* should also be avoided, although butter is acceptable in limited amounts, as is non-fat, unsweetened yogurt if you are milk-tolerant. (Unsweetened soy milk can be used in place of milk.) Also eliminate all *bread* and *yeast-raised baked products,* such as whole grain cereals, pastas, tortillas, muffins, and crackers. Other foods to avoid include *mushrooms, rye and wheat, alcoholic beverages, caffeine, white or refined flour products, packaged and processed foods, olives, pickles, sauerkraut, vinegar, mustard, ketchup, margarine, refined and hydrogenated oils, soy sauce,* and *tamari.*

Significant improvement should begin to occur within one month of following the above dietary guidelines and the steps outlined in stage 1. If little or no change is noticed, then you should probably be tested for food allergy and/or the presence of parasites. People with leaky gut syndrome make very slow progress.

Stage 3. After you have followed stages 1 and 2 for about six weeks, you will be ready to begin stage 3, which involves restoring normal friendly bacteria in the bowel through the use of lactobacillus acidophilius and bifidus supplements, commonly available at most health food stores. Good bacteria cannot fully grow back until yeast overgrowth in the bowel has been greatly diminished. Although there are many brands of these products to choose from, the majority of them are of little value, since they contain only a small amount of these living organisms. Even most freeze-dried types are deficient in adequate amounts. To ensure potency, buy refrigerated brands with an expiration date between one and ten months from the date of your purchase, and supplying between one and ten billion organisms per day. Also buy only liquid cultures or powdered forms containing whey (dairy) or nondairy varieties, as only these forms provide an ample food supply to sustain the fragile lactobacilli. Take two servings per day, morning and evening.

Be aware that many yogurt products do not contain a high amount of viable organisms by the time they reach the consumer. This is especially true of highly processed ones or those with many additional ingredients. People who are sensitive to dairy products, as well as those with chronic respiratory conditions, should not use yogurt as a consistent source of friendly bacteria. Remember to avoid those brands of yogurt that have added sweeteners.

Stage 4. The final stage in treating candidiasis involves strengthening the immune system. One of the easiest ways to do this, along with proper diet, is through the use of nutritional supplements. *In addition* to the complete vitamin, mineral, and herbal regimen listed on the table for treating sinusitis on in chapter 6, the following nutrients are recommended:

- *Biotin*—300 to 1,000 mcg three times daily
- *Flaxseed oil* (already a part of the candida diet) or other essential fatty acids (omega-3, evening primrose, or black currant oils)
- *Amino acid supplements*—balanced and broad-spectrum
- *Adrenal-enhancing supplements*
- *Pancreatic enzymes*—one or two tablets with each meal
- *Hydrochloric acid* (HCl)—one capsule with pepsin with every meal, to restore digestive function
- In addition to the preceding, be sure to drink adequate amounts of *water* throughout the day, *exercise* regularly, and get at least eight hours of *sleep* per night

Stress-reduction techniques. See the recommendations made for treating depression in chapter 7.

If, after following this program for six weeks or more, you still are experiencing little or no improvement, probably there are other contributing factors to your problem that still need to be addressed. These can include food allergy and leaky gut syndrome (both already mentioned), intestinal parasites (especially giardia), pancreatic enzyme deficiency, hypothyroidism, adrenal exhaustion, chronic viral infection, chronic fatigue syndrome, chemical hypersensitivity, and heavy metal poisoning, among other possible causes. Candidiasis can also be sexually transmitted from your regular sex partner. In all cases of prolonged candidiasis, professional care is required to address all the causes and to implement an appropriate treatment strategy.

Candidiasis remains one of the most elusive conditions to detect, primarily because it manifests such a wide variety of symptoms and because it's still a challenging diagnosis to make. The information in this chapter should help you determine if you might be suffering from candidiasis. Further information can be found in the books listed in the appendix. Once a diagnosis of candidiasis is made, making a commitment to the program outlined here can offer significant relief. You will know when you have fully recovered because you will feel better than you have in years. Don't allow your success to be short-lived, however. Try to maintain a healthy diet free of excess sugar, alcohol, preservatives, and fried, fatty foods. Also continue to nurture yourself in body, mind, and spirit, to insure that your immune function remains strong and optimally healthy.

10

Men's Conditions

Prevalence

PROSTATIC AND ERECTILE DYSFUNCTION are probably two of the greatest health concerns for American men. The most common diseases of the prostate are prostate cancer, benign prostatic hypertrophy (BPH), and prostatitis. Prostate cancer is responsible for over 40,000 deaths annually. There were about 320,000 newly diagnosed cases in 1996, compared to 244,000 new cases in 1995 and less than 85,000 in 1985. Part of this increase is due to more effective screening. Nearly one of every five American men will develop prostate cancer in his lifetime. After lung cancer, it has become the second most lethal cancer for men. BPH is an enlarged prostate that affects nearly 30 percent of 50-year-old men, 50 percent of 60-year-olds, and almost 80 percent of men over 70. Prostatitis is an inflammation or infection of the prostate usually seen in men between the ages of 20 and 50.

Impotence might well be the most common chronic condition afflicting men, with estimates as high as 30 million. Before Viagra, only about two hundred thousand men per year sought medical attention for this condition. It has been reported in the *Journal of Clinical Practice* that 52 percent of men 40 to 70 years old have some degree of impotence; it is also estimated that 85 percent of men over 70 can't get a firm erection. Impotence is defined as the inability to sustain a satisfactory erection to perform intercourse and ejaculation.

Anatomy of the Genitourinary Tract

The male genitourinary tract consists of the penis, testicles, epididymis (a tube along the back side of the testicles where sperm are stored), vas deferens (tube connecting testicle to urethra), prostate, bladder, and urethra.

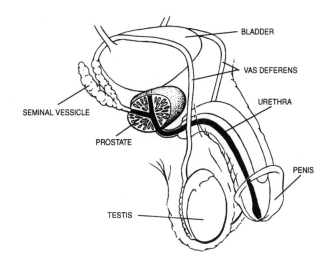

BLADDER

VAS DEFERENS

URETHRA

SEMINAL VESSICLE

PROSTATE

PENIS

TESTIS

Male Genitourinary Tract

The prostate gland, about the size and shape of a walnut, lies below the bladder and surrounds the urethra. Its primary function is the secretion of a thin, milky-white alkaline fluid during ejaculation that accounts for about 30 percent of the volume of semen. In lubricating the urethra and increasing sperm motility, this fluid enhances delivery and fertility of the sperm that originate in the testicles. In addition, the prostate also acts as the genitourinary tract's first line of defense against infection and disease.

CONDITION

PROSTATE CANCER

Symptoms and Diagnosis

The most common cancer in men over 50 years of age is prostate cancer, and it is the second most common cancer afflicting men, after lung cancer. The highest incidence is found in black males, who are 40 percent more likely to be stricken with the disease.

About 20 percent of enlarged prostates are the result of cancer. As long as it's confined to the prostate gland, the cancer is largely curable. About 80 percent of these cancers either do not metastasize (spread beyond the gland to other parts of the body) or are of the slow-growing variety, often causing little or no problem. About one out of every eight men diagnosed with prostate cancer will die from it.

Early detection of cancer of the prostate is difficult, since it often is present with no detectable symptoms. A *rectal exam*, preferably performed by the same physician on an annual basis, is a diagnostic method recommended by urologists (genitourinary tract surgeons). The doctor inserts a gloved finger into the rectum in order to touch the prostate gland, on which he or she can literally feel cancerous growths, such as bumps or nodules, or an asymmetry from one side of the gland to the other. However, one limitation of the rectal exam is that it's not possible for doctors to feel the tiniest, earliest stage, most curable tumors. Recent research at Washington University in St. Louis finds that 60 to 70 percent of cancers detected by rectal exam alone have already spread beyond the prostate.

That's the primary reason for the popularity of the "prostate specific antigen" or *PSA test*, which has been widely used during the past decade and is the biggest factor in the dramatic rise of prostate cancer diagnoses. A PSA test detects cancer much earlier than a rectal exam and measures the blood level of a protein produced by all prostate cells. In general, readings under a PSA count of 4 indicate that cancer is highly unlikely, while over 22 it's highly likely. About 70 percent of cancers detected with the PSA test are still curable—twice as many as with the rectal exam alone.

One problem with this test is that it produces almost one-third false positives (that is, results that are above 4 but turn out not to be cancer). One reason for this is that both BPH and prostatitis can increase PSA levels and indicate a higher likelihood of cancer when such a greater risk may not exist.

Conventional Medical Treatment

If the PSA is elevated, the next steps may be to take a closer look at the prostate with a transrectal ultrasound probe, and then to take needle biopsies from several regions of the gland. If prostate cancer is diagnosed early and it has not metastasized, men are usually offered two options by conventional medicine—to treat the cancer or pursue a course of "watchful waiting." Treatment usually consists of surgical removal of the entire prostate gland, a procedure called a radical prostatectomy. Although this option offers a cure (if the cancer has not spread beyond the prostate), it also presents the risk of devastating side effects:

- One to two percent of prostatectomy patients will have complete lack of urinary control.

- About 20 to 30 percent will have partial control and stress incontinence—leakage caused by any kind of physical pressure—and more than half will have minimum leakage, only a few occasional drops.

- Ninety percent of men over 50 with prostatectomies will be left impotent.

In addition to this huge risk of impotence, this surgical procedure often requires a week-long hospital stay, several weeks of dependence on an in-dwelling catheter to urinate, and an extended recovery time. A 1994 survey performed by the American Foundation for Urologic Disease found that 16 percent of prostatectomy patients would not choose the treatment again.

Other methods of treating prostate cancer include "nerve-sparing" surgery (with a 50 percent rate of impotency), cryotherapy (freezing the prostate cells with liquid nitrogen; 60 percent impotency), and radiation (cancer returns within ten years in 75 to 80 percent of patients). Other recent and promising conventional treatment options include: proton beam therapy—an experimental form of radiation with 10 to 50 percent impotency and five-year survival rates equal to prostatectomy; brachytherapy—radioactive seed pods are implanted into the prostate; and hormone therapy—antiandrogenic drugs such as Lupron or Flutamide suppress the secretion of the hormones of the pituitary gland that control testosterone production.

In light of the potential for devastating side effects and the limited evidence that treating prostate cancer actually saves lives, "watchful waiting" is becoming an increasingly popular option for men diagnosed with this cancer. This option entails frequent PSAs (at least every six months), rectal exams and an occasional biopsy, but no intervention unless the cancer becomes more aggressive. The answer to the question "Who should be treated for prostate cancer?" is not a simple one. Experts at the National Cancer Institute in Maryland point out that in addition to the false positive readings, the PSA fails to differentiate between fast-growing and less-threatening prostate cancer and can lead to debilitating treatment that may not be necessary. The presence of a few cancer cells may not be a serious problem. Oncologists estimate that by age 50, as many as four out of ten men have at least some cancerous cells in their prostate, which will cause an elevated PSA reading. But according to Thomas Stamey of Stanford University, only 8 percent of these men will eventually develop symptoms that affect their quality of life, and only 3 percent will die of the cancer. Most men die *with* prostate cancer, not *from* it.

Some physicians believe that since it usually takes about a decade for prostate cancer to cause symptoms that significantly affect quality of life, any man whose life expectancy is less than ten years (65 years of age or older) should not be treated.

This controversy about who should be treated will eventually be settled when scientists are able to develop a means of distinguishing (when the cancer is small) between a lethally aggressive and a relatively benign type of prostate cancer. This research is currently underway.

The American Cancer Society and the American Urological Association both recommend an annual rectal exam and PSA test after age 50, or by 40 if you are a higher risk man.

Risk Factors and Causes

As with other cancers, the precise cause of *prostate cancer* is unknown. But several risk factors have been identified:

- Family history
- African American heritage
- High fat diet
- Men who enter puberty later than the average male
- Environmental toxins from air pollution, chemicals, and especially cadmium (a metallic element used in batteries and found as a residue in tobacco)
- Low levels of vitamin A (one study showed that these men were three times more likely to have prostate cancer than men with the highest levels of vitamin A).

Holistic Medical Treatment and Prevention

Physical Health Recommendations. The holistic treatment and prevention program for genitourinary disease is directed at loving, nurturing, and restoring balance to the prostate gland and all the pelvic organs. This program is comprised primarily of the comprehensive approach for optimal physical fitness described in chapter 2. Those recommendations for diet, water, vitamins, minerals, and exercise can be applied to all the conditions of prostatic dysfunction and impotence. In addition, include some of the following therapeutic measures:

Diet

Several studies have found that decreasing the consumption of sugar leads to lower levels of prostate cancer. It has also been shown that cultures that consume higher amounts of red meat have a higher incidence of cancer of the prostate. In China and Japan, where *low fat diets* of vegetables and fish are the norm, the incidence of prostate cancer is extremely low. However, prostate cancer rates for first- and second-generation Japanese Americans in the United States are considerably higher than in Japan, due to their adoption of an American diet.

Drinking an adequate amount of filtered or bottled water (one-half ounce per pound of body weight every day) is not only healthy for you and your prostate but will help to eliminate constipation. This is a common problem among men and can contribute to pelvic congestion and reduced blood flow to the prostate. Also reduce or eliminate caffeine and alcohol.

Vitamins, Minerals, and Supplements

The following regimen, although designed primarily for BPH and prostatitis, can only improve the health of the prostate and therefore is beneficial for prostate cancer as well.

In addition to the daily regimen of antioxidant vitamins and minerals in the dosages listed in chapter 2, *essential fatty acids (EFAs)* and zinc are particularly helpful in reducing the size of an enlarged prostate. EFAs are found as omega-3s in cold-water fish (salmon, sardines, tuna), flaxseed oil, and soybeans and are especially high in pumpkin seeds; and as omega-6 in safflower and sunflower oils, all nuts and seeds, and evening primrose oil. Although it's good to have a balance of these EFAs, the omega-3s are most important to the health of the prostate. Omega-6s can both enhance and sustain an inflammation of the prostate (prostatitis) by increasing proinflammatory prostaglandins. Either take one to two tablespoons per day of omega-3 or the equivalent amount in capsules (six 1,000 mg capsules of flax oil are equal to one tablespoon).

Foods naturally rich in *zinc* include pumpkin seeds, nuts, and grains, in addition to a variety of animal products, including beef liver and turkey, as well as seafoods. Eating organic fruits and vegetables will help, since organic soils are likely to be richer in minerals. But since the typical American diet is zinc deficient, it is recommended that men take supplements in the form of zinc picolinate in a dosage ranging from 15 to 60 mg per day. Risks of zinc supplementation are minimal, but you should not exceed 60 mg a day without the approval of your doctor. Physicians can measure zinc deficiency with a simple inexpensive liquid oral zinc sulphate/hydrate taste test. The test, called Zinc Tally, is available through Metagenics. Because large dosages of zinc supplements compete with copper for absorption from the intestine, you should take 2 to 4 mg of copper at a different time of the day from when you take zinc. In addition to the daily regimen of vitamins and minerals in the dosages listed in chapter 2, take at least:

- *Vitamin C*—2,000 mg three times daily in Ester C or polyascorbate form with mixed bioflavonoids
- *Vitamin A* and *beta carotene*—10,000 to 15,000 I.U. of each
- *Vitamin E*—400 I.U. two times daily as natural d-alpha-tocopherol
- *Vitamin B-6*—100 mg two times daily (both B-6 and vitamin E can reduce prolactin levels; prolactin increases testosterone uptake by the prostate)
- A daily multivitamin high in *B vitamins* (100 mg) and *magnesium* (500 mg)
- *Selenium*—200 mcg daily
- *Copper sebacate*—2 mg two times daily
- *Amino acids* (*glutamine*, *alanine*, and *lysine*)—500 mg each daily in divided dosages between meals

High doses of intravenous vitamin C, B-complex, and zinc have been used with some success in the treatment of prostate cancer (see chapter 13). *Caution:* Do *not* take DHEA or any proandrogens while treating prostate cancer, as this might increase dihydrotestosterone.

Herbs

Saw palmetto (160 mg two times daily), and *Pygeum africanus* (100 mg two times daily; see the BPH herbs list for a detailed description).

Empty the Prostate

Every organ in the body works more efficiently and is healthier when it is being used regularly and when fluids are able to flow through it without obstruction. From this physiologic common sense perspective comes the recommendation of ejaculation about three times per week for both prevention and treatment of prostate cancer and BPH. A recent study in England reported that men who ejaculated five times a week had a significantly lower incidence of prostate cancer.

Professional Care Therapies

Homeopathic remedies, Chinese herbs and acupuncture, Ayurvedic medicine, bodywork (acupressure, reflexology, shiatsu), chiropractic, environmental medicine (detoxification therapy), yoga, and naturopathic and osteopathic medicine have all been used successfully in treating prostatic disorders.

Mental and Emotional Health Recommendations. Together with the medical (urologic) community, most men share the following beliefs:

- An enlarged prostate with its concomitant symptoms is an inevitable consequence of aging.

- Our ability to maintain strong erections and engage in enjoyable sexual intercourse diminishes greatly as we get older, until eventually we are unable to function sexually at all.

- There is a growing threat of prostate cancer, and if we live long enough we will get it.

Statistically, it is true that 80 percent of men over the age of 70 will develop BPH; that one out of five men will contract prostate cancer; and that most of us will eventually experience some degree of impotence. In order to enjoy optimal health, however, it is essential that we change our limiting beliefs and attitudes. To be holistically healthy and prevent these conditions that most men develop, or to treat them if you are already afflicted, it is essential that you believe it's possible to be free of these disorders. There are, after all, 20 percent of us who will not de-velop enlarged prostates; four out of five who will never have cancer of the prostate; and millions of us who are not and will not ever be impotent. Do you ex-pect to be among the fortunate few? It is overly simplistic to think that merely having this expectation is sufficient to make it a done deal, but *optimism* is a key in-gredient of holistic health, and that attitude can be greatly strengthened by prac-ticing the entire preventive program outlined in this chapter.

If you already suffer from prostate cancer or from one of the other common male conditions, then you should first determine what your goals are for treat-ment. Do you want to cure it, prevent it from getting any worse, or learn to live with it? When your goals have been established, write them down, and then re-word them into the form of affirmations. (See chapter 3 for a "refresher course" on the use of affirmations.) "My prostate is strong and healthy" is a good basic af-firmation. You can be very creative with these affirmations and think about them in visual terms.

Bioenergy

From a bioenergetic perspective the male genitourinary tract energies are related to feelings of security, survival, vitality, and one's connection to the earth and to one's "tribe," including one's family, other men, country of origin, ethnic back-ground, and/or religion. Most American men have become so urbanized and competitive that to a great extent they've lost their close connection to the earth and to their fellow male tribesmen.

Any therapeutic measure that strengthens a man's sexuality, his feeling of connection to the earth, tribal connections, and his sense of security will enhance this root energy associated with the pelvic organs and can benefit any of the four conditions discussed in this chapter. These might include:

- Visualizations that send light and energy into the prostate and pelvic area (you might see it and feel it originating deep in the earth, coming up through your legs and filling your pelvis)
- Spending more time in nature or in contact with the earth
- Feeling more connected to other men, your son, father, or brother
- Feeling greater financial security
- Emotionally healing family wounds through counseling

Working at this root level of dis-ease can empower men and ultimately cre-ate a sense of security, pleasure, and potency far greater than any other therapeu-tic measure.

In treating prostate cancer, the holistic approach can be used as a complement to the conventional treatment. Over the age of fifty, annual PSA tests and rectal exams by a urologist or primary care physician are still considered good preventive medicine for cancer of the prostate.

BENIGN PROSTATIC HYPERTROPHY (BPH)

Symptoms and Diagnosis

By the age of 50, about 30 percent of all men will experience some difficulty with urination related to enlargement of the prostate—*BPH*. The most common *symptoms* of prostatic hypertrophy are:

- Increased frequency (especially at night), urgency, and hesitancy with urination
- A reduction in the force and caliber of urination
- A sensation of fullness in the bladder after urination
- The need to urinate one or more times at night

This enlargement, caused by an abnormal overgrowth and/or swelling of the tissue of the prostate, creates a blockage of the bladder outlet (urethra). If left untreated, this can cause complete obstruction of urine flow. The following prostate scorecard was developed by the American Urological Association to help men determine if they are candidates for treatment of prostate enlargement.

A digital rectal exam performed by a physician, along with suggestive symptoms, is still considered a reliable method of diagnosing BPH.

Conventional Medical Treatment

Depending on how much trouble the symptoms are causing, urologists are treating men with BPH with pharmaceutical drugs, surgery, or just "watchful waiting." In one recent study of six hundred men with BPH who were treated with the latter approach, only 10 percent requested medical treatment at the study's completion. It was learned that men could control many of their symptoms simply by limiting fluids before bedtime, especially anything that irritates the prostate like caffeine and alcohol. Regular ejaculations (three times a week) also helped some men find symptom relief. Currently the most popular drug being used to treat BPH is *Proscar*. It works by preventing the build-up of dihydrotestosterone, a testosterone-like compound that appears to promote the development of BPH. However, recent clinical studies have shown it to be only marginally effective. Proscar also causes impotence in about 4 percent of men who take it and decreases

PROSTATE SCORECARD

Wondering if you're a candidate for treatment for prostate enlargement? This questionnaire, developed by the American Urological Association and recommended by an independent panel organized by the Agency for Health Care Policy and Research, can help you find out.

If you score in the *mild* range, generally watchful waiting is fine. A rating of *moderate* or *severe* might suggest medication or surgery. Keep in mind that doctors factor in a lot of information in deciding which treatment is appropriate for which man. This little quiz is just one part of that diagnostic process.

Circle one number for each of the following questions. Add up the seven numbers to get your AUA symptom score: _____ 0–7 = mild 8–19 = moderate 20–35 = severe	Not at all	Less than 1 time in 5	Less than half the time	About half the time	More than half the time	Almost always
1. Over the past month, how often have you had a sensation of not enough emptying of your bladder completely after you finished urinating?	0	1	2	3	4	5
2. Over the past month, how often have you had to urinate again less than two hours after you finished urinating?	0	1	2	3	4	5
3. Over the past month, how often have you found you stopped and started again several times when you urinated?	0	1	2	3	4	5
4. Over the past month, how often have you found it difficult to postpone urination?	0	1	2	3	4	5
5. Over the past month, how often have you had a weak urinary stream?	0	1	2	3	4	5
6. Over the past month, how often have you had to push or strain to begin urination?	0	1	2	3	4	5
7. Over the past month, how many times did you most typically get up to urinate from the time you went to bed at night until the time you got up in the morning?	0 (none)	1 (1 time)	2 (2 times)	3 (3 times)	4 (4 times)	5 (5+ times)

libido in 7 percent. Other commonly used drugs are the high blood pressure medications—*Hytrin, Minipress,* and *Cardura.* They work by relaxing the tiny muscles in the arterial walls of the arteries of the prostate, thus widening these blood vessels, increasing blood flow to the prostate, and relieving the prostate's pressure on the urethra. They only relieve symptoms and do not slow the progress of the condition. They also may produce side effects such as dizziness and fatigue (especially in men with normal or low blood pressure) and, in unusual cases, impotence. Flomax is a new drug that works similarly to these blood pressure medications but has a greater effect on the muscle tissue in the prostate than on the rest of the arteries in the body. As a result, there is less risk of lowered blood pressure and dizziness than with the other drugs.

If symptoms don't respond to drug treatment, transurethral resection (*TUR*) of the prostate—surgical removal of a portion of the prostate gland—is the option offered by most urologists. Although the risk of incontinence (loss of urinary control) is greater than with drugs, the relief from symptoms is also more significant. Unfortunately this surgical procedure is a choice most readily offered by urologists, who as surgeons, clearly have a bias. Of the 350,000 prostate operations performed each year, many could be avoided if physicians offered the simple and safe natural remedies described under holistic medical treatment.

Risk Factors and Causes

As men age, their hormone levels change. After the age of 50, free testosterone levels in the blood begin to decrease, while at the same time testosterone levels are increasing in the prostate gland. Within the prostate, testosterone is converted to an even more potent compound called *dihydrotestosterone*. This hormone causes cells to multiply excessively, eventually leading to prostate enlargement.

The increased uptake of testosterone by the prostate appears to be the result of another hormone, *prolactin*, secreted by the pituitary gland in the brain. Prolactin also increases the activity of the enzyme that converts testosterone to dihydrotestosterone. Since alcohol, especially beer, and emotional stress increase prolactin levels, both may be significant contributors to causing *BPH*.

Holistic Medical Treatment and Prevention

Diet

For treating BPH, prostatitis, and impotence and preventing prostate cancer, especially *avoid foods that are high in fat and refined carbohydrates*, as well as caffeine, alcohol, tobacco, and spicy foods. Each of them can negate the beneficial effects of vitamins C and E and zinc, which are all essential components of prostatic tissues and are necessary for the formation of seminal fluid. One handful per day of nonrancid raw pumpkin seeds is also helpful in treating BPH.

Vitamins, Minerals, and Supplements

See the recommendations for prostate cancer.

Herbs

Perhaps the most exciting addition to the treatment of BPH has been the extract of *saw palmetto berries (Serenoa repens)*. Multiple studies have shown that the fat-soluble (liposterolic) extract of these berries prevents the conversion of testosterone to dihydrotestosterone, thus preventing prostate enlargement. This mechanism is very similar to the way in which Proscar works, but clinical studies suggest that saw palmetto berries are more effective. In one controlled study, as many as 89 percent of men taking saw palmetto berries improved after one month of treatment. Unlike Proscar, saw palmetto berries do not cause impotence. In fact, the extract has a reputation for being an aphrodisiac. It is much less expensive than Proscar and has been used safely for many decades with no significant side effects being reported. The clinical results have been impressive in improving the symptoms of frequency of nighttime urination and urine flow rates for thousands of men with BPH. These results were usually obtained after two to three months. For the treatment of BPH, the recommended dosage for a liposterolic extract of saw palmetto berries containing 85–95 percent fatty acids and sterols is 320 mg daily (either 160 mg two times daily or 80 mg four times daily). One-half of that dosage (160 mg daily) can also be effective as a maintenance dose for treating or for preventing BPH.

The powdered bark of the tree *Pygeum africanus* has been shown to promote the regression of symptoms associated with BPH, and with no toxic side effects. Many health food stores currently have products that combine saw palmetto and Pygeum africanus—a great daily dose of preventive medicine. A saw palmetto berry a day might keep the surgeon away.

Empty the Prostate

As in the treatment of prostate cancer, it may be even more important to empty the prostate through frequent ejaculation for both prevention and treatment of BPH. See "Empty the Prostate" in the section on prostate cancer.

Prostatic Massage and the PC Muscle

Regular prostatic massage has been shown to be an effective therapy for relieving pressure and discomfort due to BPH. It is usually administered by a physician, who inserts a gloved finger into the rectum to massage the prostate directly. There is, however, a much simpler method for achieving a similar result. In addition to emptying the prostate, which also relieves pressure, you can massage your own prostate by regularly contracting or tightening your *PC* (pubococcygeus) *muscle*. When you squeeze this muscle it pushes against, or "massages," the prostate. Located on the pelvic floor between the anus and scrotum, the PC muscle can be identified by stopping the flow of urine in midstream. Once you identify this feeling of contraction, you can practice it as often as you like (other than during urination). This exercise is not only helpful in massaging and possibly reducing the size of an enlarged prostate, but it can also enhance sexual pleasure. Regular practice of PC contraction on a daily basis and during lovemaking can prolong and intensify orgasm.

To get in the habit of using the PC exercise, incorporate it into your daily routine: remind yourself to do it when the phone rings when you are seated at your desk at work, for example, or each time you stop at a traffic light. You can even coordinate PC exercises with abdominal breathing by contracting the PC muscle with every inhalation. It is recommended that you start with 10 to 15 PC contractions daily. Try to do them consecutively and gradually work your way up to 30 or more. Contractions and relaxation should be about the same length of time—two to four seconds. You can gradually increase the length of each to beyond four seconds as your PC muscle becomes stronger. As for its sexual application, a prolonged PC contraction can be used just prior to ejaculation to avoid orgasm and maintain an erection by arresting the pumping action of the multiple contractions that accompany ejaculation.

Mental and Emotional Health Recommendations. See the prostate cancer section. The imagery you use to shrink an enlarged prostate might include picturing a ball or balloon being slowly deflated. Or you might see the prostate shrinking from plum size to walnut size.

Bioenergy
See the prostate cancer section.

PROSTATITIS

Symptoms and Diagnosis

Prostatitis is usually seen in younger men (between 30 and 50) than those who suffer from BPH and falls into three categories:

1. Bacterial prostatitis—an infection of the gland that causes swelling
2. Nonbacterial prostatitis—swelling of the prostate without an infection
3. Prostadynia—a general irritation of the prostate without infection or swelling

Symptoms of chronic prostatitis, which can be intermittent and range from mild to severe, include:

- Pain or tenderness in the area of the prostate that might extend into the genitals
- Groin discomfort and lower back pain
- Difficult, frequent, and urgent urination
- Burning sensation or pain during urination
- A discharge from the penis after bowel movements

- Pain following ejaculation
- Depression

The prostate gland is also susceptible to acute infection or inflammation. An acute infection is marked by severe pain and tenderness in the area of the prostate, at times extending into the genitals, pelvis, and back. Fever, chills, and extreme fatigue might also be present with acute prostatitis. The symptoms of chronic prostatitis, as noted on the preceding list, are similar but more mild. If this chronic condition goes untreated, which it often does, there is an increased risk of transmitting the infection to a sexual partner, as well as more severe complications such as kidney infection, epididymitis (inflammation of the epididymis), and orchitis (a painful swelling of the testicles). Other possible consequences of untreated chronic prostatitis are bladder obstruction and prostate stones.

Conventional Medical Treatment

Medical treatment for both acute and chronic prostatitis consists almost exclusively of *antibiotics*. The acute condition usually responds well to the medication. The trouble with this approach is that in as many as 95 percent of chronic cases, bacteria are not the primary cause of the symptoms; and eradicating them is the only therapeutic benefit of antibiotics.

Risk Factors and Causes

Prostatitis may result from:

- A weakened immune system
- Depletion of prostatic glandular elements such as zinc, ascorbic acid (vitamin C), and proteolytic enzymes
- Increased amounts of sexual activity, particularly with multiple partners, which depletes the prostate of zinc and enzymes

Both zinc and proteolytic enzymes sterilize the urethra and protect the gland from infection. Excesses of caffeine, alcohol, and spicy foods also contribute to a lack of glandular nutrition, which ultimately adds to depletion of the prostate and lowered immune function.

Bacteria in the urine, as it passes through the urethra, can settle in the prostate. Chlamydia, an intracellular parasite transmitted through sexual contact, is also believed to be a common cause of prostatitis. The noninfective or inflammatory causes of prostatitis may be associated with autoimmune disorders, resulting from a depleted glandular environment.

Although it is a frequent but usually unconscious contributor to each of the men's health conditions discussed in this chapter, *shame* is the primary *emotional factor* contributing to prostatitis.

Holistic Medical Treatment

Diet
A less acidic and therefore less irritating urine can be produced by avoiding spicy foods, caffeine, and acidic drinks like orange juice. Drinking lots of water is also helpful—eight to ten 8-ounce glasses a day.

Minerals
Zinc is an essential mineral for a healthy prostate. Take 30 to 60 mg per day. One suggested dose for zinc in treating chronic prostatitis is 150 mg a day for two weeks, followed by 30 mg a day indefinitely. Be sure to reduce after two weeks, since this dosage can become toxic. Also remember to take copper sebacate (at least two hours apart from zinc), 1 to 2 mg daily to avoid disturbing the zinc/copper balance. (See the prostate cancer section for additional information about zinc.)

Herbs
Although it is also used for BPH, *Pygeum africanum* is even more effective in treating chronic prostatitis. The recommended dose is 50 to 100 mg twice a day of an extract standardized to contain 14 percent triterpenes and 0.5 percent docosanol. The standard course of treatment is three months, with mild gastrointestinal discomfort as the only reported possible side effect. The evergreen plant *pipsissewa* is especially effective for chronic prostatitis. It helps provide the prostate and urinary tract with increased blood flow and nutrition. Horsetail is an herbal medicine used in the treatment of acute prostate infection. *Saw palmetto berries (Serenoa repens)* enhance blood flow and nutrition to the prostate. Take 160 mg of the standardized extract two times a day. *Echinacea angustifolia*, an effective herb for treating any infection, can be a valuable part of the treatment program for both acute and chronic prostatitis. Take one dropperful three or four times a day. *Stinging nettles* may reduce inflammation and congestion in the prostate. Take 100 mg three times a day or in liquid form one teaspoon three times a day. *Cernilton*, a pollen extract from a Swedish ryegrass plant, popular in Europe (available from Cenitin America at 1 800-831-9505), can also be effective. Take two tablets three times a day.

Medications

An *antibiotic* is usually a part of the holistic medical treatment for acute and chronic prostatitis.

Exercise

Follow the suggestions for regular aerobic exercise in chapter 2, but *avoid* long bike rides and *jarring exercise* like jogging. Both can be uncomfortable for an enlarged and/or inflamed prostate gland. Swimming is probably the most gentle and effective means of exercising your entire body, but yoga and walking will also help to bring blood, nutrients, and oxygen to the prostate area.

Empty the Prostate and Prostatic Massage

Ejaculation should be eliminated during an acute infection in order to allow the prostate to renew itself and to keep the infection from spreading further. However, for chronic prostatitis, ejaculation is recommended at least every other day to help clear the prostate of infection.

   Prostate massage can help antibiotics and herbs to penetrate the prostate and enhance excretion of infected fluid. The massage may be administered either by yourself, your partner, or a physician. Consult a urologist for proper technique.

   For the remainder of the holistic medical treatment, see the BPH and prostate cancer sections.

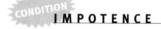

IMPOTENCE

Symptoms and Diagnosis

Impotence is defined as the inability to sustain a satisfactory erection to perform intercourse and ejaculation. Impotence may be the health problem that is most disturbing to men and for this reason might possibly be one of the most well-researched problems in medical science.

Conventional Medical Treatment

In 1998, *Viagra,* or *sildenafil,* became one of the most publicized drugs in recent history. In its first year of availability, more than a million prescriptions for Viagra were written. It is the first pharmaceutical pill found to be effective in treating impotence, or as it is known medically, erectile dysfunction. The drug increases the ability to achieve and maintain an erection when sexually stimulated. It does so by relaxing the muscles lining the arteries of the penis, thereby increasing the flow of blood into the spongy tissue (corpus cavernosum) comprising the shaft of the penis.

Depending on which research study you read, the drug is effective between 60 and 90 percent of the time. It works best for men with milder forms of impotence that are either psychological in origin or due to side effects of medication. In men with physical and physiological causes, it works less well. This would include men with diabetes and heart disease (with concomitant arterial narrowing) or those who have had prostate surgery for cancer or an enlarged prostate.

Viagra *should be avoided if you are taking nitroglycerin* or similar nitrate-based drugs for treating the chest pain associated with heart disease. Viagra and nitroglycerin can combine to lower blood pressure to a dangerously low level. There have been no deaths conclusively linked to Viagra, but during the first six months of its sale there were reports of over 60 men who died while taking the drug. The fact that 85 percent of the prescriptions filled for Viagra were for men age 50 and older, many of whom have other medical conditions like heart disease, makes it difficult to blame these deaths specifically on Viagra. Although the FDA continues to approve its sale, there is enough suspicion of serious risk that several foreign countries, including Canada, Japan, Australia, and Israel have banned Viagra.

As with any potent drug, there can be uncomfortable side effects. The most common are severe headaches, skin flushing, indigestion, diarrhea, stuffy nose, urinary tract infection, and abnormal vision (a bluish tinge that can diminish sight by up to 50 percent and last up to six hours).

If you take Viagra, you should follow your doctor's prescription strictly and not take it more frequently than prescribed or in higher dosages.

Prior to Viagra, the most successful drug treatment involved papaverine, phentolamine, or prostaglandin E-1 administered through *self-injections into the penis*. Regular use of injections improves your capacity for natural erections not only because they can enhance the efficiency of penile blood flow, but probably more because of the mental boost resulting from knowing you are capable of having erections. The most successful oral medication had been Erex, which worked about 30 percent of the time for psychogenic (emotionally caused) impotence.

The *surgical procedure* most often performed for treating impotence is penile revascularization. This is a procedure in which fresh blood from abdominal arteries is directed into the penis, bypassing the damaged or dysfunctional arteries that contribute to impotence. It might be more appropriate to call it "penile bypass" surgery. Unfortunately, it's not nearly as successful as the far more common heart bypass surgery. In one recent study, only 38 percent of those men who had the surgery were able to have spontaneous erections six months later. Another surgical procedure involves the implantation of penile prostheses.

Besides its two primary therapeutic weapons of drugs and surgery, conventional medicine has added a third—mechanical devices—for the treatment of impotence. *Vacuum erection devices*, available from most urologists for about $400, are used to assist a man who has been having trouble initiating or sustaining his erections. The vacuum pump is basically a clear cylinder; you put it over your penis, pump it up until a suction is created, and wait about three or four minutes until you develop an erection. The suction causes the blood that creates an erection to rush into the penis. Once the penis is erect, you fasten an occlusion band around the base of the penis in order to maintain the erection for as long as half an hour. Penile prosthetic devices and silicone implants are also being used for impotence.

Risk Factors and Causes

The publicity surrounding Viagra uncovered a new epidemic. Many experts believe the problem of erectile dysfunction afflicts even more than the standard estimate of 30 million men. The comprehensive Massachusetts Male Health Study found that about 52 percent of men between the ages of 40 and 70 experience some degree of impotence. The majority of men believe impotence is a natural consequence of aging, but in fact, a man's physiological ability to have erections continues into his eighties and nineties. The adage "If you don't use it, you lose it" is also applicable to our sexual capability. Masters and Johnson, authors of *Human Sexual Response*, found couples in their eighties who were still enjoying regular sexual intercourse. However, older men who had not been sexually active for a number of years, often due to the death of a spouse, were frequently impotent if they entered into a new relationship. As men age, the amount and force of ejaculation decreases, and the recovery time between ejaculations becomes longer, but their physiologic ability to have erections is still present. One simply has to continue to exercise that capability while adding some of the holistic recommendations in the following section.

The following factors contribute significantly to this epidemic in men of all ages.

Physical Causes

- Medications, especially antidepressants and drugs used to treat high blood pressure
- Alcohol and drug addiction (Many men who frequently drink or use drugs can be sexually active when they are under the influence, but become impotent when they are sober.)
- Vascular disease, including diabetes and heart disease
- Low testosterone levels
- Low zinc intake (Zinc indirectly stimulates testosterone production.)

- High cholesterol (For every 10 points above normal cholesterol levels there is a 32 percent increase in the risk of impotence.)

- Endocrine disorders, such as hypothyroidism and hypopituitary function

- Neurological conditions, such as Parkinson's disease and multiple sclerosis

Emotional Causes. Impotence most often results from a multitude of emotional causes, and is then called psychogenic impotence. The self-esteem of most men is tied to their ability to *perform*. Even one failure can be devastating and can lead to performance anxiety on the next occasion. Subsequent sexual encounters can create a downward spiral with more anxiety and less ability to perform, which eventually results in chronic impotence.

Although performance anxiety is often cited as the leading emotional cause of sexual dysfunction, other uncomfortable emotions can also cause a bout of impotence. Often ignored by men, these include depression, fear of intimacy, guilt, shame, and boredom. Louise Hay, in *You Can Heal Your Life*, describes the probable emotional causes of impotence as "sexual pressure, tension, guilt; spite against a previous mate; fear of mother."

As infants, the majority of men were traumatized through circumcision. The emotional wound inflicted by that routine surgical procedure is often much deeper than most men realize. From the time they were young boys, most men were aware that their penis was the body part most associated with shame and with the greatest fear of exposure. Yet for men this hidden appendage and its functional status have come to symbolize their masculinity and their power, because without the ability to have an erection, they are "impotent"—without power or strength.

It is difficult to ascertain its full impact, but the emerging independence of women over the past 30 years has probably had a profound effect on men. Not that it has been all bad; both men and women have needed to strike a healthier balance. But in this age of feminism and male-bashing, the burgeoning independence and power of women has left millions of men feeling guilty and emasculated—and impotent. In an attempt to behave "appropriately," many men have learned to keep their sexuality so well hidden that they've lost touch with it. They've learned to contain their sexual energy so tightly that they've squeezed the passion and vitality right out of it.

Impotence is a symptom, not a diagnosis. You cannot rely solely on Viagra to resolve the problem. Holistic treatment will help you to address the underlying causes and to heal yourself.

Holistic Medical Treatment and Prevention

Physical Health Recommendations

Vitamins, Minerals, and Supplements

For impotence, *zinc* may be the most valuable nutritional supplement. According to clinical studies conducted at the University of Rochester School of Medicine, the testosterone levels of men given zinc supplements rose dramatically. At the University of Virginia Medical School it was discovered that zinc can also diminish the pituitary gland's production of prolactin—a hormone that stops testosterone production. The dosage of zinc is 30 to 60 mg a day along with copper sebacate, 1 or 2 mg a day (take zinc and copper supplements at least two hours apart). You can also take *beta carotene*, 25,000 I.U. two times daily, *magnesium*, 500 mg daily, and *essential fatty acids* (EFAs) for treating impotence. Both *lycopene*, a flavonoid found in red fruits and vegetables, especially tomatoes and watermelon, and *arginine*, an amino acid found in nuts and animal products (all meats), are also part of the holistic treatment program for impotence.

The hormone *DHEA* has been successfully used in treating impotence. Although it is available in some health food stores, it is recommended that this treatment be administered by a physician, after obtaining blood or salivary levels of DHEA. Men with a high risk of prostate cancer should not use DHEA.

Herbs

One of the most powerful sexual stimulants ever discovered comes from a tree in Cameroon, Africa, and is called *yohimbine*. Like Viagra, yohimbine heightens potency and maintains erections by increasing blood flow to the penis. Unlike Viagra, it does so by increasing the body's production of the adrenal hormone norepinephrine, which is essential for erections. A 1987 Canadian study showed yohimbine to be especially effective for treating impotence in men with diabetes and heart disease. The overall success rate was 44 percent. A study conducted by Dr. Robert Margolis and published in the journal *Current Therapeutic Research* found that 80 percent of ten thousand impotent patients taking yohimbine reported good to excellent results. Almost 55 percent of the patients were 55 to 80 years of age. A. J. Riley, M.D., a specialist in sexual medicine, has concluded from the extensive testing of yohimbine that "it is now possible to restore usable erections for up to 95 percent of men with erectile inadequacy." Most patients using yohimbine reported that overall sexual pleasure increased with more intensive orgasms. It also decreased the latency period between ejaculations.

The FDA lists yohimbine as an unsafe herb, primarily due to the associated risks of low and high blood pressure. It can also potentially elevate heart rate and cause anxiety, hallucinations, headache, and skin flushing. However, anecdotal and physicians' reports suggest that the herb is safe. Use yohimbine, with some caution, at a dose of 100 mg daily.

Other herbs and supplements that can also contribute to enhanced sexual potency are:

- *Damiana*—2 to 4 ml, or 60 drops, daily; considered an aphrodisiac in Central and South America
- *Ginkgo biloba*—40 mg of a standardized extract three times daily; increases circulation, especially to the neurologic system
- *Ashwagandha*—300 mg daily; an Ayurvedic herb
- *Panax ginseng*—100 mg of a standardized extract two times daily; stimulates the endocrine system
- *Siberian ginseng*—400 mg of a standardized extract three times daily; supportive to the adrenal glands and helpful with high stress

Mental and Emotional Health Recommendations. Use affirmations for treating impotence. Be creative and use vivid imagery for the greatest effect. For example: "My penis is full and erect," "There is an infinite supply of energy filling my penis," or simply "My erection is hard and powerful." Mental imagery in conjunction with reciting and/or writing these affirmations is extremely helpful. In treating impotence, it helps to imagine some type of fluid (representing blood) filling an empty space (limp penis); or light filling a dark space. Or you might imagine your spouse or lover gently, slowly, and lovingly stimulating the largest erection you've ever had.

After all of the possible physical causes for impotence have been ruled out, if you're not satisfied with the progress you're making on your own, you might consider seeing a psychotherapist, or a sex therapist. Journaling is another option, which was described in chapter 3. The longer the problem persists, the more difficult it can be to treat on your own.

Social Health Recommendations. It is particularly helpful to be able to discuss your feelings about your impotence with your spouse or sexual partner. If she or he is agreeable, try being physically intimate while knowing beforehand that you will not attempt to have intercourse. This relieves a lot of psychological pressure to perform and can eventually help to restore normal function.

Men are usually reluctant to acknowledge and discuss the problem of impotence with their significant other. But their fears are almost always exaggerated, and once they "break the ice" the outcome is usually beneficial.

Being able to share feelings and spending enjoyable "play" time with your son, another young boy, your father, or a close male friend or relative, or joining a men's group, might allow you the opportunity to more closely connect and bond with other men or feel your maleness more deeply. Although there are no scientific studies linking this type of social activity to the health of the prostate, it does make good sense from a bioenergetic standpoint.

Bioenergy

See the bioenergy section for prostate cancer.

11

Gastrointestinal Disorders

Diarrhea

Constipation

Hemorrhoids

Irritable Bowel Syndrome

Inflammatory Bowel Disease—
   Crohn's disease
   Ulcerative colitis

Diverticulosis/Diverticulitis

Peptic Ulcer

Cholecystitis/Gallstones

Parasites

THE GASTROINTESTINAL TRACT

Anatomy and Physiology

THE GASTROINTESTINAL TRACT provides the means by which we chew, digest, and obtain nourishment from food and eliminate nondigestible fiber and wastes from the colon. Digestion starts in the mouth and continues in the stomach and small intestine. Most of the food's nutrients and water are absorbed through the intestinal wall while they are passing through the 26-foot-long small bowel. In the large bowel (colon), remaining water and nutrients are absorbed into the bloodstream, leaving undigested food content, toxins, and wastes for elimination. The normal transit time for food to travel from ingestion to stool passage is 12 to 18 hours.

Over five hundred species of normal bacteria are found in the gastrointestinal tract, and the number of individual bacteria is nine times greater than the number of cells in the body. Amazingly enough, the extensive system of lymph channels in the walls of the small bowel is the largest reservoir of immune function in the body. The intake of nutrients profoundly influences the balance of the intestinal bacteria, potentially favoring growth of harmful mircoorganisms and profoundly affecting the lymphatic and immune system function (see "Candidiasis," chapter 9).

The gastrointestinal tract also houses the body's "second brain," known as the enteric nervous system, located in the linings of the esophagus, stomach, small intestine, and colon. Scientists consider it a single entity—brimming with neurotransmitter proteins, produced by cells identical to those found in the brain. This complex circuitry enables the "G-I brain" (the "belly brain") to act independently, learn, remember, and *produce gut feelings.*

The Gastrointestinal Tract

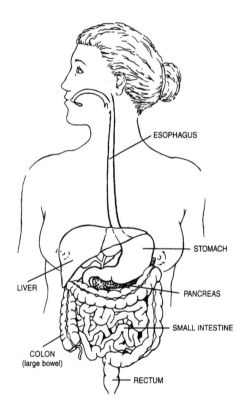

- ESOPHAGUS
- STOMACH
- LIVER
- PANCREAS
- SMALL INTESTINE
- COLON (large bowel)
- RECTUM

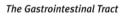

CONDITION

DIARRHEA

Prevalence and Symptoms

Diarrhea may be defined as increased liquidity, frequency, and volume of bowel movements, which interfere with the normal activities of daily living. It is often accompanied by abdominal pain, cramping, and excessive gas. Although episodes of diarrhea have been experienced by almost everyone, with little or no serious consequences, diarrhea can result in dehydration from a significant loss of water and electrolytes. Diarrhea is usually a symptom of a temporary gastrointestinal dysfunction but occasionally is a sign of serious illness. Indicators of more ominous problems are worsening diarrhea lasting longer than a week, bowel movements initiated by urgency threatening incontinence, high volume stool loss, and stools accompanied by blood or pus. Most cases of acute diarrhea resolve on their own. Up to one-half of Americans who visit developing countries develop "traveler's diarrhea" after contracting bacterial or parasitic infections.

The diarrhea of celiac disease, a malabsorption problem caused by a genetically related reactivity to gluten (a protein in grains), produces a particularly foul-smelling stool.

Conventional Treatment

Although diarrhea usually resolves on its own in two to four days, if it becomes chronic, lasting a week or more, then medical advice should be sought. Symptomatic treatment usually involves maintaining hydration and electrolytes (sodium, potassium, and magnesium) with sufficient liquids. The risk of severe dehydration from diarrhea water losses are much greater in children. A rehydration solution can be made at home (see page 254). Children are often placed on the *BRAT* diet (bananas, rice, applesauce, toast) since these foods are more easily digested and are somewhat binding. Alcohol, caffeine, milk and dairy products, and artificially flavored foods and chewing gum should be avoided. If the onset of diarrhea quickly follows the start of any new medication, it should be stopped to see if the diarrhea subsides.

Medications to slow bowel activity include absorbent medicines like Pepto-Bismol and antimotility opium-derivative drugs such as Lomotil (prescription) and Imodium (OTC). Medications containing attapulgite and kaolin (Donnagel and Kaopectate) are generally less effective. It is recommended that you wait a few hours after the onset of diarrhea before taking one of these medications. Acute diarrhea is purging the body of a toxic substance, so you need to give it a chance to complete the job. Frequently pharmaceuticals are prescribed to attack offending bacterial, fungal, or parasitic organisms demonstrated on culture or stool examination. Severe diarrhea in children may require hospitalization and treatment by intravenous rehydration with water and electrolyte solutions.

When mild to moderate diarrhea does not respond to these symptomatic treatment measures after about two weeks, more extensive diagnostic investigation is undertaken. Depending on your precise symptoms, your physician may order examination of stool samples for the presence of infectious organisms, parasites, and amounts of blood too small to be visibly detectable. Other options include referral to a specialist in endoscopy, who will introduce an instrument into the gastrointestinal tract through the throat or rectum to visually examine the stomach, small bowel, or rectum.

Causes and Risk Factors

Acute diarrhea:

- Food poisoning—contaminated drinking water or food (viruses and bacteria)
- Stomach or intestinal flu—viral infection
- Food allergy or food intolerance—especially milk and dairy products, called lactose intolerance (lactose is the sugar in milk); other common offenders are wheat, coffee, chocolate, egg, corn, soy, orange, pork, beef, chicken, peanuts, and sugar
- Anxiety
- Drug toxicity—especially antibiotics (they destroy the friendly bacteria acidophilus and bifidus); laxative abuse; excess of products containing magnesium such as antacids; corticosteroids; excess vitamin C
- Olestra-containing synthesized foods. Olestra is a synthetic fat which is not absorbed from the intestine; it theoretically can help people lose weight. It causes diarrhea in a significant number of users. Read food labels to determine its presence
- Bacterial infections—salmonella, E. coli, shigella, cholera, typhoid—potentially serious infections
- Traveler's diarrhea—usually caused by bacteria and/or parasites

Chronic diarrhea:

- Parasites—in some areas giardia is common; amebiasis
- Viruses (including rotavirus)
- Worm infestation
- Crohn's disease
- Resistant bacteria (e.g., Clostridium difficile) or candida (yeast) overgrowth after antibiotic treatment
- Ulcerative colitis
- Irritable bowel syndrome
- Diverticulitis
- Cancer of the colon
- Emotional stress—usually associated with the following issues: gut-level fear, distrust, low self-confidence, personal honor, and self-care

Holistic Medical Treatment and Prevention

Physical Health Recommendations

Hygiene

Prevention of many types of epidemic diarrhea, including food poisoning, is dependent on good personal hygiene, including hand-washing after using restroom facilities. This is particularly critical in food handlers. Effective prevention of *travelers' diarrhea* includes the following:

- Use only bottled water; do not add ice to drinks or use tap water to rinse your mouth or a toothbrush after brushing your teeth.

- Do not eat any salad or raw foods that do not have a thick peel, such as bananas or watermelons.

- Use hydrochloric acid tablets following each meal—helps to digest and inactivate parasites.

- Take acidophilus daily, one that is heat resistant.

- Take grapefruit seed extract, one tablet or capsule daily and up to six daily with acute symptoms.

- Use the herbal product Intestinalis (BioNutritional Formulas, [800] 950–8484, available through physicians), one to three tablets per day (kills parasites).

- Take Probioplex, four pills in the morning and four in the evening with acidophilus; the active ingredient is a purified immunoglobulin concentrate from whey, available from Metagenics of Eugene, Oregon.

Diet

Initially diarrhea should be treated by avoiding any solid foods and limiting intake to water, juices (fruit and vegetable, diluted two parts water to one part juice), potassium-rich vegetable broth, defizzed soft drinks, or diluted rice milk. Adults should try to drink about one pint (16 oz.) per hour. With acute diarrhea this helps to avoid dehydration while allowing the body to efficiently eliminate toxic foods, viruses, or bacteria. With chronic diarrhea due to food allergy it allows you to stay hydrated while testing for offending foods. Avoid milk if you suspect yourself to be lactose intolerant. In infants and young children, breast-feeding should be continued, and commercial rehydration solutions can be used. For children not requiring hospitalization, a homemade rehydration solution of one-half teaspoon of salt and four teaspoons of sugar in one quart of filtered or bottled water can be made up and given one-half to one ounce every 30–90 minutes. Typically rehydration solutions don't taste very good and many children may refuse them. Sports drinks like powdered Endura or Recharge are an acceptable alternative, although they're usually high in sugar and low in sodium and potassium.

As the diarrhea subsides, the liquids can be followed by yogurt (plain active culture, daily), vegetable soups, rice or barley broth, cooked fruits (crabapples), applesauce, garlic, steamed vegetables (carrots, string beans, eggplant, yams), olives, white rice, sweet rice, and buckwheat. *Avoid* fats and oils, fried foods, honey, spinach, cow's milk, alcohol, caffeine, apricots, plums, prunes, raisins, sesame seeds, and any products containing the sweeteners sorbitol, xylitol, and mannitol (commonly found in sugarless gums, vitamins, and diet foods). Pectin, found in apples, bananas, carrots, and potatoes, also helps relieve diarrhea.

The diarrhea, weight loss, and abdominal distress of people with *celiac syndrome* requires strict avoidance of grains containing gluten, including wheat, barley, rye, oats, and spelt. The avoidance of gluten is doubly important: long-term ingestion of gluten in sensitive people carries a much higher risk of colon cancer.

Vitamins, Minerals, and Supplements

Lactobacillus *acidophilus*, the normal bacterium of the bowel, is needed following diarrhea to restore the bowel flora. Powdered forms are best in dosages of one-half to one teaspoon twice daily. At 250 to 1,000 mg daily, Lactobacillus GG, a variety of Lactobacillus casei rhamosum isolated from humans, has been shown to cure 85 percent of patients with recurrent diarrhea from a resistant bacterial infection (Clostridium difficile). Supplementing with *bifidobacteria* (½ tsp. twice daily) helps control the diarrhea of poorly thriving infants 6–24 months of age. *Carob* powder, in tablespoonful doses mixed with applesauce and taken one to three times daily, can also help stop diarrhea.

In children, the addition of *zinc* has been reported to improve the effectiveness of a conventional treatment program by 30 percent, with fewer complications. The treatment of children with *vitamin A*, 100,000 to 200,000 I.U. added to infant feedings every two to three months, substantially reduced the risk for diarrhea during epidemics. The diarrhea of celiac disease responds in part to the addition of *folic acid* in doses of 30 mg daily. Additional folic acid is important in treating Crohn's disease as well.

Herbs

- *Berberine* is successful in treating the diarrhea from amebiasis, giardiasis, and E. coli. It is found in *goldenseal, Oregon grape*, and *barberry*, all used in ethnic cultures for diarrhea. Berberine has also been shown to have a toxin-neutralizing action that is helpful in traveler's diarrhea, frequently due to a toxin-producing E. coli.

- *Goldenseal* is effective in bacterial induced diarrhea. The dosage for children is one-fourth–one-half teaspoon three times daily in a 1:5 tincture; adults: one-half–1 teaspoon three times daily.

- *Garlic* has moderate antibiotic properties, especially against candida (yeast) organisms and other fungal and bacterial causes of diarrhea. Use raw or dried forms with a high content of allicin.

- *Peppermint*, 3–15 drops in water, every two to three hours.

- *Chamomile* and blackberry teas are helpful.

- *Slippery elm bark*, two capsules before meals to solidify stools

- *Gastromycin*, an Allergy Research product, three to four cups three times daily

Homeopathy

There are several homeopathic remedies for acute diarrhea, but each one is used for treating different symptoms. Common agents used for diarrhea include *aconite, chamomile, podophyllum*, and *sulfur*. Homeopathy has been shown in two studies to eliminate diarrhea more quickly than conventional treatment in childhood diarrhea.

Mental and Emotional Health Recommendations. There are several therapies that are effective in treating some types of chronic diarrhea. *Biofeedback* training is highly successful in treating irritable bowel syndrome. It is helpful as well in diarrhea in which stress plays a major role. *Meditation, yoga*, and other approaches for managing of the autonomic (involuntary) nervous system are also successful (*progressive relaxation, self-suggestion*, and *autogenics*). Psychological studies of adult diarrhea with no apparent diagnosable cause have frequently found that intense feelings and demands on other people are commonly present. The acute diarrhea associated with performance anxiety may respond nicely to counseling work to enhance self-esteem and confidence. Brief therapeutic interventions that may quickly change bowel function often involve evoking an attitude of forgiveness and letting go of the intense demands.

CONSTIPATION

Prevalence

Constipation is the most common gastrointestinal complaint in the United States. Nearly everyone has experienced to some degree the difficult and infrequent passage of bowel movements. It is a chronic problem in 2 to 3 percent of Americans, who spend more than $400 million a year on laxatives.

CASE HISTORY

E.B., a 58-year-old woman patient of mine for over 15 years, presented with diarrhea of two weeks' duration. When it did not subside promptly, she returned, and laboratory tests failed to pinpoint a specific cause. She was an anxious person with perfectionistic tendencies, and I told her I thought anxiety was playing a role in her symptoms. This met with a prompt and total denial.

Her symptoms persisted for about four months, during which she saw me twice, gradually opening herself to consider the possible role of stress in her symptoms. Her denial finally aside, we were able to come to a serious discussion in which she revealed that she had been appointed the executor of her mother's modest estate following her mother's death in a nursing home. With visible emotion she revealed that her two sisters had been very uncooperative in forwarding all the final bills and information for the many legal documents required.

She admitted to being so angry that when her sisters had come to her home in an attempt to resolve the issue, she refused to see them, leaving her husband to deny that she was home. At that point tears came, and she was visibly angry. I suggested that the anger and diarrhea were related and asked if she would acknowledge the anger and write a letter to her sisters, expressing *all her resentments,* past and present, sign it, and give it to her husband to destroy. Six months later, she told me she had written the letter early one morning, *after which she had no further diarrhea whatsoever.* The next day she had been motivated to write a reconciliation letter which she did send, eventually leading to the reestablishment of their fractured relationship.

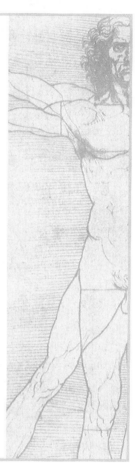

Symptoms and Diagnosis

Primary symptoms include:

- Infrequent or irregular bowel movements (BMs)—less than once a day
- Pain or strain with BMs
- Passage of small, hard stools
- Abdominal distention and bloating
- Fatigue

Constipation that lasts longer than a week for no apparent reason, and is of concern to you, might prompt you to seek a medical consultation. The physical examination will include a digital rectal exam to detect any signs of impaction, tenderness, or blood. Diagnostic tests might include: blood tests, stool analysis, X-ray studies (upper GI and barium enema), and proctosigmoidoscopy.

Conventional Medical Treatment

Conventional treatment usually involves the use of *laxatives*, of which there are three types:

1. Bulking agents—these are essentially fiber, and are often the first choice and most effective for mild constipation. Increased fiber naturally enhances proper colon function. These products, such as Metamucil, frequently contain psyllium, which is a natural plant fiber. The usual dosage is one to two teaspoons daily with water.

2. Stimulant laxatives—increase peristalsis, the muscular action of the colon. By irritating the walls of the large intestine they are effective in promoting BMs, but should only be used for short periods—one to two weeks. Long-term use can create dependency and other forms of colon dysfunction. Examples of stimulant laxatives are Ex-Lax, Dulcolax, and Senokot.

3. Stool softeners—moisten the stools by mixing water and fatty materials. They are often used in combination with stimulant laxatives. Colace and Surfak are popular stool softeners. These should also only be used for short periods while the underlying causes are being identified and corrected.

4. Adequate *water* intake is also emphasized.

Causes and Risk Factors

Constipation is primarily related to lifestyle choices and is, therefore, quite correctable even in the most severe cases.

Physical Factors

*   Foods *low in fiber*, high in saturated fats, prepackaged, and over-cooked
*   Meat, cheese, fried foods, sugar, and white flour–based foods
*   Deficiency of potassium and magnesium—both common with diuretic use
*   Calcium and iron supplements and antacids containing aluminum
*   *Inadequate water* and liquid intake
*   Excess coffee, alcohol, and soft drinks—can dehydrate the stool and irritate the lining of the colon
*   Eating too quickly, and not chewing adequately
*   The majority of prescription drugs, antacids, and chronic use of laxatives all contribute to constipation

- Inflammatory bowel disease, including Crohn's disease, irritable bowel syndrome, diverticulitis; and deficiency of vitamin B-1 and folic acid may manifest in episodes of both constipation and diarrhea
- Deficiencies of stomach acidity or pancreatic digestive enzymes
- Food sensitivities can cause constipation, with or without diarrhea
- Low thyroid function
- Physical inactivity—lack of exercise can slow transit time of stools
- Habitually postponing the urge to have a BM feeds back a weakening of the signal to defecate

Emotional Factors

- *Depression* and anxiety
- Excessive need for control
- Obsessive/compulsive tendencies
- Failing to express intense feelings
- Fear of making mistakes/need for perfection
- Grim determination to carry on in the face of an apparently insoluble problem

Holistic Medical Treatment and Prevention
Physical Health Recommendations

Diet

- Increase *fiber*—eat more raw organic fruits (plums, prunes, apricots, figs, and dates), vegetables, beans and lentils. Ground flax and sesame seeds (one to two tablespoons daily) are especially high in fiber. Have one to two tablespoons of bran (barley or oat bran) with water at mealtimes, or add bran to cereal or applesauce, two to three tablespoons.
- Increase *whole grains*, instead of eating white-flour-based products such as bread and pastry. Whole grain cereals with rice or soy milk and fruit and bran added make an excellent breakfast.
- Increase *water* intake to at least the minimum daily requirement (1/2 oz. per lb. of body weight), and drink most of it between meals to avoid diluting digestive enzymes.
- *Olive oil*, unrefined, two tablespoons daily; high-lignan organic *flaxseed oil*, one tablespoon daily.

- Reduce or eliminate sugar, milk and dairy products, coffee, alcohol, meat, fats, and spicy and refined or processed foods.
- Chew food adequately—20 to 30 chews per mouthful.

Healthy Habits to Reestablish Bowel Regularity

- Identify and eliminate the causes of your constipation (carefully review the preceding list).
- Always answer nature's call and don't repress your natural urge to have a BM.
- Sit on the toilet at the same time every day, preferably in the morning, even if you don't feel like going. Rather than straining, practice abdominal breathing while sitting on the toilet.
- Follow the dietary recommendations.
- Do regular aerobic exercise (brisk walking is fine) for 30 minutes, three to five times per week.
- Stop using laxatives.
- To reestablish regularity you might need to take an herbal laxative containing either cascara or senna at night before bed for two weeks. This may need to be done under a physician's supervision. If loose stools or diarrhea occur, then the dose of the laxative needs to be reduced until a normally formed stool is established.

Vitamins, Minerals, and Supplements

In addition to dietary fiber, *fiber supplements* can be helpful. Most come in powder form and can be added to water or diluted fruit juice. The most balanced supplements are Metamucil, Ultra Fiber (available through naturopaths and holistic physicians), or Jarrow Gentle Fiber. Add supplementary fiber slowly—one to two grams daily until you reach five grams per day. Listen to your body and watch your elimination to adjust your fiber dosage. In addition to restoring regular bowel movements, supplementary fiber can:

- Hydrate and keep the stool formed
- Feed the good bacteria and promote eubiosis—a positive bacterial balance in the gut that strengthens immunity
- Help prevent toxins from being absorbed into the body
- Reduce fat uptake, thus reducing cholesterol
- Reduce the risk of colon and rectal cancer, heart disease, and hypertension

In reestablishing normal bowel function, it is essential to create the proper bacterial balance using *probiotics*. In all cases of constipation there is an underlying bowel bacteria imbalance, called dysbiosis, which occurs when there is more of the bad bacteria than good. The beneficial bacteria are acidophilus and bifidus. It is best to take a high potency probiotic formula containing both acidophilus and bifidus in a powder form. The dosage is one-half to one teaspoon in water two times daily, morning and evening. Bifidus can also promote peristalsis.

Magnesium is essential to peristaltic function. The recommended dosage is 300 mg each evening and 100 mg with breakfast in a citrate or aspartate form. If too much is taken, it can cause diarrhea. *Potassium* (700 mg daily) should also be taken.

Vitamin C can usually soften the stool at higher dosages such as 5,000 to 10,000 mg daily. Take it as ascorbic acid with bioflavonoids in gradually increasing doses until constipation subsides.

The *B vitamins*, especially *B-1*, may be helpful in treating constipation. Pantothenate, a variation of pantothenic acid, is especially helpful for a bowel that is sluggish after surgery.

Herbs
Helpful for constipation are cascara, senna, licorice, rhubarb, barberry, psyllium, and flax. Mixtures often work better, but any one of these will work alone. Aloe vera juice (two ounces daily) also works well.

Professional Care Therapies
Homeopathic remedies include Nux vomica (especially for laxative habituation), Bryonia, Alumina, and Sulphur.

Acupuncture has been used with success in alleviating constipation.

Mental Health Recommendations. *Psychotherapy* and *biofeedback* are often effective in treating constipation. In childhood studies, improvement is significantly accelerated with biofeedback compared to conventional treatment. The relaxed state allows the autonomic nervous system, which controls the bowel, to function much more naturally and normally. Addressing depression and psychological issues is essential.

Use *eating as an excuse to relax*. Slowing down and relaxing promotes digestive secretions and peristalsis. With each meal, stop to take a moment to feel gratitude, breathe freely and deeply, chew your food thoroughly, and visualize excellent digestion and elimination.

CONDITION

HEMORRHOIDS

Prevalence

Up to 30 percent of Americans have a degree of ongoing hemorrhoid problems, and the lifetime experience is thought to be as high as 75 percent.

Anatomy and Physiology

The tissue of the anus is a cushion of blood vessels, connective tissue, nerves, and muscles. Hemorrhoids are collections of enlarged hemorrhoidal veins in the lining of the anal canal at the termination of the rectum. They are actually miniature variations of varicose veins, which can occur in the skin of the lower limbs. Internal hemorrhoids develop inside the anal sphincter muscle and cannot be felt or seen outside.

Symptoms and Diagnosis

The appearance of a hemorrhoid generates bleeding, leaving bright red blood on the stool as it passes, soaking the toilet paper and reddening the toilet water. Itching and burning sensations may or may not accompany the development of hemorrhoids but are frequently promoted as major symptoms in advertisements for OTC hemorrhoid preparations. Accompanying inflammation in the anal canal generates the discharge of mucus and often makes defecation uncomfortable. Complications include formation of a clot in the hemorrhoid, leading to a painless lump; and prolapse of hemorrhoids, a circumstance in which a bundle of enlarged internal hemorrhoidal veins from inside the anal sphincter muscle descends and presents partially outside.

Conventional Treatment

Strategies are selected to relieve symptoms and correct any underlying causes. Your physician will advise you to:

- Avoid straining, strenuous lifting and long periods of sitting
- Undertake regular exercise
- Use stool softeners and bulk laxatives
- Try zinc oxide ointment to soothe swollen, inflamed hemorrhoidal tissues
- Use OTC 0.5 percent cortisone cream for inflammation; the thinning of the anal mucosal surface with prolonged use is a disadvantage

- Relax in warm sitz baths with water temperatures 100–105 degrees F; many practitioners recommend a short cold bath to follow

Although many claims are made for OTC preparations to shrink hemorrhoids, conclusive studies are lacking.

Hemorrhoidal clots are sometimes surgically removed; they will resolve on their own in about three to four weeks. A prolapsed hemorrhoid commonly leads to surgical correction. A modified form of nearly painless management of internal hemorrhoids involves a rubber-banding procedure. In general, however, surgery is not a definitive answer in the absence of modifications in lifestyle that address the underlying causes.

Although still not used commonly, a May 1989 study in the *American Journal of Gastroenterology* revived an idea first broached in 1897, utilizing monopolar direct current treatment. The procedure works well and is usually entirely painless.

Causes and Risk Factors

The principle causes of hemorrhoids include:

- Genetic predisposition to weak blood vessel walls
- Physical conditions that put pressure on the pelvis and lower abdomen
- Pregnancy
- Long periods of occupational sitting
- Heavy lifting occupations
- Allergies leading to frequent sneezing
- Chronic cough from smoking
- Cirrhosis of the liver, which puts extra circulatory demands on the hemorrhoidal veins
- Chronic constipation is closely related to hemorrhoids; it often results in the need to strain to have a bowel movement
- Fiber deficient diets causing constipation

Holistic Prevention and Treatment

Physical Health Recommendations. *Prevention* involves:

- Adequate liquid intake
- Adequate fiber (see under constipation)
- A good aerobic exercise program

Treatment of hemorrhoids involves the following.

Diet
All the dietary changes that relieve chronic constipation (mentioned earlier) are helpful. (See p. 259)

Topical Treatment
For temporary relief use *witch hazel packs, zinc oxide ointment, cocoa butter, cod liver oil, Peruvian balsam* and *calendula ointment* for itching.

Vitamins and Supplements
- *Vitamin C*, one to two grams daily
- *Bioflavonoids* improve the elastic integrity of blood vessel walls
    1. *mixed citrus bioflavonoids*, rutin and hesperidin, three to six grams daily
    2. *hydroxyethyl-rutosides*, 500 mg twice daily, significantly reduce bleeding and hemorrhoidal symptoms in two to four weeks

Herbs
- *Butcher's broom* (Ruscus aculeatus), containing 10 percent ruscogenin content, 100 mg three times daily
- *Triphala guggulu*, 200 mg twice daily; a mainstay of Ayurvedic treatment
- *Collinsonia root* (stoneroot), a traditional native remedy that has moderate effectiveness (two capsules twice a day)

Biomolecular Options
- *Proanthocyanidins* (pycnogenol) which exert a positive effect on small blood vessels and tend to reduce swelling (50–100 mg daily).
- *Glycosaminoglycans* (GAGS) are biosynthetic agents that when taken in supplement form have been shown to be superior to flavonoids for maintenance of integrity of blood vessels and protection of their surfaces (aortic extract; dosage: 100 mg per day).

Homeopathic Remedies
Use *Aesculus, Arnica, Nux vomica* (itching), and *Sulphur* (soreness, inflammation)

IRRITABLE BOWEL SYNDROME (IBS)

Prevalence

Irritable bowel syndrome, also called spastic or mucous colitis, is said to afflict over 15 percent of the American population. Women with IBS outnumber men two to one.

Anatomy and Physiology

No accompanying structural defects are found in IBS. The symptoms are a result of hyperfunction and malfunction of the gastrointestinal tract, thought to involve the stomach, small intestine and large bowel; the neural circuitry with the brain is probably involved as well, even in the face of a totally normal anatomical picture.

Symptoms and Diagnosis

The symptoms of irritable bowel syndrome include a change from normal bowel function to periods of diarrhea and constipation, often alternating, with belching, bloating, abdominal pain, nausea, loss of appetite, flatulence, and a feeling after a bowel movement that the bowel has not completely emptied. The diarrhea, which is sometimes urgent, explosive, and scarcely controllable, may involve liquid stools with white mucous and may occur immediately after a meal or soon after awakening in the morning. Large meals tend to aggravate symptoms. Symptoms in women also tend to increase during premenstrual and menstrual phases of the cycle. Physical symptoms are often accompanied by notable depression and/or anxiety. Careful histories often establish the pre-existence of psychological symptoms, which may worsen with onset of the physical symptoms. Making the diagnosis requires exclusion of other causes of diarrhea and constipation.

Conventional Treatment

Conventional textbooks state that irritable bowel syndrome is poorly understood and that existing therapies are not known to have lasting success. Treatment includes:

- Addition of adequate fiber
- Antispasmodic drugs (Bentyl, Donnatal, Levsin)
- Drugs to stop diarrhea (Imodium, Lomotil)
- Avoidance of caffeine and excess alcohol

Risk Factors and Causes

Most authorities state that the cause of irritable bowel syndrome is unknown. The following factors are thought by many holistic physicians to be contributory:

1. Food sensitivity or allergy; the food offenders most often found, in order of frequency, include milk and milk derivatives, wheat, coffee, chocolate, citrus fruits, corn, eggs, nuts, barley, rye, oats, and potatoes

2. Intolerance of sugars—fructose, sucrose, sorbitol, mannitol, and lactose (in milk)

3. Parasitic intestinal infestation; some authorities estimate an incidence as high as 30–50 percent in IBS

4. Candida (yeast) overgrowth; in IBS patients not responsive to food elimination diets treatment with antiyeast antibiotics has been shown to result in great improvement

5. Psychological and social stress; accelerated motility of the colon occurs in irritable bowel syndrome patients experiencing stress

Holistic Treatment and Prevention

Physical Health Recommendations. Successful treatment begins with a thorough inquiry for causes and a careful history for possible triggering factors:

- Careful search for bacterial and parasitic organisms, and a digestive stool analysis utilizing a laboratory especially equipped for testing of stool specimens; specific treatment then follows for any abnormal organisms found on testing

- Systematic search for triggering factors from clues in the waxing and waning pattern of symptoms in irritable bowel syndrome may require journal-keeping recording foods and events

- Intestinal permeability functional testing for leaky gut syndrome

- Hydrogen breath test for upper gastric bacterial fermentation

Diet
Dietary improvements can include the following:

- Begin with the gradual addition of *high fiber* from raw or steamed vegetables including beans and lentils, adding one to two foods per week, making careful observation of the tolerance of each.

- Unprocessed psyllium seed powder gradually increased from one rounded teaspoonful to two tablespoonfuls daily tends to stabilize the bowel habit. Use of psyllium seed as a source of fiber bypasses the possibility that using wheat or other cereal bran may aggravate the problem if sensitivity to these grains is present.

- The intake of water should be six to eight glasses daily, sufficient to keep the urine very pale yellow most of the time.

- Thorough chewing and unhurried eating in a relaxed atmosphere is encouraged.

- Sugar is discouraged. Studies have shown that intestinal motility is prolonged by nearly *two and one-half times over normal* after introduction of a high load of sugar. This disruption of intestinal motility is one of the main problems in IBS. Sugar also encourages growth of candida (yeast), which has been implicated as an additional contributing factor in IBS.

Supplements

- Acidophilus and bifidus to reestablish normal bacterial balance
- L-glutamine, four to eight grams daily

Food Sensitivity

A food elimination and rechallenge trial should be undertaken if food sensitivity suspicion is high. You can also bypass extended food trials and simply try omitting the more highly suspect foods listed under causes and risk factors earlier. Other less common offenders include tea and onions. Chapter 19 on food allergies describes a more extensive systematic approach. Placed on an "oligoantigenic" diet limited to a few foods, IBS patients commonly feel much improved within a week. Since food additives can occasionally be a problem, organically grown foods are desirable. *Of those who follow a carefully planned exclusion diet, 75 percent experience substantial improvement.*

Herbs

Peppermint oil (one to three enteric-coated capsules twice daily between meals) is helpful. A German study found clinical improvement and decrease in pain to be twice as great from peppermint oil compared to placebo. A mixture of 20 Chinese herbs, including Artemesiae capillaris, Codonopsis pilosulae, Coicis lachyrma-jobi, Attractylodis macrocephalae, Schisandrae, and others was recently shown to be of substantial help with IBS symptoms. Herbal teas with antispasmodic properties (chamomile, peppermint, rosemary, and valerian) are soothing. Robert's Formula is also helpful in treatment (see under Crohn's disease).

Mental and Emotional Health Recommendations. Stress incidents and increased general levels of demands are frequently associated with flare-ups of IBS; these recurrences can be modified by insight-oriented psychotherapy, particularly successful when augmented by *relaxation training* and practice with *biofeedback*. Some studies have documented 75 percent improvement in physical and psychological symptoms after several months of regular biofeedback practice. *Hypnosis* is also very effective in irritable bowel syndrome. After an initial series of treatments, the best results occur in patients who periodically—one to three times a year—return for a session of reinforcement. *Self-affirmations* are particularly effective, especially when repeated in the relaxed state during relaxation, biofeedback, or *meditation*. An example: "My intestine is healed and serves me well."

Irritable bowel dysfunction has been linked to the spiritual and psychological issues of gut-level fear, distrust, low self-confidence, personal honor, and self-care. The oft-associated tendency for IBS patients to be highly invested in control and self-criticism needs to be recognized, and attempts need to be made to make alterations in the attitudes behind these cognitions and behaviors. Dealing with and resolving the issues surrounding the origin of these predisposing traits in earlier life is of high importance. Working to improve the quality of sleep also reaps significant benefits in bringing symptoms under control. Irritable bowel syndrome patients are often worriers, with special concern about work and their disease. Fun, play, and laughter can be highly therapeutic.

Professional Care Therapies

Acupuncture and energy therapies such as *Reiki, Therapeutic Touch, Jin Shin Jyutsu* and *Jo Rei* can all be helpful in treating IBS.

INFLAMMATORY BOWEL DISEASE—CROHN'S DISEASE

Prevalence

Inflammatory bowel disease includes Crohn's disease and ulcerative colitis (see following section). The incidence of Crohn's disease is estimated to involve about one hundred thousand people in the United States. A modest majority are women. Age of onset is usually between 15 and 40. Inflammatory bowel disease is over twice as common in Caucasians than in non-Caucasians and four times as common in Jews as in non-Jews. Since the 1950s, there has been a steady, remarkable increase in the incidence of Crohn's disease in the United States.

Anatomy and Physiology

Crohn's disease is a bowel disorder involving inflammation of the entire wall of the small and large intestine. When confined to the lower portion of the small bowel, it is called regional enteritis; involvement of the colon is sometimes called granulomatous colitis.

Symptoms and Diagnosis

The signature of Crohn's symptoms includes pain in the lower abdomen (usually the right side), anorexia, flatulence, malaise, and weight loss. It is punctuated by episodes of diarrhea and often accompanied by mild fever, loss of appetite, weight loss, and a general feeling of malaise or being unwell. Examination often reveals tenderness in the lower right abdomen. X-ray study of the intestines usually confirms definite abnormalities in the terminal ileum (the last one-third of the small bowel) as it empties into the colon. The risk for colon cancer increases modestly after having the disease for several decades.

Crohn's disease leads to a distorted pattern of assimilation of nutrients from the affected segments of small bowel. The levels of proinflammatory prostaglandins, including the extremely potent leukotrienes, are greatly elevated in the wall of the affected bowel. Abnormal bacteria and yeast organisms often overgrow the small intestine, creating secondary problems. Protein is not properly absorbed, and this leads to weight loss in many cases. Due to losses in diarrhea or poor assimilation through the inflamed mucosal lining, it is common to have low levels of:

- Vitamins A, E, and C
- Vitamin D
- Vitamin K
- B-complex vitamins; (a) B-12 is deficient 50 percent of the time; repletion may require injections; (b) folic acid is deficient 25–65 percent of the time; repletion may require injections
- Magnesium, potassium, calcium
- Iron; levels drop due to bleeding from inflamed mucosal lesions
- Trace minerals; zinc is deficient in 40 percent of Crohn's patients

Conventional Treatment

Drug treatment is the conventional standard of care for Crohn's. The most common drugs prescribed are sulfasalazine (a sulfur-containing antibiotic) and cortisone. Sulfasalazine helps control abnormal bacteria, and cortisone has a marked anti-inflammatory effect. Both these drugs have undesirable side effects. The anemia of Crohn's is addressed by increasing iron intake, and extra protein in the diet opposes the typical weight loss. Severe progression of the disease sometimes requires surgery to remove the most severely affected segments of small and/or large bowel and to manage the tendency for fistulas to develop (a fistula is an abnormal passage connecting the bowel to the outside or to other bowel segments;

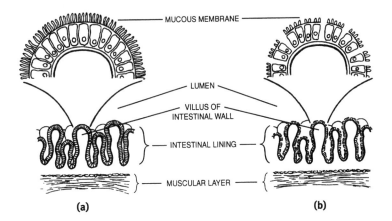

Small Intestinal Wall
(a) Normal Wall
(b) Damaged and Leaky Wall

MUCOUS MEMBRANE

LUMEN

VILLUS OF
INTESTINAL WALL

INTESTINAL LINING

MUSCULAR LAYER

(a)   (b)

fistulas to the skin drain infected secretions to the outside). It is estimated, however, that 20 percent of untreated patients experience a spontaneous remission in
any given year. In one study, 55 percent of patients receiving a placebo achieved
remission, of whom 21 percent remained in remission at the end of the second
year of the study; in another study, only 4 percent of those who had been given
prior treatment with cortisone remained in remission after two years.

Risk Factors and Causes

The causes of Crohn's disease include:

- Genetic predisposition (20–40 percent of patients)
- Possible immunological abnormalities
- The influence of stress
- Possible infectious causes
- Dietary factors

The presence of antibodies to a bacterium, Klebsiella, is found in a high percentage of Crohn's patients and patients who have rheumatoid spondylitis of the
spine (a spinal arthritis). In fact, men with Crohn's are more prone to develop
spondylitis. Some authorities believe these facts favor an infectious cause of both
diseases. Crohn's is also associated with arthritis of other joints—wrists, knees,
and ankles. Inflammatory skin nodules and canker sores are also more common in
Crohn's patients.

Crohn's disease and ulcerative colitis are extremely rare in primitive societies
not consuming calorie-dense, highly refined diets. This dietary influence is
thought to be substantial. The diets of people who subsequently develop Crohn's

disease have been documented to contain substantially less fruit, vegetables, and fiber and to include far more sugar and refined flour foods compared to those who remain healthy. One study found that the amount of sugar consumed by those who later got Crohn's disease was twice that of healthy matched controls.

Holistic Treatment and Prevention

Functional testing includes a comprehensive digestive stool analysis, permeability tests, and a search for parasites in a specially equipped laboratory.

Physical Health Recommendations

Diet

The predisposing low fiber, highly refined carbohydrate intake is thought to be very important, so the diet of choice removes sugar and refined flour and adds fiber from vegetable, whole grain, and fruit sources. You should greatly reduce or eliminate meat and dairy products to diminish levels of leukotrienes and inflammation. Increase intake of fish (for example salmon, halibut, or mackerel), with two to four servings each week.

Vitamins, Minerals, and Supplements

The recommended high potency multivitamin-mineral combination supplementation, in combination or separately, includes the following:

- *Vitamin A*, 50,000 I.U. daily during the acute phase reactivation of disease
- *Vitamin C*, one to two grams daily; magnesium, potassium, and calcium ascorbate in Ester C forms is often less irritating to the bowel
- *Mixed bioflavonoids*, 500–2,000 mg daily
- *Quercetin*, 0.5–1 gram three to four times daily
- *Vitamin E*, 400–800 I.U. daily if not included in the multivitamin; the natural d-alpha form has advantages
- *Folic acid*; poor absorption from the inflamed intestine (oral doses 1–20 mg daily)
- *Vitamin B-12*, 200 mg orally per day
- Additional *zinc* (as zinc picolinate), 50 mg daily
- *Magnesium*, 300 mg twice daily; magnesium glycinate has better bowel tolerance
- *L-glutamine*, three grams twice daily
- *Fish oil* reduces the frequency of relapses by 40–50 percent (two to three grams twice a day) or *flaxseed oil* (one tablespoonful daily).

- Adequate *protein*, which may be conveniently supplied in *amino acid* supplements that are derived from foods unlikely to be offending (milk and wheat), and requiring no digestion before assimilation; rice protein concentrate will meet this need with very low chance of allergic reaction (UltraClear Sustain, from Metagenics in Eugene, Oregon).

- *Gamma oryzanol*, 100 mg three to four times daily (derived from rice bran oil)

Recognition of possible *food sensitivities* is addressed with the institution of low antigenic diets (elemental diets) composed of a small number of foods unlikely to be offending. This dietary approach has generally met with great success. Studies show that elemental diets lead to improvement within three to four weeks, faster than the usual response to corticosteroids given at a time of recurrent acute symptoms; the improvement is sustained over longer periods of time compared to shorter remissions from cortisone treatment. Once offending foods are identified through an elimination and rechallenge procedure, they need to be omitted, often indefinitely.

Herbs

Commonly used herbs include *echinacea* (purple coneflower), *marshmallow root*, *wild indigo*, *ginger*, *Germanium maculatum*, *goldenseal*, *poke root*, and *slippery elm*. These are often combined in a traditional naturopathic formulation, Robert's Formula, and its modification, Bastyr's Formula. It is advisable to consult a health professional for a balanced program using these botanicals.

Mental and Emotional Health Recommendations. Stress plays a role in Crohn's as it does with most of the diseases in this book. You may wish to reread sections of chapter 3 to refresh your mind about the effective options for managing stress-related illness. All inflammatory conditions and immune responses improve with the resetting of a lower baseline activity level for the sympathetic nervous system that follows consistent practice of *relaxation skills*, *biofeedback*, and *meditation*. We cannot emphasize it enough: the mind is infinitely more powerful than we can imagine.

The complications of Crohn's—liver, skin, spine and joint problems, probably stemming from the abnormal assimilation of proteins due to the disease itself, need to be recognized and treated.

INFLAMMATORY BOWEL DISEASE — ULCERATIVE COLITIS

Prevalence

Two hundred to four hundred thousand people in the United States are thought to have ulcerative colitis. The incidence rate is 100 to 150 cases per one hundred thousand people. Onset is typical between the ages of 15 and 35. It strikes women more often than men, Caucasians more often than blacks, and those of Jewish descent more often than others. Like Crohn's, it is rarely seen in indigenous peoples.

Anatomy and Physiology

Ulcerative colitis is a chronic inflammatory disease of the large bowel (colon), occasionally affecting the lower part of the small bowel. The inflammation of the bowel wall is so intense that sections may be eroded, leading to ulcer-like erosions of the bowel lining surface.

Symptoms and Diagnosis

Ulcerative colitis announces its presence with bloody diarrhea, low abdominal cramps, loss of appetite, and sometimes fever. Malaise and weight loss are common. The highly inflamed and ulcerated surface bleeds extremely easily. A common pattern ensues in which phases of partial healing are interrupted by acute relapses. Physical examination reveals abdominal tenderness and often anal abnormalities, including hemorrhoids, fissures, fistulas, and sometimes abscesses. Colon X-rays demonstrate a typical moth-eaten, ulcerative mucosal pattern, and fiberoptic sigmoidoscopic examination usually reveals grossly inflamed mucosal patches with ulcerations.

Conventional Treatment

Medications are used to slow the diarrhea and suppress the inflammation:

- Azulfidine (sulfasalazine), a prescription sulfa derivative, often works well, especially in mild to moderate stages of the disease. It should not be taken by anyone allergic to sulfas.

- Olsalazine (Dipentum) is a salicylate derivative that can help maintain improvement once healing is underway.

- Instillation of retention enemas of short-chain fatty acids (sodium-acetate, -propionate, and -butyrate) done on a daily or twice daily basis is helpful.

- Combinations of aspirin and cortisone enemas have been beneficial.

- Nicotine skin patches have also been used (ulcerative colitis, for unexplained reasons, is less common in smokers).

- Low dose injected heparin (an anticoagulant) and oral sulfasalazine led to remission in eight of nine patients with poorly controlled ulcerative colitis in a 1995 study.

- Corticosteroids (prednisone) are given in very large doses to suppress the inflammation in more severe disease. The dosages of prednisone or other potent synthetic cortisone derivatives are then slowly tapered to avoid the long-term serious consequences of steroids in the body—"side effects." These effects include:

  - Suppression of the immune system

  - Overgrowth of yeast organisms in the intestine

  - Osteoporosis

  - Weight gain that spares the limbs

  - Moon-faced appearance

  - Development of prominent blood vessels in the skin

  - Wasting of muscle protein

  - Promotion of diabetes

  - Less of neuronal connections in areas of the brain

Rarely, all medical measures fail, and surgical removal of the colon or diseased portions of it become necessary life-saving measures.

Patients who have relapsing ulcerative colitis for 15 to 20 years are at a higher risk for the development of cancer of the bowel and rectum and need regular assessment because of this.

Risk Factors and Causes

The cause of ulcerative colitis is currently unknown; the following are possible contributors:

- Genetic factors.

- Infectious agents (numerous theories point the finger at viruses or bacteria).

- Nutritional factors. The inflammatory bowel diseases are seen scarcely, if at all, in indigenous cultures on whole food diets.

- Food allergies. Food sensitivity as a cause is usually not mentioned in conventional textbooks. The consistent substantial improvement with treatment by elimination and exclusion diets, or parenteral feedings (intravenous nutrition only with nothing by mouth) lends great credulity to this possibility.

- Immunity. The immune theory classifies ulcerative colitis as an autoimmune disease similar to rheumatoid arthritis and lupus erythematosus. Anticolon antibodies have been demonstrated in some studies lending support to this view.

- Psychological mechanisms appear to play a contributory role in this disease.

Carrageenan, a commonly used food stabilizer in nutrition industry, induces ulcerative colitis in guinea pigs. It may exert its damage when combined with the presence of a specific bacterium, Bacteroides vulgatus. The latter is six times more common in ulcerative colitis patients compared to normal healthy controls. *Carrageenan should be avoided in ulcerative colitis patients until further research information on this question emerges.*

Holistic Treatment and Prevention

Comprehensive testing is recommended for the functional status of the intestine and bowel (see under Crohn's disease). If pathogenic organisms (bacteria or parasites) are identified, specific treatment is as follows.

Physical Health Recommendations. Bowel rest in the acute phase of the disease is usually instituted. With severe symptoms, nutrition needs to be supplied by products that yield essentially no fiber residual, reducing the stimulation and work required by the diseased bowel. Examples are UltraClear or UltraClear Sustain by Metagenics (Eugene, OR), or Medipro by Thorne (Sandpoint, ID). In more severe cases of acute onset, intravenous feedings with nothing by mouth for a few days is necessary to sufficiently rest the bowel.

Diet

Caloric malnutrition often occurs because of poor assimilation of nutrients and declining appetite. This is more common when diarrhea is severe; optimum treatment makes use of a higher fiber diet without utilizing wheat bran.

Vitamins, Minerals, and Supplements

High amounts of micronutrient support are necessary in the acute and chronic phases of this disease. A potent, daily, megadose multivitamin-mineral preparation needs to include high amounts of antioxidant *vitamins C, E, D, K,* and *B-12* and *folic acid.* Sulfasalazine and olsalazine, if used long-term, both hasten the loss of folic acid, and extra intake is necessary. *PABA* (para-aminobenzoic acid), a B-complex vitamin manifesting anti-inflammatory and antifibrotic effects, is effective in doses of two grams four times daily. PABA is helpful in a number of autoimmune diseases, including scleroderma and dermatomyositis.

Mineral deficiencies are common in inflammatory bowel disease; anemia and iron deficiency are common because of persistent bleeding; extra losses of calcium, magnesium, potassium, and zinc occur with the diarrhea. A supplement that covers all these likely deficiencies is essential. *Daily* target intake amounts include:

- *Vitamin C* or magnesium-potassium-calcium ascorbate, one to two grams
- *Vitamin E*, 800 I.U.
- *Vitamin D*, 400 I.U.
- *Vitamin K*, 3 mg
- *Vitamin B-12*, 500 mcg
- *Folic acid*, 3–5 mg
- *Quercitin*, one-half to one gram three to four times daily
- *L-glutamine*, three to five grams three times daily for two months, then tapered to three grams twice daily
- *Elemental iron*, 50–100 mg taken with 500 mg of vitamin C and at least 100 I.U. of E for better absorption
- *Zinc picolinate*, 100 mg
- *Calcium*, 500–800 mg
- *Magnesium*, 300–500 mg
- *Potassium*, 500–700 mg
- *Gamma oryzanol*, 100 mg three times daily for four to six weeks

Also included in appropriate supplements are *mixed bioflavonoids*, which have beneficial modifying effects on the course of illness. *Omega-3 fatty acid* supplements (from fish or flaxseed, four to eight grams daily) delay but do not prevent acute flare-ups of the disease.

Partially predigested proteins, easily assimilable amino acid supplements, and low fiber elements are necessary in the acute phase of the disease. Rice protein or hydrolyzed lactalbumin are often tolerated well.

Food elimination protocols have been mentioned in connection with several gastrointestinal problems. When food sensitivity is found to be the central issue, as in some ulcerative colitis patients, and appropriate exclusions from the diet bring great and long-lasting improvement. Occasionally, the elimination of offending foods is *permanently curative*. In general, elimination of dairy products, sugar, and wheat is a likely place to start. Other more commonly found offenders are eggs, corn, cocoa, peanuts, oranges, soy, pork, beef, and chicken. Coffee, although it is a non-food, belongs on the list as well. Following a food elimination protocol is time and effort well spent.

Herbs

Herbal remedies not yet subjected to controlled studies but long in common use include *goldenseal* (two to three capsules four times a day in the acute phase) and Robert's Formula, or its modification Bastyr's Formula, from Eclectic Institute in Sandy, Oregon, or NF Formulas in Wilsonville, Oregon.

In healthy people, the mucous blanket that protects the intestinal surface contains mucins that have been found to be distinctly abnormal in active phases of ulcerative colitis yet normal in remission. Herbs that are helpful in promoting mucus secretion are *deglycyrrhizinated licorice, slippery elm,* and *marshmallow root.*

Biomolecular Options

If dehydroepiandrosterone (DHEA) levels are low, modest replacement doses are helpful, usually 10–20 mg daily for women and 15–25 mg daily for men. Injections of liposomal superoxide dismutase, one of the body's potent antioxidant enzymes, have been reported in one small research project to be helpful in both ulcerative colitis and Crohn's. When corticosteroids are necessary, a lower dose can be used in enema form, prescribed by a physician and made up by a compounding pharmacist.

Mental and Emotional Health Recommendations. Stress. Physicians familiar with many cases of ulcerative colitis see a consistent pattern, with onset often associated with some acutely stressful life event. Large studies have linked recurrences to the stopping of smoking. Why would smoking deter the recurrences of this illness? If the stress theory is accepted, one can theorize that smoking might be outlet for the expression of tension and anxiety; when that outlet is no longer available, the stress-generated responses find their way into expression in the body.

The ultimate answer lies in the incorporation of the excellent techniques that are helpful in nearly all disease: the relaxed state achieved through practice of *biofeedback, meditation, imagery, quiet contemplation, autogenics,* or *progressive relaxation. Hypnotherapy,* too, particularly in conjunction with other methods, can be of enormous assistance.

Extensive early studies of ulcerative colitis patients showed that the conversations of subjects, especially at times of recurrences, are often sprinkled with statements expressing a desire to get rid of their stressful troubles. Ulcerative colitis and diarrhea have been found in numerous studies and clinical experience to be related to high levels of anger, particularly when the patient possesses no socially acceptable skill for the expression of his or her hostility. If you have ulcerative colitis, even the chance of being able to talk about your feelings, without acting them out, may be a novel experience for you.

The *attitude* most often underlying the emotional experience of anger is hostility; indeed, ulcerative colitis patients are found to have tendencies toward hostility, conformity, and rigidity more often than comparison subjects without ulcerative colitis. Ulcerative colitis is also one of the diseases in which the initial episode is often associated with the loss of an important relationship. Appropriate counseling and personal work to help alter the psychological dynamics, attitudes, and worldview under which you are functioning have an enormous payoff, with lessening of symptoms and normalization of bowel function. Clearly, ulcerative colitis is one of the many gastrointestinal dysfunctions that are more than organ-specific problems. These dysfunctions are only local manifestations of a systemic or generalized problem, which has many aspects—mental, emotional, nutritional, hereditary, allergic, neurological, and hormonal. To approach anything resembling a cure frequently requires a comprehensive, holistic approach.

Traditional Chinese medicine, including *acupuncture*, includes inflammatory bowel disease among the problems that it can help. *Homeopathy*, too, with its individualized approach, offers stories of success.

A CASE HISTORY

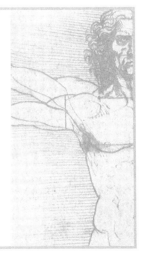

In a case history reported by stress pioneers Harold Wolff, Stewart Wolf, and W. J. Grace, a teenage patient had undergone life-preserving surgery to remove most of the colon after a long period of ultimately unsuccessful medical treatment for severe ulcerative colitis. The colostomy site had healed, leaving a rim of remaining colonic mucosa on the abdominal wall visible from the outside. During recovery in the hospital, on making a home visit and finding that a younger sister had been allowed to take over his own bedroom, the patient, with no visible or verbal acknowledgement of emotional distress, experienced a full-blown attack immediately, with intense visible mucosal inflammation and massive diarrhea. Part of the pathological picture in this disease is the intense energy of unexpressed emotion, which, when unresolved, manifests in the colon.

DIVERTICULAR DISORDERS

Prevalence

Authorities believe that one in ten people below the age of 40 have diverticula, increasing to one out of two in the over-60 group. The great majority have no symptoms. About 20 percent of patients with diverticula will develop the inflammation and infection known as diverticulitis.

Anatomy and Physiology

Diverticula are marble-sized pouches, small appendix-like protrusions of colon mucosa that herniate their way through weaknesses in the muscular layer of the colon. The resulting sac may, on occasion, become inflamed, infected, or twisted to cut off its own blood supply or may even perforate (like a perforated appendix); the condition is then called diverticulitis. Diverticula, once formed, do not disappear.

Symptoms and Diagnosis

The presence of a diverticulum is not usually accompanied by any symptoms. When inflamed (diverticulitis), diverticula give symptoms of localized pain, usually in the left lower abdomen, cramping, alteration of bowel habit, and a sense of fullness in the lower abdomen. On examination, tenderness is present; if severe infection or perforation are present, fever is common.

Conventional Treatment

Diverticulosis and diverticulitis were formerly treated by placing all patients on low fiber diets, because of concern that food particles, including small seeds, could be wedged into the diverticula themselves, provoking complications. With more understanding of the underlying causes of diverticular formation, the pendulum has swung, and high fiber diets are now standard recommendations. The predisposing *constipation* is addressed by all the dietary measures mentioned under that topic above. A high fiber diet with thoroughly masticated food is introduced very gradually after an acute episode. Antispasmodic drugs are used for relief of cramping symptoms (Bentyl, Donnatal, Levsin). Surgery for complications or removal of segments of the colon affected by multiple diverticula is necessary in some instances. There is a slight increase in the risk of cancer in people with longstanding, persistent diverticulitis.

Risk Factors and Causes

The risk factor most often associated with diverticulosis is a tendency toward constipation. When the left colon does not empty regularly, the colonic contractions work extra hard in attempting to propel the stool content forward; because the stool is poorly hydrated (partially because there is not enough fiber to attract sufficient water), it becomes hard, and contractions become ineffective. Excessive pressure within the colon is generated by these nonpropulsive contractions and "blows out" the projection called a diverticulum, usually less than one-half inch in size. The incidence of diverticulosis in persons consuming a low fiber diet is three times the incidence in those consuming a high fiber diet. A mild genetic predisposition to development of diverticula has also been observed.

Holistic Treatment and Prevention

Management of constipation is emphasized. This is the prevention as well as the treatment. Complications can nearly always be prevented by careful attention to these details.

Diet

In treatment of diverticulitis, holistic physicians, once an acute episode has passed, recommend a high fiber diet, with adequate water intake, and meticulous attention to thorough and complete mastication of all hard particulate portions of foods and seeds. Good foods to start adding after the acute episode include papaya, yams, bananas, and steamed carrots. The building of a full-strength immune system with superb nutrition, adequate supplements, and other measures, including exercise, also reduces the risks of complications.

Supplements

- *Acidophilus* and *bifidus*, twice daily
- *L-glutamate*, four to eight mgs daily
- *Gamma oryzanol*, 100 mg 3 times daily

Herbs

- *Slippery elm bark*, two capsules three times daily
- *Goldenseal*, two capsules every two hours during the day
- *Alfalfa tablets*, three to four pills before each meal
- *Aloe vera juice*, two ounces daily
- *Slippery elm* and *marshmallow teas*

PEPTIC ULCER

Prevalence

Ulcers are very common; an estimated 10 percent of the population has had or will have an ulcer in their lifetime. The ratio of men to women is about four to one. One hundred years ago the ratio was three to one, women over men. Duodenal ulcers (in the first part of the small bowel) are four times as common as gastric ulcers (stomach).

Anatomy and Physiology

The term *peptic ulcer* refers to ulcerations, or canker sore–like erosions, usually less than one-third inch in diameter, developing in the lining of the stomach or first part of the small intestine just beyond the stomach. The defect in the mucosal surface is the result of excessive erosive action of stomach acid and pepsin, a major digestive enzyme secreted by the lining cells of the stomach. The lining of the stomach is ordinarily naturally protected against ulcerative erosions.

Gastric ulcers can occur in any portion of the stomach, a pouch-like tube that, on being emptied and flattened out, has an average length of ten inches and width of four inches. Gastric ulcers are occasionally the earliest sign of gastric cancer, whereas duodenal ulcers are almost never cancerous. Duodenal ulcers occur in the first portion of the duodenum, the upper and much narrower small intestine beyond the stomach.

Symptoms and Diagnosis

The major typical symptom of duodenal ulcer is the onset of gnawing or burning upper abdominal pain about an hour after eating. Early on, ulcer pain usually first makes itself known later in the day or at night, rather than in the morning. The often associated increased acidity may also give symptoms of heartburn—the burning feeling behind the breastbone resulting from regurgitation of acid content upward into the esophagus. Patients with ulcer usually experience prompt relief with eating or with the ingestion of antacid tablets or liquid.

The diagnosis of a gastric or duodenal ulcer is made on the basis of the typical history, and confirmed by an upper G-I X-ray study or by endoscopy, the passage of a flexible tube down the throat and esophagus enabling the operator to visualize the lining of the stomach and duodenum. Endoscopy or special blood tests can confirm the presence or absence of a commonly found bacterium Helicobacter pylori. In the last ten years, a significant majority of ulcer patients have been found to carry this organism in the lining of the lower stomach. It is not totally clear, however, whether the presence of the organism is wholly causative or whether this organism may be only an innocent bystander making a modest contribution to the problem.

Conventional Treatment

The conventional management of ulcer disease mainly encompasses medications, with surgery for complications. The major classes of drugs are:

- Antacids
- H2 antagonist acid blockers
- Gastric coating agents
- Proton-pump (acid-pump) inhibitors
- Antibiotics for H. pylori treatment

The most commonly used antacids are Maalox, Mylanta, Amphojel, Digel, and Aludrox; disadvantages of these aluminum-containing medications include the displacing of calcium in the body and possible aluminum toxicity, including accumulation of aluminum in the brain, thought by some to contribute to Alzheimer's dementia. Other antacids include Tums and calcium carbonate (may cause acid rebound), Rolaids, Alka-Seltzer, and Bromo-Seltzer (contain sodium that may add a load on the heart and affect blood pressure).

Conventional treatment also utilizes drugs that block acid secretion (H2 antagonists, e.g., Zantac, Tagamet, Pepcid, and Axid). These medicines, formerly available only on prescription but now available OTC, are extremely popular. With an active ulcer, relief of symptoms is prompt and healing usually occurs within one to two months. Drawbacks include suppression of acid secretion to the point of hindering digestion, the occurrence of nausea and diarrhea, and the blocking of vital nutrient absorption, including vitamin B-12. Unusual side effects include liver damage, headaches, depression, impotence, and breast enlargement in men. Cimetidine (Tagamet) may also reduce immune defenses.

Carafate (sucralfate) is a prescription medicine that promotes ulcer healing by coating and protecting the ulcer surface.

Omeprazole (Prilosec) is the first drug of a new class of medicines called proton-pump or acid-pump inhibitors. It is a powerful inhibitor of gastric secretion and recommended for only short-term use of not more than a month due to potential side effects.

Antibiotic treatment for H. pylori reduces the incidence of relapse and lengthens the time between episodes. A higher eradication rate is achieved when antibiotic treatment is combined with bismuth subsalicylate, found in Pepto-Bismol.

Several decades ago, surgery was commonly done for recurrent and persistent ulcers. Recurrences after surgery were common. The problem with surgery in this disease is similar to that in many situations: *removal of portions of the stomach or bypassing the first part of the duodenum did not alter the underlying causative mechanisms.* The advent of the acid-blocking drugs has greatly reduced the need and enthusiasm for surgery. Today, ulcer disease becomes a surgical necessity only if an ulcer bleeds uncontrollably or perforates or if a gastric ulcer is found to be cancerous.

Risk Factors and Causes

The two major causes of ulcers are:

- Excess acidity from the stomach, overwhelming the normal slightly alkaline condition of the small intestine. Gastric secretions, with a pH of about 2, are potentially extremely corrosive.

- A reduction in the efficiency by which the normal protective mechanisms defend the gastric and duodenal mucosa against ulceration. These mechanisms include (1) the production of large amounts of mucin, which constantly covers the gastric surface like a layer of thin, uncooked egg white, as well as (2) the ability of the stomach to regenerate its entire lining within hours due to a very rapid regeneration of surface cells.

Among the factors that compromise nature's protection of the lining of the stomach and duodenum are:

- Intake of aspirin and NSAIDs (Motrin, Advil, ibuprofen, Indocin, Clinoril, Feldene, Relafen, Tolectin, Voltaren). Aspirin is a gastric and intestinal mucosal irritant and frequently causes damage and small amounts of bleeding.

- Cortisone derivatives (prednisone, prednisolone, Medrol) also reduce the resistance of the gastric mucosa.

- Coffee, caffeine (soft drinks), and alcohol also contribute to this loss of protection.

- Fried and highly spiced foods and chili powder are problematic.

- Cow's milk and its derivatives cause a marked increase in acidity in many people.

- Smoking reduces the secretion of pancreatic bicarbonates, which neutralize acid as it enters the duodenum, and accelerates the dumping of stomach contents into the duodenum. Smoking is highly associated with the incidence of ulcers, less favorable response to treatment, and doubled mortality from complications.

- Deficiencies of nutrients (see holistic treatment on page 284).

- Stress is strongly related to the risk of ulcer development. In fact, a particularly aggressive and ominous type of "stress ulcer" not uncommonly develops in patients undergoing life-threatening medical or surgical emergencies. It is common enough that physicians caring for such patients in an intensive care unit usually anticipate such an event and take steps to prevent it. The opinion of many authorities notwithstanding, the tension induced by significant and unmanaged stress is almost a universal factor in causing ulcers. The life history of patients with ulcers is often one of recurrences alternating with healing and disappearance of symptoms. Added stress often heralds a recurrence.

Ulcers may manifest complications, including:

- Sudden searing pain from perforation (similar to the perforation of an infected appendix)
- Mild bleeding manifested by dark or black, tarry-looking stools
- Massive bleeding manifested by vomiting moderate to large amounts of blood, which may have the appearance of coffee grounds. Any of these complications constitutes an emergency and must be handled as such.

Holistic Treatment and Prevention

Careful attention is paid to underlying causes and contributors to ulcer disease.

Physical Health Recommendations

Lifestyle Routines

- *Reduction of intake of drugs* contributing to ulcers. For example, over 50 percent of all bleeding ulcers requiring hospitalization are associated with the taking of NSAIDs. Less toxic alternatives are often available for the management of musculoskeletal pain and arthritis, making it possible to eliminate or reduce the need for NSAIDs (see chapter 8).
- *Smoking abatement* is assertively approached in a holistic manner, utilizing biofeedback, cognitive therapy, exercise, and acupuncture.
- *Overuse of alcohol*, often a problem in ulcer disease, is addressed with some of the same approaches that help control smoking. Part of that approach is to emphasize control and reduction of intake as a way of honoring the needs of your body; it is a manifestation of loving yourself.

Diet, Vitamins, Minerals, and Supplements

There is persuasive evidence that free radicals play a role in H. pylori–infected ulcer patients; increased antioxidant intake is a logical step in treatment. Nutrients that are helpful are:

- *Vitamin A*, 50,000 I.U. daily for treatment of an active ulcer and 10,000–25,000 I.U. daily for maintenance
- *Zinc*, 30 mg daily balanced with copper, two mg daily
- *Vitamin C* inhibits H. pylori growth in the test tube (one to three grams daily)
- *Lactobacillus acidophilus* inhibits H. pylori growth
- *Vitamin E*, 400–800 I.U. daily
- *Vitamin B-complex* (50 mg of each element) is also important
- *High fiber diet* reduces risks of recurrence about 50 percent compared to recurrences during previous low fiber diet
- Intake of *omega-3 oils* prevents NSAID-induced ulcers in animals
- Feeding of large amounts of bananas or banana plantain to animals prevents and heals ulcers. In humans, low intake of *potassium* has predicted a higher ulcer incidence; this may explain why bananas, containing potassium, yield positive benefits
- *Bioflavonoids* exhibit antiulcer activity; one gram of *catechin* five times daily reduces histamine levels and inhibits H. pylori
- *Cabbage juice* has been established in older research as helpful in ulcer healing (prepared from a blender, one to two pints four times daily). The most effective active ingredient is thought to be *glutamine*, an amino acid, which may also be used in doses of one and a half to three grams daily in divided doses

Food Sensitivities

The long tradition of utilizing milk and milk products in ulcer treatment has ceased in the light of evidence that increasing milk intake is associated with increasing the risk of ulcers. Research from the 1940s and 1950s established milk and other foods—chicken, wheat, corn, eggs, beef, tomato, coffee, tea, oranges, avocados, peaches, potatoes, barley, chocolate, grapes, peanuts, and spices—as potential allergenic or sensitizing agents in gastric and duodenal irritation. In 30 patients in whom milk sensitivity had been established by elimination and reprovocation, the application of a few drops of milk to the gastric lining introduced through an endoscope resulted in immediate swelling, erosions, and bleeding in all 30. Persons with recurrent ulcerations deserve a food elimination trial and identification of offending foods, if any are found. A nutritional plan omitting sensitizing foods is highly successful. Failing to eliminate food offenders *almost always results in continuing recurrences.*

Herbs

- *Deglycyrrhizinated licorice* (DGL) is highly successful and has been shown to have comparable effects to the H2 antagonist drugs (Tagamet, for example) in both duodenal and gastric ulcer. Anti–H. pylori activity has been shown as well, possibly explaining the lower recurrence rate with DGL compared to H2 antagonist drugs. Dosage: two 380-mg tablets three to four times daily on an empty stomach, 20 minutes before meals. The tablets should be held in the mouth for a few minutes to provide full activation by saliva. Lower doses may be used for maintenance and prevention of recurrence. The tendency for licorice to raise blood pressure is bypassed by removal of the glycyrrhizin.

- *Ginger* strengthens the mucosa of the upper gastrointestinal tract. It can be prepared as a strong tea of the blended fresh root; most health food stores carry 250-mg capsules of powdered root to be taken three to four times daily.

- *Bastyr's Formula* (modified Robert's Formula), though relatively unresearched, has a long tradition of use in naturopathic settings and a long history as a homeopathic remedy.

- Ayurvedic botanical remedies and other botanicals are used, including a mixture of *slippery elm* and *goldenseal* powder mixed in a 2:1 ratio, two capsules three to four times a day.

- *Aloe vera juice*, one to two tablespoons three to four times a day, also has a tradition of being helpful.

- *Grapefruit seed extract*, two capsules before meals for six weeks following antibiotic treatment for H. pylori tends to reduce recurrences.

Mental and Emotional Health Recommendations. Initiating a systematic stress management program is often found to be the essential element in affecting a cure. Learning *relaxation through biofeedback or meditation*, using *imagery* to modify the competitive striving often found to be present, getting regular *aerobic physical exercise*, and establishing a pattern of *sound sleep* are all important components. A perfectionism pattern frequently found in association with duodenal ulcer can be modified with action-oriented counseling incorporating insight, practice, and conscious rehearsal of new behaviors.

Spiritual and Social Health Recommendations. Since studies show the incidence and severity of ulcers to be highly correlated with a lack of positive life events, strategizing ways of enhancing loving self-treatment, improving relationships, and finding social support is important. The quality of the relationship with your physician guiding the treatment also bears on the outcome. One study in patients with bleeding ulcers found that positive results were three times as common when a medication was given with confidence and positive enthusiasm by a caring physician compared to the offering of medication by a nurse without authority or enthusiasm; in reality, both "medications" were placebos. The *belief* in the efficacy of your treatment greatly enhances the potential for achieving healing.

The upper abdominal organs, including the stomach, pancreas, duodenum, and liver, are related to the solar plexus and to issues of personal power, according to the insightful observations of medical intuitive Caroline Myss. She emphasizes that disruptions of normal function in these organs relate to issues of self-responsibility, self-esteem, oversensitivity to criticism, and fear of rejection. These observations correlate exceedingly well with conventional psychosomatic research mentioned earlier.

Professional Care Therapies

Acupuncture has success in treatment, utilizing acupoints associated with stress, anxiety, and stomach energy.

Homeopathic remedies include Nux vomica for the type-A person who gets heartburn following overindulgent eating; Ignatia for a tendency to eat foods that cause symptoms; Bryonia for after-meal tenderness worsened by movement; and Chamomilla for indigestion following anger and irritability.

The holistic interaction between you and your attending physician needs to address all these issues and underlying causes as completely as possible. Like most other conditions, ulcer is a symptom of imbalance and lack of harmony within your being, manifested locally in the stomach or duodenum. The empowerment that comes from this work can graduate you to a more comfortable individuality, contacting an inner sense of life purpose, enhancing realistic self-appreciation, and identifying with deeply held values and principles.

GALLSTONES AND GALL BLADDER DISEASE

Prevalence

Gallstones and gallbladder disease are common in Western cultures. In the United States, autopsy surveys confirm gallstones in 8 percent of men and 20 percent of women over the age of 40. About 65 percent of people who develop gallstones never have any symptoms. Estimates of the number of surgical gall bladder removals done for gallstones in the United States each year range from three hundred thousand to slightly under one million.

Anatomy and Physiology

The gallbladder is a pear-shaped sac with average dimension of three inches by one to one and a half inches, tapering to a narrow neck with a diameter of one-quarter inch. The neck connects to the common bile duct, the structure that provides a channel by which bile produced by the liver reaches the small intestine (duodenum). Bile is a moderately thick brownish liquid containing bile salts—to help with fat digestion—as well as toxins, cholesterol, and substances processed by the liver for elimination through the intestines. As bile is secreted by the liver, it is stored in the "side pocket" gallbladder between meals. When food containing fat reaches the stomach, a reflex causes the gallbladder to contract to release the stored bile into the common bile duct, which releases it to the intestine.

This healthy function may be disrupted by the formation of gallstones in the gallbladder. Gallstones consist of mixtures of cholesterol, calcium, and bile pigments. A combination of decreased bile salts or increased cholesterol leads to the formation of free cholesterol (which is not soluble in water), precipitating as solid particles that develop into stones of varying size. When stones become larger than the size of the neck of the gallbladder, they obstruct the release of bile from the gallbladder and announce their presence with pain and other symptoms.

Symptoms and Diagnosis

The presence of gallstones in the gallbladder duct (bile duct) causes pain, inflammation, indigestion, and nausea. The pain is typically in the right upper aspect of the abdomen, directly over the liver/gallbladder area, and usually has its onset after consumption of food containing fat. Pain may also be referred to the right upper aspect of the back and right shoulder. A vast majority of gallbladder system disease is associated with stones. Very rarely, pressure generated by the gallbladder's attempts to expel a stone through the duct can result in rupture, which constitutes a surgical emergency. Confirmation of the suspected diagnosis of gallstones is made by ultrasound examination. X-rays may reveal the presence of stones containing calcium, and X-ray dye studies are necessary to demonstrate noncalcified stones.

Conventional Treatment

Once the diagnosis has been confirmed, three choices face the conventional physician:

- Surgery
- Medical treatment—"watchful waiting."
- Dissolving of stones with medicines

When attacks of gallbladder disease recur, surgery to remove the gallbladder has been the predominant recommendation. Surgery has been greatly modified in recent years with the advent of laparoscopic approaches that allow for removal of the gallbladder through a very small incision, speeding convalescence and shortening hospitalization time. Disadvantages of surgery are:

1. A very small risk of operative complications

2. The 5 percent risk of incomplete removal of all stones at surgery, including those in the common bile duct

3. The significant incidence of re-formation of stones in the common bile duct weeks, months, or years after surgery (7–27 percent in five years). Symptoms of recurrent stones in the common duct (postcholecystectomy syndrome) are very similar to the symptoms of the original problem of stones in the gallbladder. This complication again shows that the *surgery does not alter the underlying process creating the presence of stones.*

There has been a shift in the philosophy of gallbladder disease management over the last decade with the realization that most patients with gallstones can be managed nonsurgically. Medical management—what is called "watchful waiting"—is becoming more acceptable; the occurrence of an obstructed gallbladder with imminent danger of rupture is quite rare. Conventional medical measures emphasize:

- A low fat diet
- Weight reduction
- Initiatives to lower cholesterol
- Maintaining adequate hydration
- Medications for relief of pain at times of recurrent attacks

Treatment with Actigall (ursodeoxycholic acid), a stone-dissolving drug, has met with only modest (30 percent) success. The drug is expensive, can be used only for non–calcium-containing stones, requires months of treatment, and has a 50 percent recurrence rate within five years.

Risk Factors and Causes

Risk factors for gallstones include:

- Being female
- Being of northern European or Native American descent

- Being over the age of 30

- Consuming a high fat, low fiber diet

- Having coexisting alcoholic cirrhosis

- Infection with the liver fluke (in the Orient)

- Consuming a high intake of sugars and low intake of calcium

- Low gastric acid levels; one excellent study showed deficient stomach acidity in 50 percent of gallstone patients

- Being significantly overweight

- Participating in weight loss programs increases risk. During weight loss, bile acid formation decreases, allowing cholesterol in the bile to become less soluble, increasing crystal and stone formation

- Excessive sunbathing (Caucasians). Compared to sun avoiders, the risk for gallstones in Caucasian sunbathers is doubled, with risk increasing to *26 times greater for those who have a history of always sunburning.* This may relate to altered calcium metabolism secondary to higher than normal amounts of vitamin D generated in the skin by the sun exposure

- Certain drugs are also problematic:

  1. Oral contraceptive agents increase gallstone risk two to three times.

  2. Post-menopausal hormone replacement drugs increase the incidence.

  3. Clofibrate and gemfibrozil used to lower cholesterol carry a moderate to high risk for gallstone formation due to higher excretion of cholesterol in the bile.

Holistic Treatment and Prevention

Prevention is more easily accomplished than curative treatment. Regular aerobic physical exercise has recently been reported to reduce the incidence of gallstones 20 percent below the levels seen in sedentary persons.

Diet
Persons on a high fiber, low fat, high vegetable and fruit diet have a significantly lower incidence of gallstones. Besides increasing the bile acid production to keep cholesterol more soluble, fiber reduces the absorption of deoxycholic acid, which also reduces the solubility of cholesterol. Avoiding a high intake of sugar decreases your risk of precipitation of gallstones.

Elimination Diets
Any individual foods that are found to cause symptoms need to be avoided. Dr. J. C. Breneman found in the 1960s that a series of his gallbladder patients were to-

tally free of recurrences while on an elimination diet permitting only beef, rye, rice, soybeans, spinach, beets, cherries, peaches, and apricots. On challenge testing, the foods provoking gallbladder symptoms (with the percentage affected) were: eggs (93 percent), pork (64 percent), onion (52 percent), fowl (35 percent), milk (25 percent), coffee (22 percent), oranges (19 percent), corn, beans, and nuts (15 percent), apples and tomatoes (6 percent). Treatment with antihistamines accelerated recovery, giving further impetus to the belief that gallbladder disease has a significant allergic factor. This approach has been highly successful in the hands of holistic physicians.

Vitamins and Supplements

- *Vitamin C*, one to three grams daily improves bile composition and reduces stone formation risk; women taking in high amounts of vitamin C supplements have reduced their risk of stones and the risk of ever needing gallbladder surgery by 25 percent.

- *Vitamin E* is also part of a complete program, since studies have found that low levels of vitamin E cause gallstones in animals.

- *B-complex vitamins* (*choline, folic acid,* and *B-12*) have been shown to have lipotropic activity, decreasing fat deposition in the liver. When used with substances that increase bile secretion (see herbs, page 292), these lipotropic agents increase bile solubility and prompt dissolution rather than formation of stones.

- *Magnesium citrate* or *aspartate*, 500–1,000 mg daily

- *Lecithin* (phosphatidylcholine), 2.4 grams twice daily, or choline 1000 mg daily, both increase the solubility of cholesterol in bile (lecithin contains choline).

- *Methionine*, an essential amino acid, has lipotropic activity.

- *Taurine*—a nonessential amino acid—prevents gallstones in mice by increasing bile acid production and should be tried in humans if gallstones are found, or if there is a strong family history.

- *Hydrochloric acid–pepsin*, ten grams after protein meals.

- *Adequate water* is essential to prevent even mild dehydration from decreasing the solubility of bile salts and increasing the likelihood of stone precipitation. Drink a minimum of six to eight glasses daily.

Herbs

Herbs that increase bile production by the liver (with dosages three times a day) include:

- *Dandelion* (Taraxacum officinale), dried root, four grams
- *Silymarin* (Silybum marianum), 100–200 mg
- *Artichoke* (Cynara scolymus), leaf extract, 500 mg
- *Turmeric* (Curcuma longa), 300 mg
- *Boldo* (Peumus boldo), dried leaves, 250–500 mg

Betaine, a plant derivative, has been shown to have lipotropic activity, decreasing fat deposition in the liver. *Peppermint oil,* five drops three times a day, is helpful in treatment of acute phases. Gallstones may also be dissolved by a combination of *natural plant terpenes* (menthol, menthone, pinene, borneol, cineol, and camphene). One such preparation, *Rowachol,* used alone, achieved dissolution of stones 42 percent of the time, which increased to 73 percent when used with the drug Actigall.

Interest in a *natural flushing* procedure has recently been revived, using the juice of a lemon and a cup of olive oil each morning for several consecutive days. A danger of this procedure is obstruction of the neck of the gallbladder. A recent report confirms numerous small stones in the stools of patients undergoing this procedure, the presence of which was identified by X-rays of the stools themselves.

One additional approach from the folk remedy tradition utilizes a *castor oil pack* applied to the skin over the right abdomen and flank. This procedure, widely applied but essentially unresearched, is used to modify pain and promote healing. A piece of cotton or wool flannel is saturated with pharmacy grade castor oil; this is applied to the affected area and covered with saran wrap and a warm heating pad for half an hour at a time. Alternatively, it can be applied without heating and left in place overnight, secured by snug clothing to keep it in place.

Professional Care Therapies

Classic individualized *homeopathy* and *acupuncture*, especially for pain, may both be helpful.

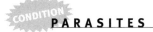

PARASITES

Prevalence

Ten percent of the population is thought to be carrying parasites. Perhaps 60 percent of people in the United States have parasites on at least one occasion in their lives. Twenty-five percent of the world's people are thought to be carrying roundworms. Research has found that randomized examination of blood specimens indicated that 18 percent of Americans had had infections with giardia. Certain parasites have a distinct geographical distribution: roundworms are most common in the Appalachian mountain regions; parasitic worm infestations are more common in the south; Lyme disease is more common in the Northeast and New England; tick-borne disease is more common in the mountainous West and Appalachian mountains; and Native Americans on Arizona reservations have a 50 percent rate of parasitic infection.

Anatomy and Physiology

Parasites are single-cell organisms (protozoa), insects, and worms that invade and feed off the human host, frequently causing harm and disease. Certain parasites can even lead to death. Worms can infect the skin and the gastrointestinal tract, pass into the bloodstream, and even invade the liver, lungs, and other tissues. Parasites may contribute to diseases of the skin, intestine, and bowel, to arthritis and rheumatoid symptoms, chronic fatigue syndrome, and AIDS.

Common parasites include:

- *Protozoa*—amoebae, dientamoebae, giardia, Blastocystis hominis, Trichomonas, Cryptosporidium and Plasmodium (malaria) organisms;
- *Insects*—head, body, and pubic lice, mites, ticks, and fleas;
- *Worms*—pinworms, roundworms, tapeworms, hookworms, whipworms, Guinea worms, and filaria.

Symptoms and Diagnosis

The symptoms of parasitic infestation vary, depending on the invading organism and the body organs involved.

Intestinal Parasites. Chronic gastrointestinal complaints with bloating, diarrhea, and a tendency toward allergies not otherwise explained deserve a careful investigation for parasites. Acute phase symptoms from a number of parasitic infections can compromise immunity and lead to malnutrition and low assimilation of vitamins and variations in blood sugar levels.

- *Giardia.* Persistent diarrhea in children suggests a need for careful checking for giardia; accompanying symptoms include rashes, hives, and food sensitivity reactions. Up to 30 percent of people with chronic fatigue syndrome accompanied by depression have been found to have giardia infections.
- *Amoebae.* Acute amoebic infections often lead to anorexia, nausea, weight loss, malaise, fevers, and night sweats. Amoebae can migrate into lung and liver tissues and can simulate most of the symptoms of ulcerative colitis.
- *Pinworms.* In children, adults, and the elderly, the most common sign of pinworms is itching of the anal area.

The diagnosis of intestinal parasites is not easily accomplished. Stool samples for suspected intestinal parasites must be carefully collected for laboratory investigation, with multiple specimens submitted and sent to a laboratory whose personnel are especially trained in parasitology. Many local laboratories do not specialize in these procedures and find parasites significantly less often than laboratories with a special interest in parasitology. Great Smokies Laboratory of Asheville, North Carolina, and Diagnos-Techs in Kent, Washington, are examples. This meticulous search is a requirement for any intestinal condition or major health problem not satisfactorily explained and successfully treated by routine tests and therapy. In suspected giardiasis, since stool examinations often miss the diagnosis, physicians can order giardia antigen tests, which measure the quantity of antibody synthesized by the immune system in the presence of the organism. A high giardia antigen level significantly raises the index of suspicion.

Skin Parasites

- *Worm* infestations can cause skin deterioration of the soles of the feet, anorexia, weight loss, and anemia.
- *Head lice* cause itching of the scalp; the crab louse infests human hair of the pubic and armpit areas; these lice can carry the infectious organisms causing typhus and relapsing fever.
- The *scabies* organism (itch mite) burrows into the outer layers of smooth skin, causing intense itching and skin disruption due to persistent scratching.
- The *Trichomonas* organism is a relatively common vaginal invader, causing a thin, milky discharge which can be spread to sexual partners (see chapter 17).

Foreign travel. Persons returning from foreign travel where parasitic exposure is more likely can return home and have no clinical manifestations of infection for a number of years. The malarial parasite is transmitted by infected mosquitoes and is a hazard for foreign travelers and occasionally for those in the southern United States; symptoms of acute infection, including fever and chills, appear within days or weeks.

Conventional Treatment

Once a diagnosis of parasitic infection is made, treatment relies primarily on improved hygiene and appropriate drug treatment. In lice infestation, the hair-bearing areas need to be inspected daily, and the nits of the lice mechanically removed. Nits are loosened by rubbing into the scalp a mix of equal portions of vinegar and rubbing alcohol. Bedding and clothing needs to be washed and changed daily, and personal items like combs should not be shared.

Prescription antiparasitic drugs are the mainstay of treatment.

- Lice are treated with Kwell and Rid Lice Killing shampoos, which contain lindane and pyrethrins/piperonyl butoxide, respectively.
- Kwell and Eurax (active ingredient crotamiton) are prescribed for scabies.
- Mintezol (thiabendazol) and Vermox (mebendazole) are prescribed for pinworms, hookworms, whipworms, and roundworms; Mintezol for threadworms; Atabrine (quinacrine) or Niclocide (niclosamide) for tapeworms; Biltricide (praziquantel) for Schistosomiasis and liver flukes.
- Aralen (chloroquine), Flagyl and Protostat (metronidazole), Humatin (paromomycin), and Yodoxin (iodoquinol) are used for amoebae.
- Atabrine, Vermox, and Flagyl are prescribed for giardia.
- Daraprim (pyrimethaprim) is used in toxoplasmosis.
- Flagyl and Protostat are prescribed in trichomoniasis.
- A variety of drugs is used for the various forms of malaria.

The warning label for Kwell states "Seizures and . . . deaths have been reported after excess dosage." This highlights the problems of potential toxicity from many of these products. Atabrine can cause seizures, albeit rarely, even at normal doses; Yodoxin in high doses can have neurological side effects; Flagyl and Protostat can cause seizures and permanent peripheral nerve damage; Daraprim, used in conjunction with sulfa drugs, can cause seizures and neurogenic side effects, and as a folic acid antagonist, can cause anemia; and prolonged use of Aralen (used for amebiasis extended outside the intestine) can cause seizures, ocular damage and deafness.

Risk Factors and Causes

Parasites may be contracted by:

- Hand-to-mouth contamination, believed to explain the high incidence of pinworms in children
- Consumption of contaminated and uncooked food
- Intake of contaminated water supplies (Cryptosporidia, Blastocystis)
- Intake of animal-contaminated mountain water infested with giardia (hikers and backpackers)

In general, the spread of parasitic infections is now more common because of increasingly crowded living conditions, a significant factor explaining the high incidence of roundworm infections the world over. Dientamoebae and giardia have been found in children and staff in day care centers. A high rate of parasitic infestation exists in Native Americans living on reservations. Consumption of uncooked ethnic foods such as sushi and sashimi increases the risk of contraction of parasites that would otherwise be destroyed in cooking. The infectiousness of Trichinella, the worm prone to infest pork and other meat sources, gives testimony to the wisdom of adequate cooking of these food sources.

Holistic Prevention and Treatment

Emphasis on *hygiene* and *environmental awareness* is an important strategy emphasized in prevention of parasitic infections.

- Since the majority of parasites enter the body through the ingestion of water and food-borne contamination, the cooking of meats until well done is essential.
- Raw meat and fish should be avoided, and they should be cut and trimmed for cooking on a different board from vegetables to avoid cross-contamination.
- Vegetables should be thoroughly rinsed; soaking organic and inorganic vegetables in salted water (one teaspoon per five cups of purified water) for 30 minutes before cooking will also help.
- If any parasites are endemic in the area in which you live, a few drops of grapefruit seed extract can be sprinkled on the vegetables before refrigerating.
- When backpacking and hiking in primitive areas, water from streams should be avoided, treated with iodine tablets, or processed through a fine-pore filter.

- Water sources in emerging nations of South and Central America, Africa, and Asia may be contaminated; bottled water is preferable if available. Reported cases even document the acquisition of parasites from contaminated water sources by merely using it to brush the teeth.

- Since pets are a source of worms and other parasites, they need to be periodically checked and treated or given prophylactic veterinary management. Pets should not lick the face of members of the family nor eat off dishes used by the family.

- As in all infections, proper hygiene and handwashing is a must after using the bathroom or working in the garden and before handling food.

Treatment of parasitic infections includes a recognition that depleted immunity induces a greater susceptibility to parasitic invasion.

Diet
Attention may be directed to deficient stomach acidity (more often found in young children and the aging population), which allows organisms to enter the intestine without being destroyed. Anything compromising the immune system should be addressed. Sugar has such effects and should be reduced or eliminated in a healthy diet. Elimination of dairy products because of the high chance of sensitivity reactions is also warranted.

Vitamins, Minerals, and Supplements
Antioxidants (beta carotene, vitamins E and C), B-complex vitamins, selenium, magnesium, and *zinc* are added to restore and enhance immune function, countering any deficiency that predisposes to susceptibility to parasitic invasion. *Lactobacilli* and *bifidobacteria* as probiotic additions (such as Probioplex Intensive Care, from Metagenics in Eugene, Oregon) also improve the intestinal climate for greater resistance.

Herbs
Herbal therapy may include the following agents with antiparasitic effects:

- Emulsified tablets of *oregano oil,* 50 mg three to four times daily (ADP-Biotics)
- *Garlic oil,* 20 mg three to four times daily; concentrated garlic extracts kill 99 percent of multiplying amoeba organisms in the test tube
- *Artemesia annua* (Chinese wormwood), 500 mg three to four times daily
- *Goldenseal* has both antiparasitic and antibacterial properties; the antiamoebic properties of *berberine,* the most active alkaloid in goldenseal, have been definitively shown in laboratory studies. Animal studies confirm its effectiveness against

the trophozoite stage of liver infestation (the active multiplication stage), destroyed by few other preparations. Berberine is active against giardia; its effectiveness in a children's study was nearly as good as Flagyl with essentially no side effects. Dosage of berberine-containing standardized extracts in tincture form (1:5) is 1½–3 tsp. three times daily.

- *Grapefruit* and other *citrus seed extracts* (Allergy Research, San Leandro, CA) have also been observed in individual case reports to be beneficial; they are extensively used in parasite treatment in foreign countries; grapefruit seed extract and garlic are recommended as prophylaxis during travel abroad.

- *Black walnut tincture* is a traditional remedy—one dropperful three to four times daily.

- *Intestinalis*, one pill twice daily, has significant utility in treating Blastocystis.

Traditional Chinese Medicine treatment for parasites utilizes:

- *Pumpkin seeds* (uncooked) and/or *quisqualis seeds* (roasted), both 10–12 daily.

- *Meliae seeds* and betel nuts are used for resistant infections, combined with a laxative or purgative to empty the intestinal tract regularly.

- Two combinations used for treatment are *Aquilaria 22* and *Artestatin;* the dose for both is three capsules 3 times a day (Health Concerns, Alameda, CA).

- For parasitic skin invasion, ground *torryae seeds* can be mixed with aloe vera gel and applied as a topical ointment.

Ayurvedic practitioners use a variety of herbs:

- For pinworms, one to two *bitter melons* per day, for 7–10 days. This oriental vegetable is cut up and eaten in frequently ingested limited amounts several times a day and mixed with other foods because of its bitterness. The presentation of the small white worms in the stool is some indication of the success of most treatments.

- Roundworms are often treated with *kamila, vidang,* and *embliaribes,* taken as a powder extract twice daily in one of the sweet juices.

- Kamila also has effectiveness for tapeworms.

- For giardia, amoebae, and Cryptosporidium, *bilva, neem,* and *berberine* are used in a combination treatment.

12

Kidney Stones

Prevalence

IT IS THOUGHT that about one-half million adults experience a kidney stone each year in the United States, about two hundred thousand of whom are hospitalized. The lifetime incidence of kidney stones in men is 10 percent, and records indicate that the incidence is increasing. The occurrence in men significantly exceeds that in women; incidence in Caucasians exceeds that in African Americans; and incidence in summer exceeds that in winter. Kidney stones are rare under the age of 30.

Anatomy and Physiology

Kidney stones consist of solid collections of calcium oxalate or calcium phosphate (85 percent) or uric acid (10 percent), which form in the urine collection system of the kidneys. Uric acid stones are more common in gout. Struvite stones (ammonium–magnesium phosphate, 5 percent) occur in patients with chronic urinary infections. The stones may vary from BB size to marble size. Tiny stones pass unnoticed, but larger ones are too large to pass through the ureters, the tubular structures that drain urine to the bladder, and block the flow of urine.

Symptoms and Diagnosis

The increased back pressure applied to the kidney with blockage of a ureter by a stone causes intense, one-sided pain in the back at the level of the lowest ribs. The pain frequently comes in waves. If a stone blocks the ureter close to the bladder, the one-sided pain may also be felt in the lower abdomen and pelvis with radiation into the genital area. Blood may appear in the urine. If infection accompanies the lodging of a stone, fever and chills often result. The diagnosis is confirmed by ultrasound or X-ray dye studies. You may be asked to strain your urine specimens during the acute phase, to "catch" the stone for analysis and identification.

Conventional Treatment

The conventional advice to prevent recurrence in those at risk or those who have had one calcium-containing kidney stone include reduction of calcium intake (milk, supplements). However, calcium restriction augments absorption of oxalate, itself a risk factor for stone formation. Vitamin C supplements are commonly cited as risk factors by conventional authorities with consequent advice to avoid them. In a meticulous review of conventional bias against nutrient treatment of disease, however, J. S. Goodwin and M. R. Tangum found *no research study whatsoever* demonstrating any hazard of vitamin C for kidney stones (published in *Archives of Internal Medicine*, November 1998). High intake of liquids, particularly water, is always advised.

Management of the acute stone incident includes medication for pain, observation to see if the stone will pass, instrumentation through the bladder to "snag" the stone and bring it into the bladder, breaking up the stone with lithotripter treatment (a shock-wave ultrasound treatment applied to the outside of the body), or as a last resort, open laser or conventional surgery to find, break up, or remove the stone.

Risk Factors and Causes

A family history of kidney stones increases your risk. In recurrent stone formers, research shows that the risk of further stones is 50 percent lower in those whose calcium intake was the *highest* versus those in whom it was the lowest; 50 percent lower in those with high potassium intake; 30 percent lower in those with high water intake; and 26 percent lower in those with moderately lower protein intake.

Kidney stones are much more common in:

- Hyperparathyroidism (excessive secretion of calcium-controlling hormone)
- Cushing's syndrome (excess cortisone production)
- Type II diabetics with insulin resistance
- Gout
- Irritable bowel syndrome
- Sarcoidosis
- Diseases that cause bone destruction
- People with recurring urinary infections
- Coppersmiths and workers in battery industries (cadmium)

- Excess intake of vitamin D
- Excessive use of antacids
- Excess weight
- High intake of phosphorous (colas), sodium (salt), sugar
- High intake of animal protein, especially purines (see following)
- High intake of oxalate-containing foods (see following)
- Higher intakes of coffee and tea (caffeine)
- Deficient liquid intake
- Deficient intake of potassium, magnesium *and calcium*
- Deficient intake of vitamins C and B-6

Holistic Treatment and Prevention

Diet

Urinary calcium and oxalate, both tending to induce stone formation, are reduced (40 percent and 50 percent, respectively) with intake of ten grams of fish oil daily. *Magnesium* keeps calcium from precipitating into crystals in the urine and reduces recurrences *85 to 92 percent.* Twenty grams of *rice bran* daily has been shown to reduce stone incidence 84 percent. Recent studies have actually demonstrated a 20 percent reduction in kidney stone risk in men getting one and a half grams of *vitamin C* daily compared to those getting less than 250 mg per day. *Cranberries* in high amounts reduce ionized calcium in the urine 50 percent.

To prevent stone formation or recurrences, you can:

- Avoid excesses of alcohol, caffeine, sugar, fat, and refined carbohydrates
- Avoid aluminum containing antacids
- Limit sodium (salt) to two grams daily or less
- Reduce animal protein and avoid purine protein (organ meats, shellfish, brewer's and baker's yeast, herring, sardines, mackerel, and anchovies)
- Avoid excess phosphorous in soft drinks by quitting or cutting down
- Abate smoking (small amounts of cadmium in tobacco)
- Reduce intakes of vitamin D–enriched food (milk, cheese)
- Reduce high oxalate foods (spinach, beet greens, parsley, rhubarb, black tea, nuts, and cocoa)
- Increase water and liquid intake to reach a urine volume of two quarts daily

- Increase fiber intake
- Increase cranberry intake (unsweetened, in capsulated concentrate form)
- Increase intake of high magnesium-to-calcium ratio foods (avocado, potato, tomato, banana, orange, barley, buckwheat, rye, oats, brown rice, cashews, sesame seeds, soy, lima beans)

Vitamins, Minerals, and Supplements (Daily Amounts)
- *Fish oil*, ten grams, or *flax oil*, one tablespoon
- *Magnesium* (preferably citrate), 300 to 600 mg
- *Vitamin B-6*, 25 mg
- *Potassium citrate* and *calcium citrate*, 500 to 1,000 mg
- *Vitamin K*, 2 mg
- *Vitamin C*, one to two grams
- *Vitamin E*, 400 I.U.

Specifically for uric acid stones:

- Reduce purine intake (see preceding list)
- *Folic acid*, 5 mg daily
- *Lemon juice* from two lemons daily (reduces blood uric acid)
- Alkalinize the urine with *citrates* (see above)

Specifically for struvite stones:

- Acidify the urine (ammonium chloride, 200 mg three times daily)
- Treat recurrent infections (see chapter 17)

Herbs:
A combination of one ounce of a 1:40 decoction of *Ammi visnaga* with 5 cc of a 1:10 tincture (Khellin) taken three times daily promotes great ureteral relaxation, facilitating passage of stones, often of large size. *Lobelia* tincture, three to four drops three times an hour, may also help relax ureteral muscles to allow stone passage.

    Senna, a natural laxative, and *aloe vera* contain athraquinones, which bind calcium and reduce the formation of calcium crystals. They can be used at levels short of what produces a laxative effect. *Cranberry juice concentrate*, three to four capsules two to three times daily—equivalent to sixteen ounces of cranberry juice, reduces ionized calcium in the urine.

Professional Care Therapies

Greater pain tolerance and ureteral relaxation can be achieved through *acupuncture* treatment. *Reflexology* has some success with inducing muscular relaxation facilitating stone passage.

13

Cancer

Prevalence

CANCER IS A very common disease of industrialized nations, currently causing slightly in excess of 20 percent of all deaths in the United States. Some one million new cases are diagnosed each year, with half a million deaths annually. The incidence of cancer has increased sixty times since 1800, and the risk of cancer for men born in the 1950s is three times higher than for men born in the 1880s. Since 1958 alone, the incidence of cancer in men has increased 55 percent. The curve of cancer incidence rises steeply after the age of 60. A number of potential contributing causes have fueled the increase.

Recent data, however, indicate that the aggregate death rate from cancer has been declining in this decade, falling 0.5 percent per year from 1990–95. The overall incidence also fell: 0.7 percent per year from 1990–95, and the trend is continuing. Incidence rates of breast, prostate, colon, and rectal cancers are all decreasing, along with that of lung cancer in men. Mortality in white women with breast cancer increased 0.5 percent annually between 1980 and 1988 and declined 1.6 percent annually from 1989 through 1992, with further declines since. Mortality in black women with breast cancer increased 2 percent per year from 1980 to 1988; the increases slowed to 0.5 percent per year from 1989 to 1992. We may cautiously assume that the long increase in cancer incidence has passed its peak.

Anatomy and Physiology

Cancer is a distorted, wild, uncontrolled growth of portions of body tissues or organs in which cells multiply rapidly without restraint, producing a family of descendants that invade and destroy the structure and function of adjacent normal tissues in the organ from which the tumor originated. Cancerous cells can travel through the bloodstream or lymph channels to lodge elsewhere in the body, starting new growths (metastases) and compromising the function of organs to which the cells spread. The initiatory phase of cancerous growth is triggered by a distortion in the DNA command apparatus of the nucleus of body cells. Many authorities believe that human beings in a single lifetime experience cancer many times and that on most occasions the immune chemical and cellular defenses defeat the new growth so quickly that no symptoms ever make themselves known. These authorities believe that we should pay more attention to the state of the immune system, which for a variety of reasons, occasionally fails to recognize and eliminate these early growths before they can become a threat. Damage to DNA in cell nuclei from free radical proliferation appears to play a key role in initiation and promotion phases of cancer.

Symptoms and Diagnosis

The classical warning symptoms of cancer are:

- The appearance of a new and growing palpable lump
- The sudden and continuing enlargement in a palpable lymph node or gland, most easily felt in the groin, underarm, and neck areas
- The appearance of unexplained bleeding from the mouth, throat, lungs, bladder, vagina, rectum, or skin lesion
- A noticeable change in size, color, or shape of a birthmark, mole, or skin blemish
- A noticeable change in function of a major organ; for example, unusual persistent diarrhea, constipation, difficulty swallowing food, or cough
- Fatigue of new onset or unexplained weight loss

Following preliminary diagnosis by the taking of a history, performing a physical examination, and obtaining certain laboratory tests and X-rays, the definitive diagnosis of a cancer depends on the obtaining of a sample of the apparent tumor by surgical or needle biopsy.

Conventional Treatment

Following the pathological description of the cancerous tissue, the standard approach is to attempt surgical excision or removal of the entire cancer or, failing that, most of the cancer.

Many patients at this juncture are then advised to undertake further therapy to destroy the remainder of the tumor or prevent recurrence from tiny amounts of tumor unknowingly left behind at surgery. *Chemotherapy*, with varying combinations of chemicals that are destructive to rapidly multiplying cells, is used to attempt to destroy cancerous tissues manifesting uncontrolled growth. Chemotherapy is highly successful in Hodgkin's lymphoma, certain testicular and kidney cancers, and childhood leukemias. However, 70 percent of women with breast cancer whose lymph nodes are free of cancer at the time of surgery are cured without chemotherapy. Generally, the record for survival in many chemotherapy regimens is not a lot better than survival in persons who reject conventional treatment. John Cairns of the Harvard School of Public Health calculated in 1985 that only about 2 to 3 percent of those dying with cancer had derived any benefit from chemotherapy. A *New England Journal of Medicine* study in 1992 concluded that most of the patients who ultimately died of their cancer would not have been cured by chemotherapy. There are many, many studies comparing one combination of chemicals with other combinations, but there is not a lot of data comparing chemotherapy with no chemotherapeutic treatment at all.

Chemotherapy destroys not only rapidly multiplying cancer cells but rapidly multiplying immune cells as well. Patients may actually die from irreversible suppression of the immune system from the chemotherapy. This suppression limits the effectiveness and potential for chemicals to destroy all cancer cells. Many combinations of chemotherapeutic drugs cause side effects, including nausea, loss of appetite, diarrhea, weight loss, hair loss, and fatigue. Additional hazards include the appearance of secondary cancers later in life arising from the free radical damage from the original chemotherapeutic and radiation treatment.

Radiation, in the form of X-ray and radioactive isotope exposure, is used to destroy localized areas of remaining cancer. Radiation, too, has side effects: inflammation in surrounding normal tissues, diarrhea when the bowel is exposed, and degrees of nausea, loss of appetite, and fatigue. In some types of cancer, including leukemias, radiation is used to destroy the blood-cell-producing bone marrow, after which the patient is given a bone marrow transplant. Patients must then take immune suppressant drugs to avoid rejection of the transplanted bone marrow.

Newer techniques used in certain cancers involve the use of vaccines and tagged antibodies made from tumor tissue itself. Conventional treatment also now encompasses chemoprevention (e.g., tamoxifen or raloxifen for women with and at high risk for breast cancer).

Immunotherapy. In late-stage melanoma patients treated with a vaccine made from irradiated, cultured melanoma cells harvested from lymph node biopsies, four-year disease-free survival of 47 percent greatly exceeded the usual surgical survival of 20 percent. Similar work is proceeding in using vaccines developed from biopsy material in lymphomas.

In 1992, both the National Cancer Institute and the National Cancer Society held press conferences announcing a change in policy that shifted interest and research funding in the direction of prevention, with emphasis on nutrition. Since that time there has been an outpouring of published data relating nutrition to cancer. (This is highlighted in the holistic treatment given on page 311.) At the same time that this change of emphasis in cancer research was announced, these groups declared that the highly touted and extremely expensive "war on cancer" had been lost. The emphasis of that research and clinical application was on surgery, chemotherapy, and radiation, which continue to be the mainstays of conventional cancer management.

Risk Factors and Causes

Physical and Environmental Factors

Genetic
The incidence of some cancers has a clear hereditary influence, among them lung and breast cancer.

Nutritional Factors
Dietary and nutritional influences are thought to cause 60 percent of all cancers in women and 40 percent in men. Both cancer-causing substances in the diet and lack of cancer-inhibiting chemicals in foods play important roles. *High fat intake*, including ingestion of large amounts of oxidized fats, those that are in the process of becoming rancid, are a source of increased free radicals, which promote DNA damage. The fat of animal meats contains hyperconcentrated amounts of pesticides, which also contribute to cancers in humans. In one review, for every additional intake of ten grams of fat per day, the cancer incidence rate increased 20 percent. A significant relationship between high polyunsaturated fat intake and the reduced incidence of malignant melanoma is apparent.

The highest intakes of *sugar* are associated with a fourfold excess risk for cancer of the gallbladder compared to the lowest intakes. Recent reports link higher sugar intakes to breast cancer as well. Cancer of the colon is also associated with high sugar intake and deficiency of folic acid.

Deficiency of fiber is directly related to increased risk of colon and rectal cancers. High levels of the *phytoestrogens* equol and enterolactone confer a lower risk for breast cancer. High concentrations of these are found in soy-containing foods.

Epidemiological studies link *excess iron* to enhanced tumor growth and increased incidence of primary liver cancer and other malignancies.

Natural Carcinogenic Factors
Not all cancer-causing substances are manmade. Cancerogenic psoralen compounds naturally occur in celery, parsnips, figs, and parsley. Aflatoxins occurring in seeds, nuts (especially peanuts), and grains, if any mold has accumulated, cause liver cancer. Cottonseed products contain a carcinogen.

Environmental Carcinogenic Factors

- *Environmental toxins* (also referred to as xenobiotics) are highly suspect (e.g., air pollutants, pesticides, herbicides and fungicides, petrochemicals, and heavy metals). Exposure to petrochemicals, burned diesel fuel exhaust, and cyclic hydrocarbons result in free radical damage to DNA and lead to cancer formation. A number of chemicals used in industry increase cancer risk, including heavy metals (lead, mercury, cadmium, arsenic), solvents (e.g., benzene), chrome and nickel ores, vinyl chloride, asbestos, chlorophenols, and bischloromethylether. Other chemical sources of cancer-causing substances are defoliants (Agent Orange in Vietnam), coal-tar derivatives in paints, food additives, and nitrosamines from nitrates in cosmetics and in food as preservatives. Chronic use of hair dyes also contributes to the incidence of cancer. After combining with organic hydrocarbon residuals in polluted sources of water, chlorination of drinking water creates cancer-causing chlorinated hydrocarbons, raising the all-cancer risk 15 percent, including 21 percent for bladder cancer and 38 percent for rectal cancer. Nations and tribes with low toxic chemical use and whole food diets have an astonishingly low incidence of cancers.

- *Radiation.* Cancer risk is increased by any sources of gamma radiation, which affects nuclear plant workers, those living downwind from nuclear test sites, and those undergoing diagnostic and treatment exposure to X-rays. Children exposed to X-rays for shrinking adenoids and thymus glands and for treatment of ringworm of the scalp in the era 1930–60 have a higher incidence of later leukemia and cancer of the thyroid.

- *Electromagnetic fields.* Higher incidences of cancer of the head and neck appear to be present with exposure to electromagnetic fields, including use of electric razors. Years of exposure to indoor fluorescent lighting appear to significantly increase the risk of melanoma. Exposure to high tension electric power lines is related to risk of leukemias (especially in childhood).

- *Sun exposure.* Skin cancer incidence is greatly increased in white and Asian persons with long-term sun exposure, particularly with a history of deep tans and bad sunburns.

- *Drugs.* Some drugs appear to enhance the risk for initiation and/or growth of cancers. In rodents, the antidepressant drugs Prozac and amitriptyline, given at doses equivalent to doses used in humans, stimulate the growth of deliberately injected melanomas. When a cancer-inducing chemical was given to a group of rats, 20 of 21 rats also given Prozac/amitriptyline developed breast cancers at 15 weeks, compared to only four of seven animals given placebos.

Antihistamines have been shown to promote growth of cancers in laboratory animals. In mice, after injection of agents causing sarcoma and melanoma cancers, clear acceleration of sarcoma growth occurred in animals injected with Claritin and Hismanal (prescription antihistamines), and acceleration of melanomas occurred in animals injected with Atarax or Vistaril (prescription medicines for anxiety and itching). These drugs appear to accelerate growth of existing cancers.

Among drugs used to lower cholesterol, the fibrates (e.g., clofibrate [Atromid-S]) and the statins (e.g., simvastatin [Zocor]) cause cancer in rodents at levels of exposure close to comparable treatment levels in humans. There are no conclusive human data because of inconsistent and conflicting conclusions and insufficient duration of followup. Routine use of cholesterol-lowering drugs should be undertaken with great caution, except in patients at very high short-term risk of coronary artery disease. Medical editorials have pointed out the significant increased risk of dying with cancer in patients treated by drugs to lower cholesterol (see chapter 10). Strong positive relationships have been found as well between use of blood pressure–lowering drugs or sedative-hypnotics and the incidence of colon cancer. Chemicals used in chemotherapy for cancer spawn secondary cancers, often years later.

Personal Habits

- *Smoking* and tobacco use significantly increase risks of cancer of the larynx, lung, breast, mouth, stomach, esophagus, pancreas, bladder, kidney, cervix, penis, lymphoma and leukemia (risks increased by 20 to 2,500 percent). In 1997 175,000 deaths were attributable to smoking and tobacco use. Passive smoking (nonsmokers living with a smoker) increases the risk of many of these same cancers. Smoking causes 85 percent of lung cancer and 35 percent of all cancers.

- Lifelong drinkers of *alcohol* increase their risk of the following cancers several times: mouth, tongue, throat, esophagus, larynx, stomach, liver, colon, rectum (especially beer), pancreas, breast, and skin (malignant melanoma). Nineteen thousand deaths per year are attributable to alcohol use.

- *Weight.* In men a 43-inch waist confers two and a half times the risk for colon cancer compared to men with a waist measure of 35 inches or less.

Physical Deconditioning

Lack of exercise and physical deconditioning play very significant promotional roles in a number of cancers.

Biomolecular Factors

Coenzyme Q10 tissue levels are considerably lower in breast biopsy specimens that turn out to be malignant compared to levels in specimens that turn out to be benign. Some cancers are clearly affected by *hormones*, such as prostate and breast cancer. In premenopausal women, *DHEA* levels are about 10 percent lower in women who subsequently develop breast cancer.

Emotional Factors

Stress. Prospective studies show increases in cancer in persons under chronic, excessive, unmanaged stress and after acutely stressful events, such as the death of a spouse. In several studies, the way people cope with stress has been correlated with cancer-related deaths and rate of cancer progression. In animals stress increases tumor development, including accelerated initiation, growth, and spread. Stress decreases antibody formation, interferon synthesis, mitogen-stimulated lymphocyte proliferation, and natural killer (NK) cell cytotoxicity; NK cells are particularly important in controlling cancers. NK cell cytotoxicity was suppressed 45 percent in stressed animals compared to controls. Stressed animals with cancer have twice as many metastases (areas of spread) as controls. In animals stressed one hour before tumor cell injection, there was a fivefold increase in metastases over controls.

Depression. A large number of studies have noticed the consistent significant relationship of depression, helplessness, and hopelessness to the onset of various kinds of cancer. Depressed patients have a much lower incidence of successful bone marrow transplant survival than nondepressed patients. Patients who express their emotions in socially acceptable ways rather than repressing them also consistently do better. Patients who believe that a lesser amount of adjustment will be necessary to cope with their disease also do better compared to those who believe the adjustment will be very high.

Hans Eysenck and R. Grossarth-Maticek have followed two thousand persons for 20 years. They conclude that psychosocial factors (personality, stress) play roles in the development of cancer: suppression of emotion and inability to cope with interpersonal stress lead to hopelessness, helplessness, and depression, which predispose to cancer. Behavioral therapy (stress management) can reduce these risks for development of cancer.

Esoteric diagnosticians and medical intuitives who are aware of energy fields also sense cancer as a disorder related to: negative emotions of fear, guilt, self-hate, or self-denial; unfinished business with others with whom we have had a significant relationship; and resistance to change. These issues cause major resistances to the evolution of emotional, psychological, and spiritual development. Accepting the fact that we experience change according to what our growth requires necessitates the development of willingness to accept ourselves, to let go of these issues over which we really have no control, and to recognize the necessity and inevitability of change in order to grow and incorporate what we need to learn in this lifetime.

Social Factors

Dr. Caroline Thomas's long-term study of 1,500 medical students showed that the strongest psychological predictor of cancer over the next 25 years was the perception of lack of closeness with parents in childhood.

Holistic Prevention

Physical and Environmental Health Recommendations

Diet

Fruits and *vegetables*. Authorities, including the National Cancer Institute and the American Cancer Society, are increasingly supportive of the potential for decreasing the risk of malignancy through consumption of increased amounts of fruits, vegetables, fiber, and antioxidants, discussed below. Besides the evidence for decreased risk with high intake of these nutrient sources, hundreds of phytochemicals are being found to have cancer-protective properties, including:

- Limonene in citrus fruits
- Allyl sulfides in garlic, onion, leeks, and chives
- Dithiolthiones in broccoli
- Isothiocyanates from cabbage, cauliflower, kale, Brussels sprouts, broccoli sprouts, collard greens, and other cruciferous vegetables
- Ellagic acid in grapes
- Protease inhibitors, phytosterols, isoflavones, and saponins in soybeans
- Caffeic acid found in coffee
- Ferulic acid (gamma oryzanol) in various grains
- Phytic acid in grains
- Glycosinolates in broccoli sprouts
- Indulges in various vegetables

Mounting evidence supports the relationship of *high antioxidant intake* in food and supplements with a decreased risk of malignancy.

- In men, for instance, a diet high in vitamin C and dark green vegetables leads to 40 percent reduction in the risk of cancer of the bladder.

- Protective effects against the risk of brain tumors has been found in children whose mothers' diet in pregnancy had been highest in fruits and fruit juice, vegetables, vitamin A, and vitamin C.

- Analysis of many colon cancer studies found the risk of colon cancer 50 percent reduced in the group with the highest intake of fiber, fruits, vegetables, carbohydrates, and folic acid.

- The risk for cancers of the mouth/pharynx, esophagus, stomach, colon, and rectum was reduced 30 to 60 percent in those with high tomato intake. Tomatoes are high in lycopene (a carotenoid) and low in beta carotene.

- Green tea drinkers lower their risk of esophageal cancer 50 percent compared to non–green tea drinkers (high catechin content).

- In men with the highest intake of onions, the risk for stomach cancer was 50 percent lower than for those with the lowest onion intake.

- Inositol hexaphosphate (phytic acid), found in cereals and legumes, has anticarcinogenic properties. This may explain the benefits of high fiber diets in preventing certain cancers.

- Bioflavonoids are natural antioxidants. Quercetin, ellagic acid, and chlorogenic acid, found in a variety of fruits and vegetables, reduce the bioavailability of cancer-causing substances in laboratory rats.

- Genistein, contained in soybeans, and isoflavones (flavonoids), in a variety of fruits and vegetables, are of great interest for their anticancer potential.

Vitamins, Minerals, and Supplements

- Taking *multivitamin/mineral supplements* anytime in pregnancy confers a reduced risk for cancer as follows: with iron, 57 percent less, calcium, 58 percent less, and vitamin C, 65 percent less. The maternal use of multivitamins *at any time during pregnancy or in the infant in the first six weeks of life* was also associated with a 44 percent reduced risk of cancer in the child.

- *Antioxidants.* In 29,600 Chinese, intake of supplements of beta carotene, vitamin E, and selenium significantly reduced the incidence of esophageal and stomach cancer compared to those not on supplements.

- *Vitamin C.* In 12,000 men age 40–59, relative risk for dying of stomach cancer was 28 percent lower in those with a high intake of vitamin C compared with low intake. Incidence of skin cancers was significantly lower in persons with greater intake of foods high in vitamin C and beta carotene; fish; vegetables in general;

beans, lentils, peas, carrots, Swiss chard, pumpkins, and cruciferous vegetables. In a study of 2,500 patients, the risk of cancer of the lung was reduced 35 percent in those with the highest intake of vitamin C, 16 percent in those with highest beta carotene, and 36 percent in those with the highest *vitamin A* in their food intake.

- *Beta carotene, vitamin A.* Subjects with the highest beta carotene levels had a 15-year lower risk of mouth cancer than those with the lowest intakes. Those men with the lowest level of vitamin A levels were three times more likely to have prostate cancer than those with the highest levels. Average vitamin A levels are significantly lower in cancer patients compared to healthy subjects.

- Two studies of heavy smokers have not confirmed lower rates of cancer in those receiving beta carotene supplements. In one of those studies, however, prostate cancer was much lower in men receiving beta carotene. Neither of these studies assessed lycopene intake. Lycopene is now known to be the most potent carotene antioxidant, several times more powerful than beta carotene and probably much more important in cancer prevention. Since all carotenes compete with one another, it is suspected that the high-dosage beta carotene supplementation significantly reduced lycopene absorption from food sources in these studies.

- *Vitamin E.* Men with the highest vitamin E levels were at 66 percent lower risk for melanoma compared to those with the lowest intakes; those with the highest zinc intake had a 54 percent lower risk.

- *Folic acid* supplements (400–5,000 mcg daily) in a large Harvard study have been shown to reduce colon cancer incidence 75 percent compared to those taking no supplements.

- *Selenium.* In a placebo-controlled trial of one thousand persons, intake of 200 mcg daily of selenium for seven years reduced total cancer mortality 51 percent compared to placebo. The selenium group experienced a 41 percent reduction in new cancer incidence, 63 percent reduction in cancer of the colon, and a 70 percent reduction in prostate cancer. High selenium intake confers a 72 percent lower risk for precancerous colon polyps. Selenium blood levels in healthy people are much higher than in melanoma patients.

Herbs

A recent Korean study showed significant reduction in all-cancer incidence in regular Panax ginseng users; the greatest differences were for stomach and lung cancer.

Environmental Factors

As much as possible, minimizing environmental hazards is obviously wise. Some steps you can take are:

- Reduce air pollution within your home with electronic air filters, HEPA filters, and a negative air ion generator.

- Stay out of agricultural areas during spraying times.

- Arrange with your doctor and dentist to minimize your exposure to X-rays.

- If you live within a block of a high tension power line, plan to move at the earliest convenient opportunity.

- Locate yourself as conveniently far away from all sources of electromagnetic fields—electric clocks, microwaves, television and video screens. Turn on electric blankets before bedtime and off as you go to bed.

- Avoid excessive sun exposure, utilizing sunscreen, hats, caps, and long sleeves.

- When handling petrochemicals and solvents, wash carefully after using.

- Avoid the personal use of pesticides and herbicides as much as possible.

- If you use hair dyes, consider stopping.

- Use full spectrum fluorescent tubes in light fixtures at work and home.

- If you are taking any of the drugs listed above under *causes* find out from your doctor whether they are absolutely necessary or could be switched.

- If you smoke, invest in the time and effort of a good abatement program, including acupuncture.

- If you have more than one alcoholic beverage daily, consider modifying your intake.

- Use roasted nuts (destroys carcinogenic aflatoxins); nuts may also be soaked raw overnight in a vessel with water containing one drop of grapefruit seed extract.

- Buy and consume organic produce if possible.

- Use filtering devices for drinking and cooking water to remove cancer-causing sources of chlorinated hydrocarbons.

The non-organic fruits and vegetables with the highest pesticide content and best substitutes include:

High Contamination	Best Alternatives
Strawberries	Blackberries, blueberries, cantaloupe (US), kiwi, grapefruit, kiwi, oranges, raspberries, watermelon
Bell peppers: green	Broccoli, romaine lettuce, peas
red	Asparagus, broccoli, Brussels sprouts, carrots, romaine lettuce, tomatoes
Spinach	Asparagus, broccoli, Brussels sprouts, romaine lettuce

High Contamination	Best Alternatives
Cherries (US)	Blackberries, blueberries, cantaloupe (US), grapefruit, kiwi, oranges, raspberries
Peaches	Cantaloupe (US), red/pink grapefruit, nectarines, oranges, tangerines, watermelon
Cantaloupe (Mexican)	Cantaloupe (US), watermelon
Celery	Broccoli, carrots, romaine lettuce, radishes
Apples	Bananas, cantaloupe (US), grapefruit, kiwi, nectarines, oranges, pears, tangerines, watermelon
Apricots	Cantaloupe (US), red/pink grapefruit, nectarines, oranges, tangerines, watermelon
Green beans	Asparagus, broccoli, Brussels sprouts, cauliflower, peas, potatoes
Grapes (Chile)	Grapes (US, May to December in season)
Cucumbers	Carrots, broccoli, romaine lettuce, radishes, others not in left-hand column

Source: Environmental Working Group, 1718 Connecticut Ave NW, # 600, Washington, D.C., 20009.

Exercise

Animal studies link increased physical activity with a 25–100 percent retardation in growth rate of experimental sarcomas, adenocarcinomas, hepatomas, and mammary carcinomas. If you walk an hour each day, you reduce your risk of colon and rectal cancer by 50 percent compared to sedentary people. *Intense physical activity has been associated with an all-cancer relative risk of 0.27 for men and 0.55 for women.* In other words, consistent high intensity physical activity reduces cancer risk 73 percent in men and 45 percent in women! Intense activity in these studies meant running more than four hours per week or walking more than 12 hours per week.

Mental and Emotional Health Recommendations. Since depression is associated with cancer incidence, it seems reasonable to take steps to modify it if possible. In fact, the studies of Eysenck and Maticek in eastern Europe did show that intensive proactive and interactive therapy (they called it "creative novation behavior therapy") reduced risk for cancer over 15 years of their study. Behavioral and cognitive therapy can be of enormous help.

Holistic Cancer Treatment

Physical Health Recommendations

Diet

Macrobiotic diet. Analysis of case studies indicates that a strict *macrobiotic diet*, an extension of a vegetarian diet, is likely to be more effective in long-term cancer management than diets offering a variety of other foods.

Raw fruit and vegetable juices are widely recommended as part of supportive treatment in cancer; it is an easy way to take in over 95 percent of the vital phytonutrients that support the immune system. Organic fruits and vegetables are much preferred.

Vitamins, Minerals, and Supplements

Supplemental *antioxidants* exert anticarcinogenic, immunostimulant, and antimetastatic effects and act to inhibit cancer at each stage of its development. Since it is known that platelet aggregation, a free radical–mediated function, encourages implantation of bloodstream-borne cancer metastases, increasing antioxidant intake becomes important. Reasonable daily doses of antioxidants in treating cancer are 500 mcg *selenium*, 800 I.U. *vitamin E*, and four grams *vitamin C*. In a 12-year followup of three thousand subjects in the Basel study, overall cancer mortality was significantly associated with low levels of vitamin C and *carotenoids*. *Beta carotene* (25 mg daily, or 125,000 I.U. daily), regresses oral (mouth) precancerous lesions. *Vitamin A* has been shown to reduce the incidence of new primary tumors and increase the tumor-free interval in heavy-smoking patients "cured" of lung cancer.

Lycopene, a carotenoid, substantially inhibits the growth of lung cancer cells in the test tube, and has been shown to reduce progression of prostate cancer (with a dosage of 15 mg daily). Lycopene is four times more potent than alpha carotene and ten times more potent than beta carotene. Lycopene is a major tomato carotenoid.

Linus Pauling and Ewan Cameron reported benefits of *intravenous vitamin C* in "terminal" cancer patients in 1971. Ascorbic acid is preferentially toxic to tumor cells in test tube studies and clinical human research. The cytotoxicity of ascorbic acid has been shown to be related to pro-oxidant generation of hydrogen peroxide. Normal cells have a ten to one hundred times greater content of catalase compared to tumor cells; this defends them against this toxic pro-oxidant effect of the vitamin C. Vitamin C can thus induce cytotoxicity in tumor cells with negligible toxic effects to normal cells. Many tumor cell types are completely destroyed in laboratory tests by concentrations of 5–40 mg per dl of ascorbic acid, a level that can be achieved by an intravenous infusion of 60–100 grams of vitamin C over ten hours. Dr. Hugh Riordan and the authors of this book have documented a number of cases of arrest of advanced tumor growth. This demonstration of the cytotoxicity to tumor cells by high concentrations of ascorbic acid goes far beyond the previously understood immunostimulatory properties of ascorbic acid.

In laboratory rats exposed to radiation, those given *vitamin E* had significant increased protection against radiation damage to normal cells, including precancerous cell changes.

Two recent reviews confirm the benefits of high-dose antioxidants during chemo- and radiation therapy in both reducing toxicity of treatment and enhancing treatment effects.

Patients under treatment for cancer of the bladder were randomized to therapy with either an RDA level multivitamin-mineral daily or a megadose multivitamin-mineral containing RDA levels of vitamins and minerals plus vitamins A (40,000 I.U.), B-6 (100 mg), C (two grams), E (400 I.U.), and zinc (90 mg). *The five-year cancer recurrence rates were 91 percent for the RDA vitamin group and 41 percent for the megadose group.* And in a study of lung cancer patients on standard chemotherapy and radiation therapy, supplements *enhanced survival 40 to 60 percent* and reduced toxic side effects as well, compared to normal experience. Daily dosages included:

- *Vitamin A*, 15,000–40,000 I.U.
- *Beta carotene*, 10,000–20,000 I.U.
- *Vitamin E*, 300–800 I.U.
- *Vitamin B-1*, 150–750 mg
- *Vitamin B-2*, 15–50 mg
- *Vitamin B-6*, 200–1,140 mg
- *Vitamin B-12*, 30–1,600 mcg
- *Niacinamide*, 150–400 mg
- *Vitamin D*, 400–1,000 I.U.
- *Vitamin C*, two to five grams
- *Pantothenate* (B-5), 50–300 mg
- *Biotin*, 0.3–10 mg
- *Calcium*, 500–1,000 mg
- *Magnesium*, 250–500 mg
- *Potassium*, 120 mg

- *Manganese,* 97–194 mg

- *Zinc,* 27–46 mg

- *Copper,* 3 mg

- *Chromium,* 1.6–3.1 mg

- *Selenium,* 1.7–3.4 mg

- *Vanadium,* 468–936 mg

- *Tungsten,* 2.2–4.5 mg

- *Essential fatty acids,* 5–65 gm

Side effects of radiation and chemotherapy were also considerably reduced compared to normal experience.

Selenium facilitates immune activity and has anticancer activity in animals and in cancer cells in the test tube.

Twenty-one smoking patients with precancerous changes in the bronchial lining given oral doses of *folic acid* (10–20 mg daily) and *vitamin B-12* (750 mcg daily) for a year significantly decreased cancerous development in the precancerous cells compared to no decreases in the controls.

Recurring precancerous colon polyps are up to 85 percent reduced in those taking vitamin A (30,000 I.U.), vitamin C (one gram) and vitamin E (or d-alpha-tocopherol acetate, 70 mg daily). Adequate *calcium* also significantly reduces risk. Risks are worsened with intake of red meat, total fat, and saturated fat.

Gamma linolenic acid. Twenty-one end-stage cancer patients who had undergone maximal conventional treatment and were classed as untreatable were given 9–18 grams daily of evening primrose oil, high in gamma linolenic acid. Most experienced marked subjective improvement.

Algae. In 87 tobacco chewers with diagnosed leukoplakia oral lesions (precancers of the lips and mouth), taking one gram daily of Spirulina fusiformis, a blue-green microalgae, completely regressed the cancerous changes in 20 of 44 subjects; partial regression occurred in 5 of 44.

Glutamine. Forty-three patients admitted to a bone marrow transplant unit receiving standard nutrition plus glutamine (an amino acid) had significantly less infection and recovered faster after the transplant procedure. Appropriate doses are one to two grams daily. Glutamine added to chemotherapy regimens in laboratory animals with cancer eliminates the toxic effects of drugs like methotrexate and inhibits cancer growth in mice.

Probiotics. The toxicity of chemotherapy routinely disrupts intestinal bacterial balance; restoring L. acidophilus and bifidus organisms in the intestine promotes normal intestinal function during treatment.

Herbs

Genistein, an isoflavone from fruits and vegetables, was found to inhibit the growth of stomach cancer cells in test tube experiments. Other flavonoids—*flavone, luteolin,* and *daidzein*—also arrested the cancer cells. Human squamous skin cancer cells in test tube experiments were significantly inhibited by various concentrations of quercetin. Reasonable doses are 400 mg twice daily. *Tangeretin,* a naturally occurring flavone in citrus fruit, causes cancer cell death in promyelocytic leukemia cells in the test tube. So large amounts of citrus fruits are encouraged. *Maitake mushroom extracts* have immune-enhancing and anticancer properties, well shown in animal studies, and are now being used in the United States (three capsules three times daily). *Silymarin* (80 percent standardized extracts) have utility in preserving liver function during chemotherapy treatment with 5-fluorouracil and other agents (140–210 mg two to three times daily).

Biomolecular Options

Anticoagulants reduce the rate of metastases in cancer patients. Some reports have catalogued great reductions in cancer patients who were coincidentally anticoagulated for other reasons. This report has not led to widespread utilization of this observation.

The ability to synthesize the adrenal hormone dehydroepiandrosterone (DHEA), declines markedly over the third through sixth decades of life. The levels of DHEA in patients with a wide variety of cancers are found to be generally low. *DHEA* has been used with benefit as treatment in some types of cancer.

A body compound, *urea,* (two to two and a half grams four to six times daily) has been found to increase survival in patients with far-advanced cancer of the liver, both primary and metastatic.

Two cases of far-advanced metastatic lung cancer have been reported to go into remission when given *cimetidine (Tagamet);* case histories of far-advanced melanoma have been reported in which administration of cimetidine resulted in dramatic regression of tumor in two of three patients.

Glutathione, an antioxidant synthesized by the body, added intravenously to chemotherapeutic cisplatin regimens for advanced ovarian cancer decreased toxicity and significantly improved prognosis.

There is some preliminary evidence that *melatonin* may be helpful in the treatment of cancer. Patients with brain metastases from solid cancers who received melatonin (20 mg daily) in addition to supportive care tripled their aggregate survival time in one year of treatment. Clear improvement in quality of life and performance status was present in 30 percent of the melatonin patients compared to none of the controls. Melatonin (10 mg daily) prevented metastases in 40 percent of patients with far-advanced cancers.

Coenzyme Q10 (100 mg daily) added to treatment prevented the heart toxicity usually developing with adriamycin chemotherapy. In women with breast cancer, advanced liver and metastatic disease has successfully been treated with 400 mg daily.

Exercise

Physical activity appears to be helpful in the treatment of cancer after diagnosis. In human studies, increased physical activity in the cancer patient increases appetite, conserves lean tissue, improves functional capacity, slows the clinical course of cancer, pushes back the time of death, and improves the quality of life.

Mental and Emotional Health Recommendations. *Relaxation training.* Only nine hours of relaxation training has been shown to significantly reduce cancer pain and use of narcotics and tranquilizers. Hypnotic suggestion also greatly enhances the management of pain in cancer.

Patients with malignant melanoma who were enrolled in an intervention group did better than those in a "routine care" group. The intervention group met one and a half hours weekly for six weeks. Group processes and interventions included *health education, cancer education, enhancement of illness-related problem solving skills, instruction and practice in relaxation skills, psychological support, and promoting interaction between patients and health care professionals.* Psychological and immunological testing at six months compared to baseline showed significant improvement in immunity compared to controls, and anxiety and depression were significantly less as well. Imagery enhanced the effects of relaxation on immunity. In a six-year followup, the risk of dying was 33 percent less and the risk of recurrence 50 percent less in the intervention group.

Social Health Recommendations. In a landmark study of late-stage female breast cancer patients, a one-year weekly *support group* including relaxation training greatly enhanced quality of life and more than doubled the survival time of these women. Patients with a solid support system of relatives, spouses, and significant others have a better prognosis, as do married men and men with a confidant.

Professional Care Therapies

In well-controlled animal studies, cancer progression has been shown to be inhibited with energy treatments by *healers* using therapeutic or healing touch, Reiki, or similar hands-on techniques.

Holistic Cure

Mental Imagery. In many of the reports of persons recovering from cancer, especially advanced cancer, patients have used imagery of their immune systems overcoming or defeating the cancer cells and imagery of themselves returning to health. Authoritative research confirms that the success of imagery is highly related to the vividness and effectiveness visualized in the imagery. Guided imagery therapy with skilled professionals can be very helpful and meaningful.

Spiritual Factors and Beliefs. Several thousand case histories of documented "spontaneous" recovery from cancer have been summarized by Brendan O'Regan of the Institute of Noetic Sciences. In many case histories, the "fighting spirit," will to live, and belief in recovery appear to be very important prognostic factors. Most patients who recover from life-threatening cancer have made a radical change in some aspect of their lives—in diet, exercise, attitude, relationships with family members, or sense of connection with God. Other characteristics frequently observed to be present in persons who cure their cancers include full acceptance of their disease and using the occasion of the disease as an opportunity to gain some sense of meaning and purpose in their lives. This introspective journey of self-discovery is often so important to them that many actually feel gratitude for the "gift" of cancer.

Confidence and belief in the program of cancer treatment undertaken seems to be essential in successfully treating cancer. Self-confidence and confidence in the treating physicians are also essential elements. It is very important for patients to participate in decisions regarding their own treatment.

Alternative Programs. Radically alternative cancer treatments named for their innovators include the Hoxsey, Gerson, Contreras, and Kelly programs. These centers operate primarily in Mexico, utilizing methods that are not approved by the FDA in the United States. Other approaches have been developed by Stanislaw Burzynski, M.D., Ph.D., (*antineoplastron therapy*); and biochemist Gaston Naessens (anticancer formula *714x*). Dr. Joseph Gold has pioneered *hydrazine sulfate* therapy, and there is documented evidence that this compound appears to benefit cancer patients by restoring better nutritional support to their healthy cells. The success of these programs is difficult to assess, since no comprehensive statistics are available. However, there are apparently enough successful treatments that they should not be lightly dismissed.

14

Cardiovascular Disease

Heart Disease—
  Coronary Artery Disease
  Angina
  Arrhythmias
  Congestive Heart Failure
Hypertension
Stroke
Hyperlipidemia

Prevalence:

CARDIOVASCULAR DISEASE is the leading cause of mortality and disability in the United States, accounting for 30 percent of all deaths. Heart disease, strokes, and vascular diseases claim seven hundred thousand lives lives each year, and an estimated 56 billion dollars is spent each year for the care of affected patients. Arteriosclerosis (hardening of the arteries), the primary cause of mortality from heart attacks and strokes, though a twentieth-century disease, has declined since 1968, with a 50 percent fall in the incidence and death from heart attacks and a 60 percent decrease in strokes.

Anatomy and Physiology

The cardiovascular system consists of the heart, arteries, and veins. The heart is a hollow-chambered, muscular organ the size of a large fist, functioning to move blood to the lungs for oxygenation and then pump blood under high pressure through the arteries to the rest of the body. A specialized set of coronary arteries allows the heart to pump blood to itself. Certain arteries, including those leading to the heart, brain, kidneys and lower limbs are particularly susceptible to the deterioration process called arteriosclerosis (atherosclerosis). This insidious process progressively thickens the walls of the blood vessels to the point that the passages of the arteries can no longer supply blood to the organs they serve. When an artery is completely blocked, part of the organ which has had its blood supply cut off undergoes rapid death. The result in the heart is a heart attack (myocardial infarction), in the brain a stroke, and in the lower limbs, a pregangrenous condition.

The Heart

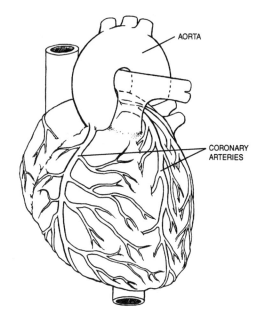

AORTA

CORONARY
ARTERIES

HEART DISEASE—CORONARY ARTERY DISEASE (CAD)

CONDITION

Prevalence

Heart attacks were rare before 1920 but now lead the list of causes of mortality in the United States. Twenty percent of all deaths are related to heart attacks, taking the lives of 530,000 people each year. Sixty million Americans are thought to be living with some degree of coronary artery disease. The good news about heart disease is the steady decline in heart attacks since 1968. Both major improvements in lifestyle habits and better care of those with arteriosclerotic vascular problems have contributed to the 50 percent decline in heart disease mortality.

Symptoms and Diagnosis

Coronary artery disease gives no symptoms in early stages. The underlying arteriosclerosis (hardening and thickening of the arterial walls), which is the basis for most coronary disease, may begin in childhood or adulthood, triggered by a combination of many factors. A significant fraction of heart disease patients become aware of their disease with the sudden chest pain of a heart attack (myocardial infarction). The pain is typically severe, centered in the front of the chest and slightly to the left of the mid-line, and often radiated to the left arm, neck, chin, or upper left side of the back. These symptoms should trigger an immediate call to your physician and emergency services. When coronary disease announces its presence less dramatically, the pain, resembling the description of a heart attack but much more mild and usually related to physical exertion and occasionally to stress, is called angina pectoris (see below). The diagnosis of an acute heart attack is confirmed by tests in the hospital, including blood tests, electrocardiograms, and X-ray studies of the coronary arteries.

Conventional Medical Treatment

Since heart problems are the leading cause of death in the United States, identifying people at risk is a high priority. All the classic risk factors are considered, and a careful family history is obtained. When a history of exertional chest pain, rhythm disturbances, or shortness of breath is elicited, coronary heart disease is confirmed by finding abnormalities in exercise electrocardiograms (stress tests), angiograms, or radioisotope heart scans. Laboratory blood tests confirm evidence of problems and increased risk with elevated cholesterol, LDL-C ("bad" cholesterol), cholesterol/HDL-C ratio, lipoprotein (a), and triglycerides; and decreased HDL-C ("good" cholesterol).

Preventive measures include, if appropriate, stopping smoking; substantially improving diet with decreased intake of saturated fat and cholesterol and increased fruits, vegetables, and whole grains; bringing blood pressure under control with drugs; and improving cholesterol levels with drugs.

Drug Treatments. A wide array of commonly used *drugs to lower cholesterol* is described under hyperlipidemia, below. After a decade of lowering cholesterol with the first generation of these drugs, research showed only mildly improved prognosis in heart disease but *increased* total mortality from all causes. A 1992 study in the journal *Circulation* reviewed 19 studies of aggressive lowering of cholesterol with drugs, and in 18 of them found an increased incidence of chronic lung disease, pneumonia, influenza, hemorrhagic strokes, cirrhosis of the liver, digestive diseases, alcohol dependence, suicide, leukemias, lymphomas, and cancers of the liver and lung. There was a tendency for these alarming associations to manifest in persons whose cholesterol was lowered below 160 mg per dl. Though disputed by some authorities, depression appears to be more common in people with low blood cholesterol. A 1991 study in the *Journal of the American Medical Association* followed 1,200 men with known risk factors for heart disease. The group treated intensively with blood pressure–lowering and cholesterol-lowering drugs reduced cardiac risk factors 46 percent compared to the group treated more casually. Ten years later, however, there were 45 percent more deaths in the intensively treated drug group compared to the casually treated group. A review of research in laboratory rodents published in January 1996 in the same journal established a conclusive pattern of carcinogenicity for clofibrate and the statin drugs in concentrations comparable to blood levels achieved in humans at standard doses. In fact, the manufacturer's literature for the widely prescribed drug gemfibrozil says: "There was no difference in mortality between the clofibrate-treated subjects and . . . placebo-treated subjects, but twice as many clofibrate-treated subjects developed cholelithiasis (gallstones) requiring surgery." Gemfibrozil is chemically very similar to clofibrate.

Use of the newer *statin drugs to lower cholesterol* has demonstrated a lowered incidence of heart attacks and lowered overall mortality rate, even in those whose cholesterol levels were normal at the outset. Some caution is advised, however, based on the fact that disadvantages of earlier generations of cholesterol-lowering drugs came to light only after 10 years of use. Results need to be evaluated over the long term. Makers of the statin drugs recommend blood tests every six months to monitor any elevation in liver enzymes that may occur. Warnings are also given about rare cases of muscle damage, especially when a combination of drugs is used, and about very cautious use in patients with any degree of kidney failure.

At the time of threatened or actual heart attacks, *clot-dissolving drugs* are used to restore circulation. *Aspirin* is commonly used to inhibit the predisposition for clots to form easily, reducing the incidence of first and second heart attacks. *Anticoagulation*, used in the 1960–1970 era, is again becoming more popular, utilizing low doses of the anticoagulants heparin and Coumadin.

Surgery

Cardiologists utilize *angioplasty* to dilate narrowed portions of coronary arteries, sometimes leaving in place a stent to prevent the recurrence of constriction, which often occurs; cardiac surgeons perform *bypass operations*, fashioning new arterial channels around areas of constriction. Up to one-third of bypasses are found to be closed off in a matter of months or years. Arteriosclerosis in the bypass segments develops quickly, being found in one-third of patients one year after surgery. A last surgical option in end-stage coronary heart disease is a *heart transplant*. The estimated cost, when a donor heart is available, is about $350,000. In one study, after vigorous medical treatment, 40 percent of those initially qualifying to be on a waiting list for a donor heart no longer met the criteria for transplant when a heart became available.

These operative procedures do not halt the incessant progression of the arteriosclerosis.

Risk Factors and Causes

The presence of a diagonal *earlobe crease* (see illustration), though not a true risk factor, is a reliable indicator of increased risk. Another associated marker for CAD risk is *short stature*. Men who are less than six feet one inch tall have a 35 percent higher risk of heart attack than taller men. The explanation for these two associations remains unclear.

Ear Crease

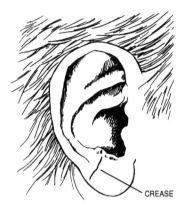

CREASE

The triggering cause for a heart attack is the interruption of blood supply to a segment of the heart; by far the most common triggering event is the formation of a *blood clot* in an already markedly narrowed arteriosclerotic artery. Severe *coronary artery spasm* triggered by stress can be responsible for loss of blood supply, even in the face of only minor arteriosclerotic changes.

Coronary artery disease, which can lead to heart attacks, results from a combination of a number of risk factors. The *classic risk factors* are:

- Genetic predisposition
- High blood pressure
- Elevated blood cholesterol
- Smoking
- Diabetes

Genetic factors play a role in heart disease, particularly in fairly uncommon but devastating patterns in which members of certain families mishandle cholesterol metabolism. In these family patterns males can have heart attacks in their twenties. A much more common and less threatening genetic pattern is seen in *hyperhomocysteinemia*, a defective handling of two amino acids, methionine and cysteine. Some, although not all, authorities believe this may explain up to 20 percent of the incidence of heart attacks and strokes. *Elevated levels of fibrinogen*, a blood clotting element in the body, are also partially genetically determined. Elevated fibrinogen levels are related to stress, excessive blood clotting, obesity, diabetes, high blood pressure, depleted good cholesterol, elevated bad cholesterol and triglycerides, and kidney disease. High blood fibrinogen is a potent, independent risk factor for arteriosclerotic diseases.

High blood pressure adds to the risk of damage to the delicate inner lining of the arteries. An entire section (hypertension) below is devoted to this widespread problem.

Elevated cholesterol is unequivocally related to the incidence of heart attacks and strokes. A high ratio of total cholesterol to good cholesterol significantly increases risk; elevated levels of triglycerides and deficient levels of good cholesterol are also independent risk factors. Elevated free radical populations in excess of antioxidant defenses promote the oxidation of low-density lipoprotein cholesterol, triggering the deposition of cholesterol and cellular debris that thickens the walls of the arteries, eventually blocking the flow of blood (see under hyperlypidemia below).

Smoking became rapidly accepted in American culture with the advent of mass-produced cigarettes in the early 1920s. By the 1960s, 46 percent of adults smoked regularly, at the time cardiovascular disease reached its peak. The gradual drop in smoking to 24 percent of the adult population by 1998 is probably one of the principal explanations for the decrease in heart disease and strokes. Passive exposure to smoke in the environment also carries a high risk; in some diseases it is nearly as great as the risk for the smoker.

Since the 1960s, *diabetes* has been recognized as a risk factor for arteriosclerotic diseases. Type II (adult) diabetes, with a strong genetic component, leads to several biochemical changes, including higher compensating levels of corticosteroids, increased biochemical stress, and production of high levels of free radicals. The presence of diabetes accelerates premature degeneration of arterial walls, inducing circulatory deficiencies which promote the principal complications of diabetes itself. Because some studies have shown that up to fifty percent of men having heart attacks have none of the classic risk factors, *additional risk factors* have been investigated. These include physical, mental, emotional, and spiritual factors:

- Nutrition: deficient fiber, fruits, vegetables, antioxidants, omega-3 oils, and water; and too much saturated, oxidized and hydrogenated fat and sugar.
- Deficiency of Coenzyme Q10, L-carnitine, and DHEA
- Insufficient water intake
- Obesity
- Sleep deficiency
- Deconditioning syndrome

- Air pollution

- Stress

- High degrees of hostility and the negative emotions of depression, anger, and anxiety

- Loneliness and social isolation

Physical Factors. *Nutritional* considerations loom large in heart disease and strokes. The *decreased intake of whole grains, fruits, and vegetables* and the increase in use of refined and bleached wheat flour one hundred years ago set the stage for the rise of heart disease. In the early 1970s, these nutritional shifts in society were recognized to relate to development of deficiencies or lower intakes of essential nutrients that play roles in prevention of arteriosclerosis—*vitamins E, C, B-6, and B-12 and beta carotene, folic acid, zinc, magnesium, chromium, and selenium.* Copper deficiency can also contribute to arterial aneurysms.

Accompanying this shift to refined flour was an increase in the intake of fats and sugars. The increased fat came from greater consumption of animal meats and cow's milk derivatives high in *saturated fats.* This shift is thought to be significantly associated with the rapid rise in arteriosclerotic disease in the 1940–1970 era. Since the 1970s, per capita intake of these caloric sources has slowly declined. Also contributing to the increase in fat consumption was the belief that vegetable sources of polyunsaturated fats would not contribute to heart disease and strokes. Unfortunately, most of these oil sources were converted into fats that are solid at room temperature (hydrogenated cooking fats, margarines, and peanut butter). Time and research have shown that these foods contain *trans fats*, which are as bad if not worse than saturated fats as causes of arteriosclerosis. On the other hand, quality fats containing *omega-3 fatty acids* are a mitigating factor in heart disease. Greenland Eskimos, with a very high percentage of their calories coming from animal fats, have a low incidence of heart disease, probably because of the high intake of omega-3 fatty acids from fish.

Recent research has reconfirmed data from the 1980s showing that *sugars* are a significant risk factor for heart disease. A 1992 editorial in the *Journal of the Royal Society of Medicine* declared that there "is more evidence of sugar as a cause [of coronary artery disease] than there is for dietary fat and cholesterol." The intake of excess loads of sugar promotes hyperinsulinemia, leading to a compensatory shift in body hormones and chemicals, spawning a variety of problems, including diabetes, heart disease, gout, and hypertension. This condition has been called syndrome X by some authorities. Fat intake has modestly declined since the 1970s, while sugar has steadily increased. Intake of fruits, vegetables, and whole grains improved steadily through the 1980s and 1990s. This shift is the most encouraging aspect of our nutritional picture in the United States today.

A very recent study has found that men drinking two glasses or less of *water* daily had twice the risk of death from heart attacks and strokes compared to those drinking five or more glasses daily. Women drinking two glasses or less per day experienced half again the fatality rate. Regular and excessive *alcohol* consumption contributes to hypertension, and *caffeine* and coffee intake appear to contribute to heart attacks, although not all authorities agree on this.

Accumulating evidence also points a finger at deficiencies of biochemicals synthesized in the body as contributors to risk of heart attacks. These include *Coenzyme Q10*, a quintessential cellular enzyme, and *L-carnitine*, a nonessential amino acid. Coenzyme Q10 levels in patients with heart disease are lower than levels in healthy people. L-carnitine is essential in cellular energy production and is easily lost from heart muscle cells in patients with coronary artery disease. In men over 50 years of age, deficient levels of testosterone and *DHEA* (dehydroepiandrosterone) are also commonly found in those with heart disease.

Obesity is a risk factor in both men and women. Risk for coronary heart disease in women is twice as great in women having a waist circumference of 38 inches or greater or whose ratio of waist to hip circumference is 0.76 or higher. The risk of heart attack is also greater in men with *sleep deficiency.*

Other physical risk factors include the "deconditioning syndrome"—a fancy name for the *lack of physical fitness* that comes with an excessively sedentary lifestyle. Men exercising at high levels experience an incidence of heart attack that is 50 percent lower than that of men who exercise the least. The increase in exercising Americans has been a major factor in the reduction of heart attacks in the last 30 years.

The *pollution of air* in most of our major cities also is a risk factor. The risk is especially high in industries that require workers to be exposed to solvents and petrochemicals.

Mental and Emotional Factors. *Stress* is a risk factor for heart disease and strokes, as well as for most degenerative diseases. The incidence of heart attacks, strokes, and sudden cardiac deaths is higher on Monday mornings than any other time period in the week. Stress also speeds arteriosclerosis (see hyperlipidemia section).

Negative attitudes and intense negative emotions increase risks for heart attack. On experiencing the *grief* of the loss of a loved one, the risk for heart attack is 14 times greater than normal for the first 24 hours following the death. This decreases to only a twofold higher risk 30 days later. The presence or absence of *depression* is the best predictor of survival in men after a heart attack; depressed patients are *six times* more likely to die within 18 months compared to those not depressed. Type A behavior, identified in the 1970s and typified by a pervasive attitude of *hostility*, has been shown in repeated studies to be an important predisposing risk factor for heart disease. Medical students exhibiting high levels of hostility were found in the next 25 years as physicians to have four and one-half times the incidence of heart attacks compared to those with low hostility. Hostility generates high levels of *anger* and *anxiety*, which also contribute to heart attacks. Within two hours after a time of intense anger, risk for having a heart attack increases by two and a half times. The experience of intense emotions coupled with an inability to express them (type D behavior) is also identified as a significant risk factor.

Spiritual and Social Factors. Numerous studies and case histories confirm the fact that people who have positive belief systems, a sense of purpose, and an awareness of a transpersonal cosmic connection with a universal power overcome a variety of genetic, physical, and biochemical predispositions to disease. The shallow experience of many people in this arena is a risk factor for heart disease as well as a variety of other diseases.

The stress of *loneliness* and *social isolation* multiplies all risks of heart disease and significantly worsens prognosis after heart attacks. Men appear to be much more affected than women; this may reflect the fact that men have far fewer supportive relationships than women. Widowed, separated, and divorced men, all of whom have lost opportunities for experiencing intimacy, are especially at risk. Heart energies are related to unconditional love and forgiveness. The self-criticism frequently surfacing when these spiritual energies are blocked leaves us with fear and the feeling of vulnerability. We remain caught in the cycle of resentment, with superimposed feelings of added anger about being powerless. The result has been described by one observer of these issues in cardiac disease as "*the hardened heart.*"

Holistic Prevention and Treatment

The holistic approach to heart disease utilizes the comprehensive evaluation discussed under conventional treatment. Added emphasis is given to the risk factors beyond the classic ones—smoking, hypertension, elevated cholesterol, and diabetes. A simple clinical measure of arteriosclerosis used by many holistic physicians is the ankle-arm index. A ratio of less than 0.9, determined by dividing the systolic blood pressure at the ankle by the systolic pressure in the arm, is highly suspicious for the presence of significant arteriosclerosis. The holistic approach gives heavy emphasis to prevention by challenging all patients to modify their lifestyle to minimize identified risk factors. Even in those rare persons who are heir to a genetically determined progressive cholesterol build-up, lifestyle modifications can offset part of the poor prognosis.

Physical Health Recommendations

Diet

Initiatives include increasing the intake of *whole foods*, including vegetables, fruits, whole unrefined grains, legumes, beans, nuts, seeds, fiber, vitamins, minerals, and essential fatty acids. Only 8 percent of Americans meet the governmental nutritional standard of at least two fruit and three vegetable servings daily. Increasing *fiber* to a reasonable level of 15 grams per day requires most Americans to double or triple their intake. Fiber is found in the same whole foods. While increased fiber intake decreases both bad and good cholesterol, its effect on good cholesterol is much less. Consumption of more *fish* and *fish oils* increases omega-3 essential fatty acid intake. Men eating at least an ounce of fish daily were found to have a 20-year mortality 50 percent lower than that of non–fish eaters. If two to three fish servings per week is not feasible, omega-3 oils can be obtained from fish oil capsules in doses of two grams twice a day. *Flaxseed oil*, two to three teaspoons daily, supplies large amounts of omega-3 oils as well. *Garlic* and *onions* contain active ingredients that tend to lower cholesterol, blood pressure, and risk of certain cancers. *Alfalfa* has been demonstrated in animal studies to regress atherosclerotic plaques and help restore normal structure within arterial walls.

If your body stores of the carotenoid *lycopene* are at highest levels, your risk of heart attack is reduced 50 percent compared to people with low levels. Food sources are watermelon, guava, pink grapefruit, tomatoes, tomato juice, catsup, and dried apricots. *Reduction* of saturated and unsaturated hydrogenated fats (meats, whole milk products, margarines), refined (white) flour products, sugar, caffeinated beverages, and alcohol is also high priority. *Oxidized fats*—those that are becoming rancid and prerancid—are to be avoided as much as possible. While many authorities have recommended reduction of high cholesterol foods such as egg yolks, the evidence for any benefit is marginal. Unless your family has a high genetic predisposition, reasonable egg consumption is not an issue. *Sugar* is a more important factor than many authorities believe. Substituting sugar for starch in the diet significantly raises triglycerides and reduces good cholesterol; and sugar intake in the United States has been rising steadily for 50 years.

Vitamins, Minerals, and Supplements

As a result of incorporation of many of these dietary options, the intake of antioxidant-producing nutritional elements is greatly increased. Basic to the arteriosclerotic process within arterial walls is the multiplication of free radical populations, outstripping the capacity for antioxidants to neutralize the damage. Scores of studies have found that few Americans meet all the RDAs (recommended dietary allowances) for vitamins and minerals. In many instances, intakes are up to 50–70 percent less than the RDAs, which may be marginal in many instances; children, teenagers, and the elderly have especially bad intake records. To assure adequate intake of nutrients that oppose the acceleration of arteriosclerosis, review the recommended table of supplements in chapter 2.

There is strong evidence that increased intake of antioxidant nutrients plays an important role in preventing coronary heart disease.

- Healthy volunteers consuming *vitamin E* supplements (400 to 1,200 I.U. daily) showed significant decreases in susceptibility to oxidation of LDL-C, thought to be the inciting event in the genesis of the arterial wall deterioration. In an extensive study of twelve European male populations, low levels of vitamin E explained 62 percent of the risk of dying of a heart attack compared to high cholesterol, which explained 17 percent. A 50 percent reduction in nonfatal heart attacks was achieved in a six-month period in men taking vitamin E supplements (400–800 I.U. daily) compared to men taking a placebo.

- Subjects with a higher intake of *beta carotene* have a lower incidence of heart disease over the next 10 to 20 years. If you do not get high amounts of *lycopene*-containing foods (see under diet), supplements are available; a reasonable dose is 50 to 75 mg daily.

- Ingestion of *vitamin C* before a high fat breakfast prevents the vasospasm (constriction of the arteries) caused by the fat; it decreases vascular resistance in smokers, improves circulation, and, given with mannitol (a sugar alcohol) during a heart attack, has been shown to double one-year survival. Vitamin C (500 mg daily) cuts the rate of restenosis (recurrent arterial narrowing) after angioplasty 50 percent.

- *Niacin (B-3)* in pharmacological doses of 500–1,500 mg daily and occasionally increased to 3,000 to 4,500 mg daily, decreases serum cholesterol 20 percent and triglycerides 40 percent and increases HDL (good) cholesterol 33 percent. In contrast, Mevacor, the prototype of the newer statin drugs, raised HDL-C by 7 percent. A disadvantage of niacin is marked flushing of the skin about 20 minutes after ingestion. This is a nuisance and not of medical significance; it is reduced by taking the niacin with food. Slow release or time release forms are to be avoided because of potential liver toxicity. Newer products that contain inositol hexaniacinate are essentially free of the flushing reaction and achieve equivalent results with very few other side effects. The dosage is 500 mg three times daily with meals, increased after two weeks to 1,000 mg three times daily.

- *Pantethine* (a form of pantothenic acid, vitamin B-5) is rapidly depleted in hearts with deficient oxygenation. Used in pharmacological doses of 300 mg three times a day, it has been shown to lower total cholesterol and triglycerides while increasing HDL-C (high density lipoprotein cholesterol).

- Levels of *vitamin B-6* (pyridoxine) are significantly lower in heart attack patients compared to healthy people. The relative risk for heart attacks in those with the lowest levels of pyridoxine is estimated to be five times higher. Every additional milligram of vitamin B-6 daily reduces the risk 6 percent.

- The *homocysteinemia* genetic risk factor mentioned earlier is easily neutralized and totally eliminated with daily intake of adequate *folic acid* (400-800 micrograms), *vitamin B-6*, (100 mg) and *vitamin B-12* (1,000 micrograms). Every additional 100 micrograms of daily folic acid intake cuts the heart attack risk 6 percent. Another biosynthetic substance, *betaine*, derived from the B-vitamin choline, is also therapeutic in doses of three grams twice a day.

- *Magnesium* in replacement doses (400 mg daily) raises HDL-C by up to one-third and reduces total cholesterol up to 14 percent. Intravenous magnesium treatment as early as possible during a heart attack improves survival 25 percent.

- *Iron* is essential in the chemical promotion of arteriosclerosis. Some authorities have shown that excess stores of iron accelerate the process, but not all recent studies have confirmed this finding. Nonetheless, donating blood one to three times a year and taking supplements without iron to reduce excess iron stores seems reasonable. We discussed excess iron and cancer in chapter 13.

- The *clotting process*, the precipitating event in most heart attacks and strokes, is initiated when blood cells known as platelets stick to one another, causing a chain reaction of 25 chemicals to produce a clot, or thrombus. This process is accelerated in many diseases, stress, and excessive emotional experience that releases epinephrine (adrenaline). This excessive platelet stickiness, or adhesiveness, is opposed and reversed by aspirin, adequate amounts of *magnesium, vitamins C, E*, and *B-6, choline, garlic, omega-3 oils*, physical exercise, and certain herbs. Bromelain, a proteolytic enzyme of the pineapple plant, also inhibits platelet aggregation (stickiness). Some studies have found vitamin E 20–50 percent better than aspirin for this purpose.

Herbs

- *Commiphora mukul* (gugulipids), an Ayurvedic herb, reduces platelet adhesiveness (stickiness) and increases clot-dissolving activity. One study showed a 20 percent reduction in cholesterol, 30 percent reduction in triglycerides, and 35 percent increase in good cholesterol in 16 weeks with a daily dose of 2.25 grams twice daily. Purified derivatives have few side effects.

- Although studies disagree, *garlic pearls*, 12 grams daily, have been shown to reduce cholesterol 12 percent and triglycerides 17 percent and improve HDL-C 13 percent in three weeks. Another study documented reduction of total cholesterol 12 percent in three months on 800 mg of concentrated garlic powder daily. A recent study showing no improvement compared to placebo was criticized because of the selection of the garlic preparation itself.

- *Ginger*, using one gram of powdered product daily, has been shown to lower cholesterol and decrease platelet aggregation.

- *Hawthorn berry extract*, one-fourth to one-half teaspoon twice daily of the solid gel, acts to protect arterial walls (from Scientific Botanicals in Seattle, WA).

- *Catechin*, 400 mg twice a day, is therapeutic.

- *Ginkgo biloba*, 40 mg three times daily, improves circulation.

Biomolecular Options

- *L-carnitine* is a nonessential amino acid found in small amounts in food and supplied largely from synthesis in the body. Pharmacological doses of four grams daily were shown in one study to improve one-year survival after heart attack tenfold compared to control patients on placebo. L-carnitine is rapidly depleted in hearts that are oxygen deficient; usual helpful dosages are one to three grams daily.

- *Coenzyme Q10*, also produced by the body, has antioxidant properties that exceed those of vitamins C and E and beta carotene. In doses of 100 mg daily, it improves treadmill performance in patients with coronary artery disease, improves circulation through the smallest blood vessels, markedly improves symptoms in mitral valve prolapse, and, in animals, protects against the free radical injury occurring after blood is released into an organ that has been deprived of oxygen during experimental surgery.

- *Glycosaminoglycans (GAGS)*, compounds composed of sugar and protein molecules produced by the body, help maintain the integrity of collagen, a common connective-tissue protein. *Mesoglycan*, a glycosaminoglycan derivative, is found in high amounts in alfalfa. Dosage: 100 mg daily.

- *DHEA* is also available in health food stores. Studies generally demonstrate benefits, especially in those in whom deficient levels have been found. It is wise to have your DHEA levels checked and take appropriate dosages, usually 15–25 mg daily or less, prescribed by a physician. In research, men with a low DHEA were three times more likely to die from arteriosclerosis over a 12-year period than those whose levels were high.

- Low *testosterone* levels are also found in men who later develop coronary heart problems. Cautious doses of testosterone (200 mg weekly by injection) have been shown to increase treadmill performance and electrocardiographic abnormalities. Since testosterone may increase prostate cancer risk, this needs to be an individualized decision made with your physician.

- *Chelation* treatment involves the intravenous injection of chelating agents which remove from the body heavy metals such as lead and mercury and intermediate metals such as iron and copper. It is standard conventional medical treatment for acute and chronic heavy metal poisoning. Chelation with EDTA (an amino acid–like compound) for the last 25 years has been offered by a small number of physicians in the United States for the treatment of arteriosclerotic disease. Considered unscientific and unproven by conventional authorities, numerous case histories and before/after treatment studies have shown benefit, especially in advanced disease. Since the inception of formalized guidelines for use were adopted in 1972, no deaths in treating over half a million patients have been recorded. The mechanisms of action are not thoroughly understood. One of the likely possibilities was emphasized in a review in the *New England Journal of Medicine* in April 1989 that pointed out that all the changes by which arterial wall cells deteriorate to incorporate cholesterol "depend on a common initiating step—the peroxidation of polyunsaturated fatty acids in the LDL lipids. The modification of LDL by cells is totally inhibited by antioxidants," and the "*oxidative modification* is absolutely dependent on the concentrations of iron and copper in the medium and *is therefore completely inhibited by EDTA* or other metal chelators" (emphasis ours). No large placebo-controlled studies have demonstrated unequivocal benefit. A very recent study showed that kidney function improved in patients undergoing EDTA chelation treatments. Unapproved by the FDA, chelation is currently legal in most states by legislative action, largely based on enthusiastic testimonials and successful case reports.

Exercise

Physical exercise constitutes an essential companion to the nutritional initiatives just emphasized. Fortunate you are if you were raised in a family that exercised. Consistent aerobic exercise, discussed in chapter 2, increases good cholesterol about 10 percent and markedly decreases triglycerides. Numerous studies confirm a 15 percent reduction (improvement) in cholesterol/HDL-C ratios with faithful exercise.

In persons with advanced heart disease, the prescription for exercise must be very cautiously and gradually increased. For sedentary persons who have several other risk factors for heart disease, sudden heavy exercise carries a one hundred-fold increased risk of heart attack; all exercise must be approached gradually and increased slowly. Exercise decreases the tendency for platelets to adhere and form clots. Mortality rates from heart attacks and strokes are 60 percent lower in the most fit compared to the least fit. A gentler form of exercise, yoga, has been shown in research to increase the ability of the body to dissolve clots. Levels of fibrinogen, a risk factor, are 10 percent lower in exercising men than in sedentary men.

Mental and Emotional Health Recommendations. Since stress has powerful effects on the cardiovascular system, you need to address the issue by seeking opportunities to gain experiential and cognitive skills to manage it successfully. *Biofeedback* training is highly successful in creating a gradual and substantial change in the functioning of the nervous system.

Learning and practicing *meditation* accomplished the same thing. A very recent study showed significant reversal of atherosclerosis of the carotid arteries in the neck in patients meditating twice daily for 9 months. *Progressive relaxation* is another closely related skill in which patients learn the art of spontaneous muscle relaxation. Levels of catecholamines (adrenaline-like substances), cortisone, and cholesterol all decrease substantially when these skills are acquired and practiced. Some studies have shown over a 12 percent drop in cholesterol with less than a year's practice of meditation. The time required for practice varies upward from ten minutes daily. Nearly all patients who faithfully practice their skills make substantial progress. Anger, anxiety, and depression, all contributors to cardiovascular disease risk, tend to greatly recede with regular relaxation practice. Preoperative *hypnosis* has been shown to substantially improve relaxation states after coronary bypass surgery, accompanied by significant decreased use of pain medications. *Counseling* of a proactive nature is also highly successful in dealing with emotional issues and strategizing to modify the negative attitude of hostility in the positive direction of greater unconditional love. Dr. Dean Ornish utilized daily meditation practice with positive imagery and twice-weekly group counseling sessions as part of his program, which accomplished actual reversal of the arteriosclerotic process within a year. Exercise and vegetarian diet were important elements of his program as well.

Spiritual and Social Health Recommendations. Factors in treatment include evoking a willingness to honor others and yourself by investing in *forgiveness*, which restores the flow of unconditional love and reduces the demands on others and yourself—demands that define the stress you experience. The energy of the heart in the spiritual sense is related to all the emotional and attitudinal issues known to be important in the genesis of heart disease, including hostility, resentment, anger, grief, and loneliness. It also encompasses the positive energies of forgiveness, unconditional love, compassion, hope, and trust.

A major 1988 study authored by Dr. Randolph Byrd found that the death rate, complication rate, incidence of congestive heart failure, and need for mechanical respiration were all substantially reduced in hospitalized heart attack patients for whom regular organized *prayers* were offered compared to those for whom organized prayers were not offered. *Meditation*, besides its physical benefits, often leads to remarkable and sometimes dramatic insights, creative answers, shifts in belief, and a sense of equanimity about life that is as effective as any medication or nutrient.

Relevant *social health* factors that increase survival and shorten hospitalization time after a heart attack include the ongoing *support of family and friends.* The odds of dying within six months after a heart attack is one-third as great among patients who have many social relationships and an intimate connection to a spouse or small circle of significant others compared to patients who are lonely and isolated.

CONDITION
HEART DISEASE — ANGINA

Prevalence

Angina occurs in 50–60 percent of patients as a warning of coronary artery disease. It is quite common and is a warning of serious coronary artery disease.

Anatomy and Physiology

Angina is due to inadequate circulation to the heart and occurs as a result of blockage of one or more coronary arteries by arteriosclerosis, or as a result of spasm in those arteries (Prinzmetal's variant angina) triggered by stress or high levels of adrenaline-like chemicals. Most anginal pain initially occurs when patients are physically exerting themselves; occasionally it presents when patients are physically quiet but acutely stressed, or at night when the blood pressure drops from daytime highs.

Symptoms and Diagnosis

Angina is a pain with a squeezing quality perceived in the chest, often radiated to the left shoulder, neck, chin, and occasionally the left upper back. The pain typically appears with exertion, exposure to cold weather, or stress. The manifesting of anginal pain should trigger a prompt and thorough diagnostic investigation. A suspected diagnosis is confirmed by the tests mentioned under coronary heart disease.

Angiography is a test commonly performed for progressive symptoms of angina;

about a million such procedures are done each year. As described under coronary artery disease, angioplasty or coronary artery bypass surgery are often recommended when serious narrowing is found. Dr. Thomas Graboys, a controversial cardiologist, published in the *Journal of the American Medical Association* in 1992, a study in which noninvasive tests found that 134 of 168 patients for whom angiography had been recommended did not actually need it. Followed for four years, the annualized mortality in this group was 1.1 percent, much lower than the mortality rate of bypass surgery (5–30 percent) or angioplasty (1–2 percent). Only 15 percent eventually needed angioplasty or coronary bypass.

Conventional Medical Treatment

Conventional suggestions include physical exercise and dietary modification emphasizing low cholesterol and low fat intake.

Vasodilating medications commonly prescribed include nitroglycerin tablets taken sublingually for quick relief and long-acting oral nitrates (Isordil, Sorbitrate), patches (Nitro-Dur, Transderm-Nitro), and ointment (Nitro-Bid) for treatment and prevention of anginal pain. Other drugs used in angina include *beta-blockers* (Tenormin, Inderal, Lopressor); and *calcium channel blockers* (Calan, Cardizem, Procardia, Isoptin, Norvasc, Adalat).

Risk Factors and Causes

The major cause of angina, arteriosclerosis, is triggered by all the factors mentioned under coronary artery disease.

Even in coronary arteries with very little arteriosclerotic narrowing, however, constrictive vasospasm can be so intense that the blood supply is cut off long enough to lead to a heart attack. This *vasospastic arterial constriction* is triggered in states of magnesium depletion; by nicotine from smoking and chewing tobacco; and by low blood sugar (hypoglycemia).

Compared to healthy adults, *free radical activity* markers are much higher in advanced, unstable angina patients and moderately higher in stable angina patients. All the circumstances that induce more intense free radical responses (see chapter 2) will apply to the balance of factors favoring angina. Lack of antioxidant defenses to neutralize free radical effects also increases risk.

In depressed patients surviving a heart attack, the risk for development of angina during recovery is three times as great as the incidence in patients who are not depressed. Thirty percent of patients undergoing angiography for angina-like chest pain have normal coronary arteries; this same group has high levels of *anxiety*. Higher levels of anxiety are also linked to a much higher incidence of subsequent, serious heart disease complications. High levels of *anger* are also related to increased incidence of angina.

Holistic Treatment

Physical Health Recommendations

Nutritional Supplements

- Adequate *pantethine*, a form of pantothenic acid (vitamin B-5), as discussed under coronary heart disease, is important in preventing angina.

- The nonessential amino acid *L-arginine*, one-half to one gram three times daily, is beneficial; arginine is the molecule from which the body makes nitric oxide, one of the body's powerful vasodilators.

- Adequate intake of *magnesium*, up to 500 mg daily is essential. Crescendo angina and unstable angina, ominous varieties of the problem, respond well to 10- to 20-minute intravenous injections of one to two grams of magnesium.

- *L-carnitine*, 500–1,000 mg twice daily, substantially increases maximal possible workload, delays onset of pain in angina patients, and improves the electrocardiogram in treadmill testing. Carnitine also greatly reduces the need for conventional drugs.

- *Dimethylglycine*, one teaspoonful of the liquid preparation taken 30 minutes before exertion, decreases angina and improves oxygen uptake and exercise tolerance, including exercise at high altitudes.

- *Coenzyme Q10*, 150 mg per day, reduces the frequency of anginal attacks by 50 percent and nitroglycerine use by 33 percent and improves exercise tolerance by 40 percent.

- Chelation was discussed in coronary heart disease.

Herbs

- A 1951 *New England Journal of Medicine* study had high praise for *Khellin*, an Ammi visnaga derivative (40 mg) taken five times daily before and between meals and at bedtime for three to eleven months; it was highly effective in reducing the frequency and severity of anginal episodes, even improving exercise tolerance and the appearance of the electrocardiogram. Khellin possesses outstanding vasodilating properties.

- *Hawthorn (crataegus)*, used in many cardiac conditions, also has vasodilating properties and is helpful in angina in doses of a 1:5 tincture, 1–1½ teaspoons (250 mg) three times a day.

- *Bilberry* (Vaccinium myrtillus) contains an anthocyanoside that improves circulation and reduces small blood vessel damage (standardized extract, 240 mg three times daily).

Exercise

An experimental calisthenic exercise group has been shown to increase (improve) time-to-onset of angina *70 percent* in a year compared to a group treated with drugs improving only 30 percent.

Mental and Emotional Health Recommendations. Biofeedback, relaxation practice, and meditation all benefit angina patients, reducing tension and modifying free radical loads.

Spiritual and Social Health Recommendations. *Beliefs.* Studies of the placebo effect have shown 82 percent relief of angina from drugs and procedures that were later shown to have *no therapeutic effect whatsoever.* Placebos are effective because of the belief in their effectiveness. Your beliefs are a central factor in your spiritual life and have an enormous effect on your real-time experience. Your holistic physician and knowledgeable counselors can help with these issues.

In a recent study, education about the nature of angina and practical relevant advice given in a regular *supportive group* setting for angina patients had a much better outcome than those handled with "routine" conventional care. The greatest differences came in greater exercise and substantial nutritional improvements in the support group.

High levels of *spousal love* and social support greatly improve the prognosis for fewer complications and longer survival. Garnering support means asking for what you need, being willing to graciously accept offers of help, and expressing your feelings about what is going on without ruminating about it.

HEART DISEASE — ARRHYTHMIAS

Prevalence

Arrhythmias, or rhythm disturbances of the heart, are the major cause of sudden unexpected death, which takes thousands of lives in the United States each year. About half of these occur in the absence of any discernable heart disease, even at postmortem examination.

Anatomy and Physiology

The human heart, normally beating regularly at rest at an average of 50 to 100 beats per minute, delivers about one-plus teaspoons of blood into the arterial system with each stroke. The heart maintains its own intrinsic rhythm, which is influenced by the hypothalamic part of the brain through the autonomic nervous system. In children and fit, healthy adults, this rhythm is very slightly irregular, varying with respiration. The electromagnetic energy field of the heart is very large, exceeding the electromagnetic field of any other organ in the body.

Rhythm disturbances are the manifestation of abnormal conductance patterns of electrical messages through the heart. While most rhythm disturbances are not life threatening, they can be fatal. Arrhythmias are a common cause of death in heart attacks, frequently occurring before emergency medical help can be mobilized. The chemical receptor sites in the heart respond almost immediately to neurotransmitter chemicals such as adrenaline and hormones of the endocrine system.

Symptoms and Diagnosis

The presence of a rhythm disturbance of the heart may be signaled by fainting, sudden collapse, the sensation of rapid heartbeat, or the feeling of pressure in the chest with breathlessness. While many arrhythmias are mild and not a cause for alarm, others can be life threatening. Complaints of heart rhythm disturbances are not always easy to confirm and may require 72-hour periods of observing the heart with a special monitor used during normal daily activities.

Conventional Treatment

Once a significant heart rhythm disturbance has been confirmed, a variety of drugs may be prescribed. Names of commonly used drugs include Cardioquin, Norpace, Mexitil, Procan, quinidine, propranolol (Inderal), Brevibloc, Calan, Cardizem, phenytoin, and digoxin.

Paroxysmal atrial tachycardia, an episodic, extremely rapid heart rhythm, may be interrupted by performing the Valsalva maneuver (exhaling vigorously against a closed glottis) or putting intense thumb pressure on the soft palate in the roof of the mouth to the point of pain.

Conversion with electrical current stimulation (cardioversion) is selectively used to reestablish normal rhythms in atrial and ventricular tachycardias. Rhythm disturbances in which the heart beat is unreliable or excessively slow (bradycardias) may be treated with implantation of temporary or permanent pacemakers.

Risk Factors and Causes

Physical Factors. *Heredity.* Genetic family patterns play a role in an uncommon rhythm disturbance called long Q-T intervals.

Nutritional factors. Arrhythmias may result from copper, magnesium, potassium, or selenium deficiencies. Stress elaborates chemical and hormonal changes that deplete the body of magnesium and potassium, which are further decreased in persons taking diuretics (water pills) for heart failure or high blood pressure. A

1987 study found magnesium levels in the heart muscle of patients with ventricular tachycardia to be *65 percent lower* than levels in healthy controls. Diets high in saturated fat are associated with increased incidence of sudden death from sustained ventricular fibrillation or malignant arrhythmias. Hypoglycemia can trigger rhythm disturbances. Caffeine is consumed in common beverages daily by a majority of those in the United States. Two cups of coffee a day (300 mg) can provoke heart rhythm disturbances in susceptible people, and six to eight cups daily provokes at least minor abnormalities in a majority of beverage drinkers.

Sensitivities. Heart rhythm disturbances can be caused by *environmental* and *food sensitivity reactions.* In about 25 percent of problems occurring because of sensitivities, the offender turns out to be food related. The most common arrhythmia caused by food is paroxysmal atrial tachycardia (fast heart rate), but sinus tachycardia, sinus bradycardia (slow heart rate), and ventricular tachycardia have all been reported. The most likely food offenders are listed under hypertension. It is estimated that one-quarter of all heart rhythm disturbances are triggered by allergic and sensitivity responses.

Hormonal causes. Among the endocrine causes of rhythm disturbances is *thyrotoxicosis,* involving release of excessive amounts of thyroid hormone (hyperthyroidism). High cortisone production from adrenal gland disease or high doses of cortisone-like drugs (prednisone) contributes to risk. A wide variety of prescribed medications, as well as street drugs, including cocaine and narcotics, can lead to abnormal rhythms as well.

Mental and Emotional Factors. *Stress* is clearly frequently related to the onset or recurrence of heart rhythm disturbances. Tension, anxiety, and *fear* resulting from unmanaged stressful experiences and even from imagined stressful experiences can trigger serious and even fatal cardiac arrhythmias. Threatened muggings in which the intended victims were not actually touched have been reported to result in fatal arrhythmias, for instance.

Belief systems are also clearly related to occurrence of arrhythmias. One case history reported a patient susceptible to an arrhythmia that consistently happened during exercise after he had stepped over a barrier 44 times. When the technician deliberately miscounted the crossings, his rhythm disturbance occurred when he heard the technician say 44 but when he was actually on crossing number 56.

Holistic Treatment

Physical Health Recommendations

Diet, Minerals, and Supplements

- *Pantethine*, a form of pantothenic acid (vitamin B-5), favorably impacts arrhythmias in animal studies. It also markedly improves cholesterol ratios (300 mg three times a day).

- *Magnesium* levels fall 35 percent during surgery. Administration of extra magnesium after bypass surgery reduces the incidence of arrhythmias 50 percent. A wide variety of benign and threatening rhythm disturbances responds to a 2-gram dose of magnesium given intravenously, followed by a slow drip of magnesium over hours or days. Intravenous magnesium has been shown to be slightly more successful as an antiarrhythmic compared to the drug verapamil (Isoptin) in treatment of supraventricular tachycardias, while producing zero percent side effects, versus 21 percent from the drug, and magnesium appears to be the initial treatment of choice versus the drugs Brevibloc or Cardizem for ventricular arrhythmias, with significantly lower cost and fewer side effects. Oral doses are 400–800 mg daily.

- The intake of *selenium* is beneficial to the myocardium even in the absence of demonstrable deficiency. In persons with arrhythmias who are prone to exhibit arrhythmias, persons with intractable arrhythmias who are on long-term weight-reducing diets, or persons who have anorexia nervosa or require intravenous supplementation, selenium should be included as a supplement. Up to 850 micrograms daily as a supplement is tolerated with no toxic effects. Prime food sources include whole grains, seafoods, shellfish, Swiss chard, turnips, Brazil nuts, meat, and milk.

- In primates, high polyunsaturated fat intakes are associated with decreased susceptibility to ventricular fibrillation and arrhythmias. So it is reasonable and wise to increase omega-3 essential fatty acid intake (two to three grams twice a day).

- Reduction of processed sugar and refined flour intake forestalls the tendency toward low blood sugar that can provoke arrhythmias.

- *Coenzyme Q10*. In recovery from injuries and surgery, administration of coenzyme Q10, 100 mg daily, leads to a significantly lower incidence of ventricular arrhythmias compared to controls. In patients receiving Coenzyme Q10, reductions in ventricular premature beats of 50 percent were reported. Adenosine, a "second messenger" nucleic acid derivative produced by the body, rapidly and effectively terminates paroxysmal atrial tachycardia more rapidly than the drug verapamil when given intravenously.

Herbs

- *Hawthorn berry*, 1:1 fluid extract (¼ tsp. three times daily)

- *Cactus grandiflora*, 1:5 tincture (15–25 drops two to three times daily); helpful in heart palpitations

- A 1:1 combination of *hawthorn* and *cactus* in tincture form, 30 drops three times daily

Mental and Emotional Health Recommendations. Relaxation learned through *biofeedback*, *autogenic training*, or *meditation* can be enormously helpful in preventing both mild and serious rhythm disturbances. The centeredness achieved by the development of meditative practices permits the handling of greater amounts of acute and chronic stress at a much "lower price" of greatly reduced baseline sympathetic nervous system reactivity, less tension, and much lower increases in catecholamines (adrenaline) and cortisone with any kind of stress.

HEART DISEASE — CONGESTIVE HEART FAILURE (CHF)

Prevalence

Two to three million Americans are afflicted with congestive heart failure (about 1 percent of the population). It is the most common reason for hospitalization in those 65 and older. Slightly under a million new cases are diagnosed each year.

Anatomy and Physiology

Congestive heart failure, or cardiac insufficiency, refers to the circumstance in which the heart pumps blood inadequately to the body. It represents an inability on the part of the heart to meet its workload. Congestive heart failure tends to be progressive, with a very significant shortening of life expectancy.

Symptoms and Diagnosis

Symptoms of congestive heart failure include shortness of breath with exertion and when lying flat, the appearance of edema or swelling, particularly in the lower limbs, and progressive weight gain from retention of water in body tissues. Congestive heart failure tends to be progressive, with a very significant shortening of life expectancy. Heart enlargement is usually present, most often due to an attempt on the part of the heart itself to compensate for poor pumping action. A healthy heart increases pumping action output (stroke volume) in response to exertion; sick hearts have no reserve to meet this kind of demand.

The clinical diagnosis made from the typical history is confirmed by physical findings of retention of liquid in the lower limbs and lungs, enlargement of the heart, more labored respiration, and, in advanced conditions, loss of full oxygen saturation of the blood. Laboratory confirmation can be accomplished with an X-ray of the chest showing heart enlargement or an echocardiogram demonstrating compromised blood ejection from the left ventricle.

Conventional Treatment

Management of congestive cardiac insufficiency begins with a standard regimen of dietary sodium limitation. Drugs are prescribed primarily from the following classes of pharmaceuticals:

- Derivatives of *digitalis* (digoxin, Lanoxin) increase the strength of heart contractions.
- *Diuretics* assist in removing edema fluid in the body occurring as a result of poor heart action (Hydrodiuril [hydrochlorothiazide], Dyazide, and Lasix.
- *Angiotensin converting enzyme inhibitors* (Zestril, Capoten, Vasotec, Monopril, Prinivil, Lotensin), add another dimension to drug treatment, reducing the load on the heart.
- Selective *beta-blockers* are also used as a fourth line drug (Coreg).

Cost considerations also become a factor. The estimated cost of gaining one additional year of life with treatment with one of the angiotensin inhibitor drugs is $9,700. Inevitably, end-stage cardiac failure frequently demands high-cost hospital treatment, adding intravenous medication and bed rest to previously used outpatient regimens.

Side effects of pharmaceuticals used to treat congestive heart failure and contributing causes are also common. Commonly experienced untoward effects of pharmaceuticals include digitalis toxicity, a higher than expected death rate in those on chronic diuretic treatment (associated with loss of potassium and magnesium), and sexual impotence with many classes of cardiac drugs. One diuretic, furosemide, tends to deplete thiamine, a B-complex vitamin known to be essential for adequate heart function. An April 1999 review from the journal *Cardiology* confirmed an increased risk of renal cell carcinoma (an uncommon kidney cancer) in users of diuretics compared to non-users.

Conventional treatment also emphasizes the control of predisposing conditions, including high blood pressure and coronary artery disease. Anticoagulation is sometimes undertaken to reduce the formation of clots within the heart chambers, which occur more often in congestive heart failure.

Risk Factors and Causes

Congestive heart failure may be secondary to heart deterioration from:

- Arteriosclerotic coronary artery disease
- Hypertension
- Constriction of scar tissue surrounding the heart (constrictive pericarditis)
- Degenerative lung disease
- Primary deterioration of heart muscle fibers themselves, called cardiomyopathy, a particularly lethal cause of progressive congestive failure, may develop for reasons often unknown; identified causes include excessive alcohol consumption, after-effects of viral infections, toxic side effects from drugs, including cancer chemotherapeutic agents, and deficiency of selenium in the diet

Congestive heart failure may also develop without any of these recognized contributing factors.

Physical factors

Nutritional Factors

- Excess intake of sodium, primarily as salt, predispose susceptible persons to congestive heart failure.
- Loss of potassium and magnesium are highly suspect in the majority of arrhythmic deaths, the most common cause of the sudden death that most often ends the life of a congestive heart failure patient, whether their condition has been stable or progressive. Low blood potassium is commonly recognized and treated, but low magnesium levels are not. These minerals are removed from the body in times of excess stress and as a result of treatment with diuretic drugs.
- Individuals with subclinical selenium deficiency may show no overt signs of cardiomyopathy but nonetheless experience subtle reductions of myocardial contractility and excessive excitability responses to normal and abnormal stimuli.
- Congestive heart failure is clearly a free radical–mediated problem. The degree of heart failure is positively and progressively correlated with increasing levels of free radical activity markers; the degree of failure is negatively correlated with levels of antioxidant enzymes. Deficiency of antioxidants may soon be considered a risk factor for congestive heart failure.
- In heart disease, Coenzyme Q10 is easily displaced and lost from heart muscle cells. This leads to depleted strength of heart muscle cell contractions, tending to

lead to heart failure. Low levels of Coenzyme Q10 are predictive of heart failure; Coenzyme Q10 in cardiomyopathy patients has been found to be 20 percent below that in healthy people.

- Persons with heart failure are consistently found to have significantly lower levels of the nonessential amino acid taurine, which is mostly synthesized in the body.

- Lower levels of L-carnitine, another amino acid, are also found in heart failure.

Environmental Factors
Environmental toxins contribute to congestive heart failure. Acute exacerbations requiring hospitalization in large cities are related to times of increased carbon monoxide concentrations due to pollution and weather variations.

Emotional Factors. *Anger.* One of the sophisticated ways of assessing the degree of congestive heart failure is the measurement of the efficiency in pumping blood, called the left ventricular ejection fraction (LVEF), which has been shown to decrease 7 percent during times when patients with established coronary artery disease recounted incidents in which they had responded with anger. This recollection eroded LVEF significantly more than physical exercise (2 percent), mental arithmetic testing (0 percent), and a speech stressor experience (0 percent).

Issues of congestive heart failure are symbolic for the emotional congestion of maintaining unfulfilling relationships and situations when one's "heart is not in it" and in failing to resolve overwhelming feelings of grief—the "broken heart."

Social Factors. *Quality of relationships.* From an intuitive energy diagnosis standpoint, the weakening of heart function is captured in the symbolism of "my heart's just not in this anymore." This may be related to the lack of quality in personal relationships or in the aspects of one's workplace and occupation. The result is the emotional congestion of depression and a sense of detachment from one's life that drains energy from the essential heart functions.

Holistic Prevention
Since coronary artery arteriosclerotic disease and hypertension are significant contributing causes of congestive heart failure, all the issues in prevention of those two conditions apply here. Aggressive treatment of a rare condition called constrictive pericarditis will frequently prevent the complication of heart failure; conventional treatment with cortisone is frequently successful in this condition; in stubbornly resistant cases, administration of colchicine, a drug used for gout, is strikingly successful.

Prevalence of free radicals is found in a greater portion of patients with congestive heart failure compared to healthy subjects. The supplying of adequate nutrients, including antioxidants and minerals, amino acids, and biosynthetic agents, may be central to the prevention of congestive heart failure. Much more basic research will need to be completed to resolve these questions.

Holistic Treatment

Physical Health Recommendations

Vitamins, Minerals, and Supplements

- *Antioxidants.* Since congestive heart failure is in part a free radical problem, it is no surprise that antioxidant agents, including *vitamins A, C,* and *E,* as well as biosynthetic agents (produced by the body) with antioxidant properties contribute to both preventing and controlling congestive heart failure. The addition of vitamin E, 400 I.U. daily, to treatment of heart failure patients has persuasively shown additional dimensions of improvement.

- *Magnesium* and *potassium*, consistently lower in patients with congestive heart failure (only partially due to diuretics), deserve consistent replacement. Potassium supplements are commonly conventionally prescribed. It may take up to six months to restore magnesium body stores with oral doses, which should be 400–800 mg daily. Intravenous magnesium markedly benefits most patients with congestive heart failure within three months. Improvement continues to manifest for up to a year in 85 percent of patients. *Magnesium is contraindicated in patients with cerebral hemorrhage and in patients in severe renal failure.* Magnesium is a natural calcium channel blocker.

- *Thiamine*, 200 mg daily for 6 weeks, has been shown to improve indices of congestive failure up to 20 percent. Thiamine is readily depleted by diuretics. Cost is insignificant, risk is nil, and benefits are great.

- Based on current research, five glasses of *water* or more each day are highly recommended.

- *Polyunsaturated fat* increases in the diet are associated with improved pumping action from the left heart in primates.

- *Taurine*, an amino acid, taken 2 grams 2–3 times daily for 4 weeks, has been observed to substantially improve the state of heart function in advanced congestive heart failure. Side effects are extremely rare.

- *L-carnitine* is a nonessential amino acid helpful in congestive heart failure. Given as a 4-gram intravenous injection, it is even helpful in cardiogenic shock, a sudden, acute, life-threatening state of poor heart output. Oral doses of L-carnitine, 2 gm daily, restore energy metabolism, improve treadmill performance in CHF patients, and markedly reduce the need for drugs, with improvement usually appearing within a month of starting treatment. A review of the research found *no studies with negative results* in treatment of congestive heart failure with L-carnitine (1,500–2,000 mg daily).

- *Coenzyme Q10.* The lower the Coenzyme Q10 blood levels in patients with heart failure, the more severe the failure. Given Coenzyme Q10, 100–150 mg daily, the heart pumping efficiency of far-advanced cardiomyopathy patients increases 50 percent, manifesting in extraordinary clinical improvement. Studies show the two-year survival on continuous doses of Coenzyme Q10 to be 85 percent contrasted to the usual experience of 50 percent. Patients in congestive heart failure receiving Coenzyme Q10 have been shown to require hospitalization only 20 percent of the time compared to 48 percent for those taking a placebo.

- *Dimethylglycine* (see under arrhythmias).

- *Hawthorn berry* (see under coronary artery disease).

Exercise

Patients with severe heart failure engaging in appropriate low-grade aerobic exercise with walking and bicycle exercise for a year improved all measures of heart activity, breathing capacity, and quality of life as well. A carefully crafted exercise prescription should be obtained from your physician. T'ai chi, a gentle Chinese movement art form, often does nicely.

CONDITION

HYPERTENSION

Prevalence

Hypertension, or high blood pressure, is very common in the United States. Among adults, an estimated twenty percent of the white population and thirty percent of the African American population have blood pressures above 165/95 mmHg. Thirty percent of the entire population will eventually face hypertension. Hypertension is essentially unknown among members of emerging nations and remote tribes worldwide.

Anatomy and Physiology

Hypertension is a result of the narrowing or constriction of arteries throughout the body. Arteriosclerosis (hardening of the arteries) contributes to this change, but the major factor is the constriction of the muscular layer of the smaller arteries (arterioles). This vasoconstrictive process occurs normally in vast areas of the body when the arousal (fight-or-flight) reflex is triggered, in order to supply more blood to the muscles used in the physical activity. As constriction occurs, the blood vessels increase their resistance to the flow of blood, and the heart works harder, sustaining a higher blood pressure to force more oxygen-bearing blood into the tissues supplied through the constricted arteries. High blood pressure sustained over long periods of time takes a gradually increasing toll in malfunction of the heart itself, leading to heart attack and congestive heart failure, and accelerates arteriosclerotic damage to the blood vessels throughout the body, leading to stroke, kidney failure, and loss of circulation to the legs. Elevation of either the systolic or diastolic pressure readings carries an increased risk of premature death.

Symptoms and Diagnosis

Hypertension commonly gives no obvious symptoms and is discovered unexpectedly at the time of an examination; many Americans have the problem without knowing it, although ringing in the ears and headache may occasionally signal its presence. The latest guidelines for hypertension are as follows: high to normal pressure: 130–139/85–89 mmHg; stage 1 hypertension: 140–159/90–99 mmHg; stage 2 hypertension: 160–179/100–109 mmHg; stage 3 hypertension: 180–209/110–119 mmHg. These levels are based on an average of at least three readings with the patient at rest and free of acute stress.

Conventional Medical Treatment

Questions surrounding verification of the actual presence of hypertension lend themselves to no easy answers. The general standard requires the finding of at least three elevated random blood pressure readings to make a diagnosis of hypertension. Certain persons elevate their blood pressure only in the presence of a doctor or nurse; this is the so-called "white coat effect." Blood pressures rise when people speak; recorded pressures should reflect the nonverbal state. Careful documentation in hospitalized patients has shown a rise of as much as 25 mmHg in blood pressure as the doctor enters a room to check a patient. The taking of repeated blood pressures at home by patients themselves or by family members will usually reveal this discrepancy. A blood pressure that is elevated only in the doctor's office should not be treated by drugs.

Most physicians begin treatment of hypertension with suggestions to reduce dietary salt, lose weight, begin or increase exercise, and cease smoking. Conventional treatment also usually involves prescription medications. The classes of drugs used, with a few of the commonly used drugs in each category, include:

- Alpha adrenoreceptor blockers (Minipress)
- Alpha adrenoreceptor central inhibitory stimulants (Aldomet, Catapres)
- Beta adrenergic blockers (Inderal, Tenormin, Lopressor)

- Angiotensin converting enzyme receptor inhibitors (Zestril, Capoten, Vasotec, Monopril, Prinivil, Accupril, Lotensin)
- Angiotensin II converting enzyme (ACE) inhibitors (Cozaar, Diovan)
- Diuretics (Dyazide, Lasix, Hydrodiuril [hydrochlorothiazide])
- Rauwolfia derivatives
- Vasodilators

Drugs from two different classes can often be combined with a low dosage of both to minimize side effects and achieve better blood pressure control.

The question of when to treat hypertension continues to be a matter of disagreement. The majority of physicians start treatment for readings at 150/90 mmHg, with a few authorities concluding that drug treatment is not justified until levels reach 170/105 mmHg. The latter experts cite large studies that confirm that drug treatment in mild and moderate hypertension lessens heart disease risks but often decreases longevity due to the serious side effects of the drugs themselves. Studies have shown that the heart attack rate in men at risk for heart problems is higher in groups treated with cholesterol-lowering drugs and antihypertensives compared to those treated with exercise and dietary measures. Robert Eliot, a widely recognized research cardiologist from the University of Nebraska, has stated it unequivocally: "*There is no reduction in sudden death or heart attack incidence with drug management of blood pressure.* There is a decrease in the incidence of strokes" (our italics). Diuretics have long been known to have downside effects by removing potassium from the body; less well known but no less important is the fact that diuretics also remove magnesium and zinc from the body. Recently calcium channel blockers have been shown to be linked to a higher death rate and complications of clotting because they increase a body chemical called thromboglobulin. Other side effects impacting quality of life are persistent cough with ACE inhibitors and impotence and decreased libido reported in nearly all classes of drugs just mentioned. The side effects are the most common reason patients fail to take their antihypertensive medications at all, or fail to take them regularly.

Advertising by the American Heart Association insists that an antihypertensive drug, once started, must be continued for life. This is untrue. Many persons on drugs, having made important lifestyle changes as outlined below, can safely go off their medications.

Risk Factors and Causes

Ninety-five percent of cases of high blood pressure have no conventionally identified cause. A number of factors, however, are quite obviously related.

Physical and Environmental Factors

Habits

An increased risk of high blood pressure, especially the malignant variety, is incurred by *smoking* and *tobacco use*. Nicotine from tobacco chewed or smoked is a vasoconstrictive agent, aggravating the blood vessel narrowing that is the immediate cause of the hypertension. *Alcohol* in modest or great amounts is strongly related to the risk for high blood pressure, and *coffee* and caffeine lead to mild elevations in some but not all studies. *Overweight* persons have a higher risk of developing hypertension. Increased demands on the heart and changes in hormone chemistry are thought to explain the risk.

Genetic

Familial susceptibility makes offspring significantly more vulnerable to influences of excess sodium and loss of potassium. The genetic factor is relatively small compared to learning experiences and other lifestyle factors.

Diet

Since *vegetarians* have consistently lower blood pressures than carnivores who also eat meat, the latter practice probably contributes to hypertension. Even utilizing the balance of foods in the government food pyramid nudges people toward a more vegetarian diet. The better forms of animal protein are deep-sea, cold-water fish, consumed at up to three to five meals per week.

Sugar. In laboratory rats, groups consuming 10, 15, and 20 percent of total calories as sucrose for 14 weeks had significantly higher systolic blood pressure than rats consuming no sucrose. Sucrose in western diets averages more than 20 percent of calories. It is also important to avoid high glycemic index foods (see chapter 2). Studies in humans also suggest that increased salt retention and elevated blood pressure occur with higher intake of sugars.

Nutrient deficiencies. Deficiency in calcium, magnesium, potassium, and zinc from the diet is known to contribute to high blood pressure. Excess sodium, chiefly from salt, raises blood pressure in the one person out of six who is sodium sensitive. Dehydration, as with coronary artery disease and congestive heart failure, increases risk.

In hypertension there tends to be a deficiency of taurine, a nonessential amino acid obtained in small amounts in food and also synthesized in the body.

Food sensitizing agents. High blood pressure can be a response to food sensitivities. The probability that food sensitivities will play a role is greater in persons with a family history of allergies, those with food cravings or habitual ingestion of great amounts of a few foods, and those whose hypertension seems to come and go. Careful history taking and food elimination and reexposure trials can identify offending sensitizing foods. The most common food offenders include chocolate, corn, nuts (especially peanuts), pork, coffee, milk, wheat, rice, beef, shrimp, seafood, chicken, and apples. Caffeine is known to elevate blood pressure and should be avoided by anyone who has even occasional elevated readings.

Environmental

Hypertensive patients have higher blood levels of lead (gasoline, paint, drinking water) and three times higher amounts of cadmium (batteries and cigarettes) than nonhypertensive persons. All toxins, including these heavy metals, provoke increased levels of free radicals in the body, and hypertension is on the long list of diseases linked to this problem. Hypertension is more common in persons exposed to inhalant sensitizing agents, including chemical odors (natural gas, gasoline fumes, chlorine), air pollution, auto exhaust, soft plastic, cleaning chemicals (Lysol, phenol), perfume, polyurethane, tobacco smoke, polyesters, fiberglass, Naugahyde, new carpeting, formaldehyde, pesticides, pest strips, and foam rubber. The probability that inhalant sensitivities will play a role in hypertension is greater in persons with a personal or family history of allergies and those whose hypertension varies by the season or geographical location. Careful history taking can often identify offending sensitizing agents.

Exercise

If you are sedentary, you increase your risks of hypertension about 50 percent. Since tension accruing from stressful experiences is dissipated during physical exercise, you may simply miss the opportunity to wind yourself down. The elevated blood pressure that occurs with athletic or vigorous physical exertion is much less damaging because it does not remain sustained after the exertion is terminated. The gradual rise in blood pressures that accompanies aging occurs much less often in people who remain physically fit.

Mental and Emotional Factors. *Stress.* The fight-or-flight response is triggered by all stressful phenomena that are perceived to be threatening and require adaptation. Documented types of stress tending to lead to elevation of blood pressures include public speaking and performance tasks, worksite pressures, critical time-related requirements, as with air-traffic-controllers, and ongoing family conflicts. Other research-confirmed factors include increased life dissatisfactions, impatience, and type A behavior, which includes increased hostility and anger. Imagined stresses also can raise blood pressure as much as can those experienced in reality. Elevated blood pressures also develop in subjects who suppress or repress emotions while maintaining a calm exterior appearance (type D behavior). A 1996 study within the black community found that the risk of hypertension among African Americans is aggravated by experiences of racial discrimination and unwillingness to challenge unfair treatment.

Attitude and emotional states. Two basic types of elevated blood pressure reactions have been identified. The first is seen in persons whose sympathetic nervous system overreacts to stressful stimuli with overt and visible emotional disturbance. The second is seen when suppression or repression of strong emotions is accompanied by a calm exterior appearance. Blood pressure surges under stress are very much greater in emotionally defensive personalities than those with low defensiveness. Persons prone to more angry moods have significantly higher blood pressures at night than persons who are predominantly happy and pleasant. Anxiety-prone men and women are more prone to hypertension. Hypertension is seen by medical intuitives as related to frustration and anger, often linked with inflexibility.

Holistic Prevention

Maintaining proper weight, participating in a regular aerobic exercise plan, and engaging in some form of regular relaxation or meditation practice are the paramount issues in reducing the risk of developing hypertension. Avoiding exposure to sources of lead and cadmium is imperative, including the filtering of drinking and cooking water. Abatement of or reduction in smoking decreases blood vessel constriction and reduces the intake of cadmium.

Improvement in nutritional habits, including maintaining a very modest intake of sodium (salt) and consuming adequate essential minerals (potassium, magnesium, and calcium) and antioxidant vitamins, are also important steps in prevention. Higher intakes of polyunsaturated fatty acids are associated with decreased blood pressure and better heart pumping action.

Management of stress which elevates blood pressures involves relaxation training, reduction in hostile, negative attitudes, and decreasing anger. All the appropriate steps in hypertension treatment that follow can also be incorporated into a program for prevention.

Holistic Treatment

Conventional authorities state that careful attention to lifestyle changes can control blood pressure 40 percent of the time to the point that medications can be eliminated. The holistic perspective is much more enthusiastic. Our experience has shown that optimizing all lifestyle factors can achieve normalization of blood pressure, while eliminating drugs, 85 percent of the time.

Physical Health Recommendations. Stabilizing weight to within 5–10 percent of the ideal is substantially helpful in persons with hypertension. Blood pressures usually drop promptly as *weight loss* occurs. Ideal weights can be determined by normal tables, by measurements of abdominal girth, by calculations based on measurement of fat layers, and by using the Body Mass Index (see Chapter 16). Percentage of body fat should be below 18 for men and 24 for women. *Limiting alcohol* to one drink or less per day is also an important initiative, since excess alcohol is a major contributor to hypertension. Reduction or elimination of smoking is an obvious necessity; if you have tried and failed to quit before, you may wish to utilize acupuncture, which is often very helpful in a total program of nicotine abatement.

Diet

- *Whole foods.* Initiatives include increasing the intake of whole foods, including vegetables, fruits, whole unrefined grains, legumes, beans, nuts, seeds, fiber, vitamins, minerals, and essential fatty acids. Such a diet lowers systolic pressure 12 mmHg and diastolic 6 mmHg. Vegetarians have lower blood pressures than consumers of combined animal and vegetarian food sources (omnivores). You do not have to be vegetarian to begin to reap the benefits of increasing fruits to three servings a day and vegetables to four or five servings a day and using only low fat milk and dairy products.

- Reducing *total and saturated fat* intake lowered systolic blood pressure 12 mmHg and diastolic blood pressure 6 mmHg in one large trial in hypertensives. These decreases are substantial and comparable to the results of many drug regimens. Meals with deep-sea fish supply essential fatty acids helpful in blood pressure control.

- Increasing *linoleic acid* intake lowers blood pressure. Hypertensives are deficient in chemical compounds whose source is linoleic acid. Sources high in linoleic acid include sunflower, sesame, and pumpkin seeds and their oils; safflower, evening primrose, grapeseed, and canola oils; corn, wheat germ, soy, and rice bran, and their oils; walnuts, peanuts, and brazil nuts, and their oils.

- Intake of more than 24 grams of *fiber* daily compared to less than 12 grams daily decreased the incidence of high blood pressure 57 *percent* in a study of 30,000 men. Excellent examples of fiber include psyllium seeds, guar gum, apple pectin, and oat bran.

Vitamins, Minerals, and Supplements

Including adequate daily amounts of the following supplements (if you are not totally sure that you are getting them from food) gives assurance that optimum daily intake is met:

- *Vitamin C.* In a number of research studies, average pressure decrease with vitamin C intake above 250 mg daily is 7 percent. Vitamin C acts to oppose the arterial constriction caused by smoking, promoting arterial flexibility and dilation.

- *Vitamin E*, 600 mg.

- *Beta carotene*, 30 mg.

- *Zinc*, 45 mg.

- *Vitamin B-1*, 10–20 mg.

- *Calcium.* Men consuming more than one gram of calcium daily compared to those ingesting less than one-half gram daily have a 20 percent lower incidence of hypertension.

- *Magnesium.* Men consuming more than 400 mg daily of magnesium compared to those taking in less than 250 mg daily have a 50 percent lower incidence.

- Men consuming more than 3.5 grams daily of *potassium* compared to those ingesting less than 2.5 grams daily have a 55 percent lower incidence.

- *Avoiding excess amounts of sodium* is also important. As an adult, you need only 1.5 grams of sodium daily, which can be achieved without salting most foods and by avoiding many commercially prepared foods, including pickles, canned foods, preserved meats, and fast foods.

- Nine grams of fish oil (high in omega-3 oils) daily for six weeks has been shown to reduce diastolic blood pressure an average of five mmHg.

- *Taurine* supplements lower blood pressures; six grams daily has been shown to lower systolic pressure 10 mmHg and diastolic 5 mmHg in seven days, with no effects seen in subjects with normal blood pressures. Taurine indirectly decreases sympathetic vasoconstriction, the primary cause of hypertension. Reasonable doses are one to one and a half grams daily.

- *Coenzyme Q10*, 100 mg daily, in one group of men reduced average systolic blood pressure 10 mmHg and diastolic pressure 8 mmHg.

- *Phosphatidylserine* (100 mg three times daily) tempers excessive sympathetic nervous system activity, which elevates blood pressure.

Herbs

- In a study of patients with pressures 190–240/70–150 mmHg treated with *hawthorn berry* (Crataegus oxacantha), blood pressure decreased in all cases, resulting in pressures ranging from 110–175 systolic and 55–100 diastolic. In the 1:5 tincture form, 1–1½ teaspoons is taken daily.

- *Garlic* and *onions* both have blood pressure lowering properties. In some studies, liberal use of fresh garlic has lowered systolic blood pressure by 20 to 30 mmHg and diastolic pressure by 10 to 20 mmHg.

- *Mistletoe* (Viscum album), as a whole plant, 1:1 fluid extract, lowers blood pressure in 0.5 ml doses. Extended use and intake of doses exceeding the equivalent of four grams per day of the crude herb are not recommended.

- When anxiety prominently accompanies or contributes to hypertension, *kava kava* works well to neutralize this factor (30 percent kavalactone content, 150 mg three to five times daily).

Exercise

Blood pressures respond favorably to physical activity, including walking, running, gardening, and other steady vigorous activities. If you have hypertension and start exercising, there is a good chance that you can reduce or eliminate your medications. Low and moderate intensity exercise is as good as high intensity exercise and is especially effective in mild to moderate hypertension. In severe hypertension exercise is effective, but higher intensity is required. You will see results within a few weeks of starting an exercise program. One recent study demonstrated marked drops in mild to moderate hypertension in women when they engaged in vigorous stair-climbing for two and a half minutes seven times a day. Search for an activity you enjoy that is compatible with your schedule. *Any amount of exercise begins to reduce risk.*

Environmental Measures

Since water supplies can carry heavy metal toxins, even including small amounts of lead from soldered copper pipes, using a water filter should be considered an important initiative.

When other measures do not yield improvement and control of blood pressure, review of possible environmental and food sensitivity causes of hypertension is warranted. Once offensive foods have been identified, strict avoidance of the most sensitizing foods, rotation diets to permit mildly or moderately sensitizing foods, and careful environmental controls for inhalant substances can bring noticeable improvement.

Mental and Emotional Health Recommendations *Biofeedback* training leads to significant reduction in systolic and diastolic blood pressures, with improvements still present three years later. Systolic pressures (upper number) typically fall 15 to 20 mmHg from baseline readings, and diastolic (lower number) 8 to 12 mmHg. Cortisone levels fall as much as 20 to 25 percent, tending to postpone a number of degenerative diseases. Biofeedback does not lower readings in persons with normal pressures.

Hypnosis has been found to lower blood pressures an average of 16 to 20 mmHg, equivalent to the effect of many drugs. Results persist through months and years of followup.

Meditation. Regular meditation consistently decreases both systolic and diastolic blood pressures compared to those of nonmeditators. Hypertensive African Americans practicing meditation for three months have been shown to achieve great reductions in blood pressures compared to a group practicing progressive muscle relaxation and much greater reductions compared to a lifestyle modification education group. Some meditation studies have demonstrated twice the benefits of drug treatment in long-term followup. One of the greatest advantages is the freedom from the risk of side effects with drug treatment. Regular practice of *qigong*, a gentle Chinese moving meditation and martial art, has also been shown to lower blood pressure and prevent stroke.

Beliefs. An Australian study reported in 1982 the experience of 1,100 patients acting as placebo comparisons for a larger number of patients being treated with drugs. Their average initial blood pressure was 158/102. The group received a daily placebo, reducing average pressure to 144/91 at the end of three years. Forty-eight percent fell to normal with diastolic pressures below 80 mmHg. Drug-treated patients were only slightly better off than placebo subjects. *There was a profound placebo effect persisting for three years.* Placebo effects depend on beliefs, which tend to evoke images to which the nervous system responds. What we believe and expect engages the brain and nervous system to act consistently with what we believe. If our beliefs and images are positive, decreased fight-or-flight responses operate the nervous and adrenal systems at a lower baseline, thereby lowering blood pressure.

Spiritual and Social Health Recommendations

Social Health
Animals. Systolic and diastolic blood pressures recorded in children while reading aloud are significantly lower while reading in the presence of a friendly dog. Similar reductions occur in the elderly with animals present.

Bioenergetic Therapy
Ninety-six hypertensive patients age 16–60 were exposed to a series of long-distance treatments by a healer. Forty-eight were randomly selected to receive the treatments, and the remainder acted as an untreated control group, all continuing

their usual drug treatment. Neither the patients nor the attending physicians knew who received the treatment and who did not. Each healer engaged in relaxation, followed by attunement with a Higher Power or Infinite Being, followed by visualization or affirmation of the patient being in a perfect state of health, followed by an expression of thanks to the Source of all power and energy. The systolic blood pressure significantly improved in 92 percent of the treated group versus 74 percent of the control group.

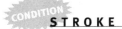

STROKE

Prevalence

Strokes cause 6 percent of all deaths in the United States and are the leading cause of mortality after heart attacks and cancer. Approximately 550,000 persons suffer a stroke each year in this country, with 30 percent mortality. Major improvements in lifestyle and better care of those with arteriosclerotic problems have contributed to a 60 percent decline in stroke mortality since the late 1960s. Unless significant interventions are undertaken, however, the risk for a second stroke within five years is 40 to 60 percent.

Anatomy and Physiology

A hemorrhagic stroke occurs when a rupture occurs in an artery in the brain, allowing blood under high pressure to escape from the artery and damage brain tissue. The much more common thrombotic stroke occurs when a blood clot forms in a partially obstructed artery, shutting off blood supply to a portion of the brain. A clot may also travel from the heart and lodge in a cerebral artery, causing similar damage.

Transient ischemic attacks (TIAs) involve a temporary loss of blood supply to a small portion of brain tissue, thought to be due to temporary spasm in an already partly compromised small artery or to tiny clots which form and are quickly dissolved. Since there is no permanent damage resulting from TIAs, they are not threatening in and of themselves. They are, however, a warning sign to which you and your physician should respond by establishing the diagnosis with appropriate tests. Profound hypoglycemia with transient paralysis has occasionally been mistaken for a TIA. The severe vasoconstriction of the warning phase of a severe migraine can also give minor stroke-like effects.

Symptoms and Diagnosis

Classic stroke symptoms present with a one-sided weakness or paralysis that may involve the leg, arm, or face and neck, or any combination of the three. If the brain damage is left-sided, loss of speech occurs. Strokes may also be manifested in loss of consciousness, loss of touch sensations, or sudden death.

Conventional Medical Treatment

The immediate treatment for a stroke includes life support if necessary, followed by extensive rehabilitation to regain all possible function and build compensating strengths and skills for remaining deficits. Recently, acute treatment has begun to include the same *clot-dissolving drugs* used in heart attacks. Great caution and judgment is required: clot-dissolving drugs in hemorrhagic strokes will aggravate the damage.

Conventional preventive measures for those with hypertension and arteriosclerosis are carried out as described under hypertension and hyperlipidemias. *Aspirin* is commonly recommended for prevention of strokes and recurrent strokes; there is a small hazard of increasing risks for hemorrhagic strokes.

Risk Factors and Causes

The most important risk factors for stroke are *hypertension* and *arteriosclerosis*. All the risk factors that play roles in these two problems, discussed above and below, are also risk factors for stroke. Certain factors deserve special emphasis.

There is a strong positive correlation with *alcohol* intake and the risk for stroke, especially for those under the age of 40. A British study found that alcohol intoxication was three times more common prior to a stroke than it was in healthy people. In the uncommon instance of strokes in those under the age of 20, alcohol was the cause in 40 percent. Smoking increases stroke risk only 6 percent in those over 65 but a stunning 80 percent in those under 65.

High levels of adrenaline-like neurotransmitters are associated with stroke risk and higher death rate in strokes. These compounds result from high levels of tension secondary to poorly managed physiological and psychological *stress*.

High blood sugars are also a risk factor for strokes, even in stages before diabetes can be recognized. There is also a relationship with obesity. Marginal deficiencies of vitamin C and other antioxidant vitamins are also contributing risk factors.

Street drugs, including amphetamines, increase risk of hemorrhagic stroke. The risk increases several times with oral contraceptive use; this risk is greatly exaggerated in smokers and increases with the length of time of use. Sedentary lifestyle raises risks for stroke as it does for coronary artery disease.

Caroline Myss and others skilled in energy analysis relate incidence of stroke to a need to control, lack of trust, and feelings of vulnerability.

Holistic Prevention and Treatment

All the elements of prevention and treatment of cardiovascular diseases discussed under coronary artery disease, angina, congestive heart failure, and hypertension apply to lowering of risk of stroke and reducing the risk of repeat strokes.

A few measures specifically more applicable to stroke should be mentioned. Research reports credit five weekly servings of *carrots*, daily ingestion of *spinach*, and at least five servings of *fruits* and *vegetables* daily with substantial lowering of the risk of stroke. Interestingly, such foods increase potassium intake; adding supplemental potassium to the diets of stroke-prone rats reduces their incidence of stroke. *Ginkgo biloba* may also have a special use in preventing stroke and recurrent stroke in those with high risk factors.

In the intensive rehabilitation work of recovering from a stroke, a unique, gentle variety of bodywork known as *Feldenkrais* often works well. The brain-retraining aspect of rehabilitation appears to be enhanced with this therapy.

There is strong evidence that persistent use of *acupuncture* in rehabilitation after stroke has notable long-term benefits for greater recovery and greater functionality in regard to activities of daily living.

In the whole picture of incidence, rehabilitation, adaptation, and prevention of recurrence of strokes, a major shift of lifestyle is usually necessary. Central to that process is a shift in beliefs and attitudes, which may be assisted by especially understanding holistic physicians or counselors.

CONDITION
HYPERLIPIDEMIA

Prevalence

The prevalence of elevated blood lipids, including cholesterol, is estimated at about 15 percent of the adult population. A Minnesota survey showed that the incidence of new cases has dropped from 17 percent to 14 percent over the last 15 years.

Anatomy and Physiology

The presence of arteriosclerosis is associated with abnormalities in cholesterol and blood fats, including triglycerides. Elevated levels of total and bad cholesterol and lipoprotein (a) make significant contributions to the hardening-of-the-artery process. The bad cholesterol fraction is carried in the bloodstream in the low density lipoprotein (LDL) molecule; LDL functions to transport cholesterol and triglycerides to the body tissues for use in metabolic processes, among which are the conversion of cholesterol into the major hormones of the body, including estrogen, progesterone, testosterone, and cortisone. LDL-C is particularly suscep-tible to oxidative degeneration in the free radical process. This damages the deli-cate arterial lining and converts monocytes into tissue macrophages, which begin to take up oxidized cholesterol, accelerating the degenerative process.

Lipoprotein (a) is a molecule related to LDL that likewise participates in the degenerative process as a separate risk factor for arteriosclerosis; some authorities believe it is a more important factor than LDL-C. Triglycerides, too, are a sepa-rate risk factor for arteriosclerosis when elevated. Good cholesterol is carried by the high density lipoprotein molecule (HDL), which transports cholesterol back to the liver for disposal from the body. A deficient level of HDL-C is also a risk factor for arteriosclerotic complications.

As the cells of the arterial wall take up oxidized cholesterol, platelets, and red and white blood cells, a degenerative substance known as plaque forms to thicken the walls, gradually blocking off the blood-carrying passage over a period of years. Eventually the passage becomes so narrowed that complete blockage occurs with the formation of a blood clot, a process also driven by free radical formation. The two most common results are a heart attack or a thrombotic stroke.

Symptoms and Diagnosis

The presence of arteriosclerotic changes in the arteries of the body is not accom-panied by any symptoms. Physical examination can reveal early manifestations of hardening of the arteries in the retina of the eye. The presence of significant ath-erosclerotic change can be strongly suspected even in the absence of all symptoms by a decreased ankle-arm index (see under holistic treatment). The diagnosis can be confirmed by various tests, including blood vessel dye studies of coronary or cerebral arteries, and by ultrasound of accessible arteries, usually the carotid ves-sels in the neck.

Conventional Medical Treatment

The conventional response to discovery of elevated cholesterol, elevated choles-terol/HDL cholesterol ratio, or high triglycerides usually includes the designing of a program to begin or increase exercise, make nutritional changes, cease smok-ing if appropriate, and take a pharmaceutical lipid-lowering agent.

Drugs commonly used to artificially lower blood cholesterol levels include Colestid, Questran, Atromid-S, Lopid, Lorelco, and niacin (vitamin B-3) deriva-tives (Nicobid, Nicolar). A new class of pharmaceuticals now in the broadest use, HMG-CoA-reductase inhibitors, includes Mevacor, Pravachol, Zocor, Lipitor, Baycol, and Lescol.

The issues surrounding attempts to lower lipids were discussed above under

Cross Section of Arteries
(a) Normal Wall
(b) Arteriosclerotic Wall

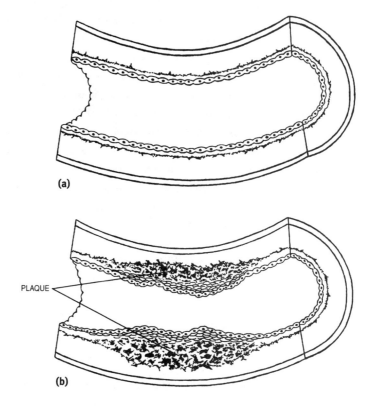

(a)

PLAQUE

(b)

Coronary Artery Disease. A 1991 study in the *Journal of the American Medical Association* detailed the aggressive treatment of 1,200 business executives with high risk factors for heart disease with cholesterol-lowering and antihypertensive drugs, which lowered the calculated cardiovascular risk factors 46 percent compared to casually treated controls. Through ten years of followup, however, the mortality in the aggressively treated group was 45 percent higher and cardiovascular mortality 140 percent higher than the controls. Aggressive treatment is not always better treatment.

Holistic and conventional physicians alike agree with the wisdom of lowering cholesterol to 200 mg/dl, LDL cholesterol to 135 mg/dl or lower, lipoprotein (a) to below 30 mg/dl, and triglycerides to below 150 mg/dl, and increasing HDL-C to above 40 mg/dl. The major difference is in the choice of approach.

Risk Factors and Causes

Physical factors. *Genetic factors* play a predominant role in 5 to 7 percent of those with lipid abnormalities, exclusive of homocysteinemia problems, discussed below. The presence of these hereditary forms of lipid problems can usually be detected by a thorough family history, laboratory determinations, and the tendency for the abnormalities to be resistant to usual treatments.

Homocysteinemia is a separate identified genetic risk factor not only for coronary heart disease, but also the underlying atherosclerosis. Elevated homocysteine levels are more common in coffee drinkers (according the *American Journal of Clinical Nutrition*, January 1997).

Smoking and hypertension risks are discussed under heart disease. Diabetes is a known risk factor; elevated sugar levels, insulin levels, and insulin resistance function to promote constriction of arteries. Hypothyroidism is an identified risk factor as well. Patients with low thyroid function have consistently higher lipid blood values, including lipoprotein (a).

Nutritional factors:

- Diets high in saturated and oxidized fat, trans fats, and sugar are risk factors.

- Alcohol, sugar, and high glycemic index foods tend to raise triglycerides, especially in hereditary hyperlipidemias.

- Deficiencies of antioxidant vitamins and the minerals on which the body's own antioxidant enzymes depend (zinc, copper, manganese, selenium, magnesium) can be considered risk factors.

- Diets low in calcium, chromium, essential fatty acids, and fiber have also been shown to promote arteriosclerosis.

Physical inactivity is highly associated with lower good cholesterol levels, higher triglyceride levels, and higher blood pressure.

Food reactivity to milk, grains, and sucrose has also been implicated as a risk factor.

Emotional Factors

- Finnish studies have shown that arteriosclerosis progressed *twice as fast* in the major arteries of the neck in men with high levels of *hostility and distrust* compared to men with low levels of these attitudes.

- Atherosclerosis has been shown to progress at a rate 20 percent faster in patients who have prominent feelings of *hopelessness* compared to those who do not harbor strong feelings of hopelessness.

- The *stress* of participating in frustrating cognitive tasks for only 20 minutes has been shown to significantly increase blood pressures, pulse rate, cholesterol, blood thickness and blood viscosity, all risk factors for arteriosclerosis.

Holistic Treatment

Physical Health Recommendations. When symptoms and signs of subclinical *hypothyroidism* are present, cautious and carefully monitored supplementation with small doses of prescribed thyroid medication is often remarkably helpful in altering lipid levels.

Diet

Because *coffee* raises homocysteine levels and *alcohol* raises triglycerides in susceptible persons, their use should be very carefully monitored and reduced to the point at which they are having no significant influence on lipid levels. Coffee in amounts greater than four cups daily adversely affects cholesterol through the effects of caffeine and by other mechanisms. Good cholesterol increases with alcohol intake; red wine, with high phenolic content, appears to be one good source. Because of the wide array of adverse effects of alcohol, including its contribution to cancers, diabetes, and accidents, very modest intake is advised; you need to make it a matter of total abstention if you have a predisposition toward addictions.

The great majority of the cholesterol in the blood at any given time has been made by the liver. Therefore, manipulating the amount of cholesterol in the diet has a very limited effect, especially if fat intake is in a low to moderate range. Cholesterol in food that has been heated is at least partially oxidized; oxidized cholesterol is toxic to the body, whereas unoxidized cholesterol is not. Excessive restriction of whole egg intake is not warranted. Limiting or *eliminating hydrogenated polyunsaturated trans fats* is a high priority (margarine, hydrogenated cooking oils, hydrogenated peanut butter). While butter containing saturated fat is not desirable, margarines are worse. *Monosaturated fats* such as olive oil resist free radical deterioration. Inclusion of liberal amounts of *alpha linolenic acids (fish, fish oil, flaxseed oil)* and *gamma linolenic acid (evening primrose and borage oils)* also favorably affect lipid levels. See under Coronary Artery Disease for dosages. Added *fruit, vegetable, and whole cereal grain fiber* lowers cholesterol. Certain whole foods have been noted for their ability to lower lipid levels. They include *soy, yogurt, carrots,* and *nuts.* Many of these whole food suggestions were combined in 1997 research in which subjects lowered cholesterol 33 percent, cholesterol/HDL-C ratio 21 percent, and lipoprotein (a) 24 percent with dietary changes. *Vegetarian diets* are associated with consistently lower blood lipid levels.

Vitamins, Minerals, and Supplements

The extensive array of suggestions for increasing micronutrient and antioxidant intake in *foods and supplements* in the coronary heart disease section should be followed by anyone with elevated lipid levels, whether or not they have evidence of heart disease.

- Added supplements of calcium have been shown in one study to reduce serum cholesterol 25 percent and triglycerides 35 percent after one year (400–1,200 mg daily).

- *Chromium*, 200–500 mcg daily, reduced cholesterol 8–10 percent in several studies.

- *Vitamin C* blood levels are inversely related to cholesterol and triglyceride blood levels. Increasing vitamin C beyond one gram daily has a modest and steady influence in lowering cholesterol and triglycerides.

- *Inositol hexaniacinate*, 500–1,000 mg three times a day, achieves impressive cholesterol-lowering and good cholesterol-raising effects.

- The *antioxidants* are essential: *vitamin E, beta carotene,* and *Coenzyme Q10.*

- *Pantethine* (vitamin B-5) impressively lowers cholesterol in doses of 900 mg daily.

- In one subtype of hereditary cholesterol problem, *L-carnitine* normalized very high levels of cholesterol in 90 percent of patients and in another subtype reduced triglycerides to normal in 100 percent of patients. L-carnitine is rapidly depleted in hearts that are oxygen deficient; usual helpful dosages are one to three grams daily.

- Extracted forms of *mesoglycan*, a glycosaminoglycan derivative, are available as a supplement that lowers total cholesterol, raises good cholesterol, prevents clot formation, and protects arterial linings from damage when taken at doses of 100 mg daily.

- Red rice yeast (*cholestin*), a natural supplement from China, impressively lowers lipid levels, 600 mg one to three times a day. It contains a low concentration of lovestatin, the active ingredient in Mevacor, a prescription drug.

Herbs

The most effective herbs are *gugulipids* and *garlic*. Fresh garlic preparations work much better than aged garlic. Products that are standardized to contain a daily dose of at least 4 mg or 10 mg of the active ingredients allicin or allini, respectively, are reliable. *Artichoke* (Cynara scolymus, 500 mg of the extract daily) increases cholesterol elimination from the liver through the bile; 20 percent reduction in cholesterol and 15 percent reduction in triglycerides has been demonstrated.

Exercise

Appropriate exercise lowers cholesterol 10 and 25 percent in men and women, respectively, decreases cholesterol/HDL-C ratios 15 and 50 percent, respectively, and increases HDL-Cs 10 and 20 percent, respectively. The sex differences may stem from the fact that more women were probably deconditioned at baseline in this type of study.

Mental and Emotional Health Recommendations. As previously mentioned, substantial reductions in cholesterol have been achieved with *meditation.* A shift in *attitudes* toward the *positive,* lessening hopelessness, depression, hostility, and cynical distrust, carries with it a substantial gain in improved lipid profiles. Some *holistic practitioners* and *counselors* can be helpful in gaining the insight, evoking the motivation, and following through with the practice of the techniques and approaches that make a permanent change in the biochemistry and functioning of the body.

15

Neurological Disease

Tension Headaches

Migraine

Multiple Sclerosis

Attention Deficit Hyperactivity Disorder (ADHD)

Alzheimer's Disease

Tinnitus

CONDITION TENSION HEADACHE

Prevalence

HEADACHES ARE AMONG the most common of human afflictions. For the majority, a headache is a passing annoyance that fades with a little aspirin and an opportunity to relax. For an estimated 45 million Americans, however, a headache is a chronic and recurring affair, seriously interfering with activities of daily living. The incidence in men and women is about equal, and there is an even distribution across all age groups from teenagers to the elderly.

Anatomy and Physiology

Tension headaches are thought to be generated by sustained excessive contractions of the scalp and neck muscles. Accessory muscles also frequently involved include those of the jaw and face. The actual pain is thought to derive from prolonged muscle contractions that trap pain-producing chemicals in the muscles themselves, similar to pain in your arm that you can experience by keeping a tight fist for five minutes without letup. Other structures that can contribute to the headache pain pattern include the temporomandibular (jaw) joint, teeth, and inner ears.

Symptoms and Diagnosis

In tension headaches, the pain is usually described as a steady, constant, pressure-like dull ache involving the entire head from the neck muscles to the temples. The temples and muscles of the upper back and neck may be quite tender, even when the intensity of the headache is mild. The intensity is occasionally severe enough to interfere with sleep. Headaches are more common in women during premenstrual and menstrual days of the cycle, in people who are fatigued or depressed, and in those who are short on sleep. Most tension headaches are not associated with a serious underlying disorder and will go away on their own. Most people, because the pain is bothersome, will take steps to get relief.

Conventional Medical Treatment

The most commonly suggested medications are NSAIDs (e.g., ibuprofen), aspirin, or acetaminophen (Tylenol). All three can have harmful side effects. When recurring headaches are accompanied by depression, antidepressants are frequently suggested and prescribed.

Risk Factors and Causes

Tension headaches are thought to be caused by tightening of the muscles of the scalp and neck, the result of exaggerated poor postural positioning of the head, or by excessive tension triggered by stress. They can be initiated by the facial muscular tension of eyestrain, holding a constant posture for a long time (as in word processing), reading with the head in a constant position, tensing the jaw in anger, grinding the teeth at night, or even chewing gum for a long period of time. The more common causes and triggers include:

- Stress
- Anxiety and depression
- Fatigue, lack of sleep, and overwork syndrome
- Deficient exercise pattern
- Eyestrain
- Sinus problems
- Poor posture
- Muscle tension
- Recent root canal treatments
- Temporomandibular (jaw) joint dysfunction
- Cervical spine mechanical problems
- Hypothyroidism and low adrenal function
- Premenstrual syndrome

- Carbon monoxide exposures

- Artificial sweeteners (up to 14 percent incidence in aspartame, or Nutrisweet, users)

- Trichloroethylene (industrial chemical) contamination of the water supply has been associated with a 50 percent incidence of headache

Holistic Treatment

Physical Health Recommendations

Vitamins and Minerals

Because tension headache is so often related to increased stress, replacement of micronutrients that are depleted in times of stress is essential. The most critical are the antioxidant *vitamins C* and *E, beta carotene, B-complex,* and the minerals *magnesium, potassium, calcium, zinc, manganese,* and *selenium.* Magnesium (aspartate or glycinate, up to 750 mg/day) is especially critical because of its antispasmodic action. A megadose multivitamin-mineral product can encompass many of these needs. *Omega-3 oils* (with a daily content of EPA, or eicosapentaenoic acid, 350 mg, and *DHA,* or docosahexaenoic acid, 250 mg) are also helpful.

Herbs

- *Valerian root* (1:5 tincture, 1–1½ tsp., or powdered extract [standardized extract of .8 percent valeric acid], 200 mg, two to three times daily) has a calming effect.

- *Passionflower* (Passiflora incarnata) (1:5 tincture, 1½ tsp., or powdered extract, 300 mg, three times daily) has mild sedative and analgesic properties.

- *Kava kava* (Piper methysticum) (45–60 mg of kavalactone content three times daily) has a calming effect.

- *Myoplex* (Metagenics in Eugene, OR) combines the preceding agents.

- Intranasal instillation of *capsaicin* (cayenne) has been shown to greatly relieve symptoms in chronic and episodic tension headache.

Exercise

A well-conceived regular exercise program lessens the incidence of tension headache, presumably through the dissipation of tension during the vigorous movement of the body.

When tension headache is related to intense working conditions, you will benefit from taking one-half to five minute minibreaks to stretch and shift posture, taking deep breaths while sighing on the outbreath, shrugging the shoulders to the ears and letting them drop, and using the mind's eye for a minute to sense yourself on your next refreshing vacation.

Mental and Emotional Health Recommendations. Learning and regularly practicing biofeedback or any other systematic relaxation approach achieves a 50 to 80 percent reduction or elimination in both tension and migraine headache severity and frequency. You can achieve the same results by learning and practicing regular *meditation. Hypnosis* also has significant success with headache. *Self-hypnosis* has been shown to be particularly helpful in children and teenagers. These approaches to the process of change are enhanced by other stress management tools, including imagery and repetition of affirmations.

Professional Care Therapies

Acupuncture in skilled hands can be very effective in acute tension headache and can be intermittently used for prevention. *Therapeutic Touch* has been shown to provide a substantial, sustained improvement in headache patterns. Other energy therapies have success as well.

Aromatherapy. An aromatic combination of peppermint oil, eucalyptus oil, and alcohol applied to the temples and forehead relaxes scalp muscles and noticeably reduces the intensity and shortens the experience with headache; use five to ten drops of each two to three times/day. Rosemary oil (one part oil to ten of vegetable oil) rubbed into the temples and forehead has also been used with success.

Manipulation. Chiropractic adjustment compared to antidepressant drugs is significantly better in long-term headache management. *Craniosacral osteopathic treatment* has substantial benefits in helping people cope with tension symptoms.

Homeopathy. Definitive prescribing can be sought from experienced practitioners. Symptomatic remedies include Aconitum, Arnica, Belladonna, Bryonia, Gelsemium, and Nux vomica.

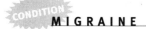

MIGRAINE

Prevalence

About 7 percent of men and 20 percent of women have experienced at least one migraine headache. Cluster headaches, though much less common, are six times more common in men than women. Though more difficult to diagnose because the presenting symptoms are more obscure, migraine does occur in children.

Anatomy and Physiology

Migraines are the most common presentation of what are known as vascular headaches, a category that also includes cluster headaches. They are thought by most authorities to occur as a result of spasm in the arteries at the base of the brain triggering the visual "aura," followed by rather sudden relaxation and dilation of the same arteries that trigger the phase of throbbing pain. Blood flow to the brain during the early vasoconstrictive phase of a migraine episode is severely compromised, so much so that ministroke-like effects are occasionally seen as a residual.

The platelet cells of the bloodstream behave differently in migraine sufferers compared to healthy subjects. Serotonin, a neurotransmitter with many functions, including contributing to blood vessel relaxation, is stored in blood platelets; in migraine subjects, the platelets tend to stick together more easily, releasing significantly more serotonin compared to those without this problem. An unusually high percentage of migraine sufferers also have mitral valve prolapse, a condition that theoretically may damage blood platelets as they pass through the mitral valve of the heart, possibly contributing to the pathological cascade of events in migraines.

Symptoms and Diagnosis

The classic migraine headache is one-sided and is frequently heralded by the onset of an "aura" of visual disturbances consisting of bright spots, zigzag lines, blind spots, or temporary loss of part of the visual field on the side involved. The pain is often severe and incapacitating. Untreated, the throbbing or pounding pain can last for hours or days and is often severe enough to also induce nausea and vomiting. It is often accompanied by excruciating sensitivity to light that forces the sufferer to seek shelter in a darkened room. Typical age of onset is before age 35. The symptoms in children tend to be nonspecific, with nausea, malaise, vertigo, and abdominal pain being more common than headache itself. Migraine episodes recede with advancing age, and postmenopausal women have a much lower incidence.

Cluster headaches are also one-sided, presenting as a steady piercing pain located behind one eye or in one temple. Cluster headaches also strike people in their twenties and thirties, typically having their onset at night or early in the morning.

Conventional Medical Treatment

Prescriptions are written for migraine from a number of drug classes, including narcotics, antidepressants, vasoconstrictors, beta-blockers, muscle relaxants, and 5-hydroxytryptophan (5HT) agonists. Zomig (zolmitripan) and Imitrex (sumatriptan) are 5HT agonists—that is, they mimic 5HT activity. These drugs require long-term treatment for at least 60 days for potential results to appear. Ergotamine drugs (Ergomar, Wigraine) are the most commonly used class of pharmaceuticals in acute migraine; ergotamine is vasoconstrictive, preventing the dilation phase reaction thought to trigger the pain. Midrin is also a commonly used vasoconstrictor. Beta-blockers (Inderal) also have a place in drug treatment. Problems may arise from habituation to some drugs, whereby stopping the vasoconstricting (ergotamine) or analgesic medicine triggers a rebound headache and a perceived need for more medication. This is an addiction pattern. Methysergide, a modified ergotamine compound, is given for long periods of time for prevention of migraine. Long-term uninterrupted use may lead to fibrotic changes in the abdomen and chest, causing vascular and kidney problems. *Drugs have no impact on reducing the frequency of migraine episodes unless continually taken.*

Because high tyramine (an amino acid) in foods can trigger production of high amounts of norepinephrine and encourage constriction of blood vessels, avoiding tyramine-containing foods is often suggested; these include cheeses, pickled herring, fermented sausages (pepperoni, salami, bologna), overripe avocados and fruits, red wine, sherry, and red wine vinegar.

Risk Factors and Causes

Migraines can be caused or triggered by:

- Genetic predisposition. About one-half of people who experience migraines have a positive family history. There is considerable evidence that migraine-prone persons have low baseline levels of serotonin.

- Food sensitivities (see holistic treatment).

- Histamine-containing and -releasing foods (see conventional treatment).

- Chemicals (nitrates, monosodium glutamate, nitroglycerin, Aspartame).

- Migraine sufferers have levels of blood magnesium well below levels in healthy people (predisposes to greater arterial constriction).

- Withdrawal from caffeine (caffeine constricts arteries).

- Smoking.

- Sleep problems (too little or too much).

- Fatigue and exhaustion.

- Weather changes, barometric changes, sun exposure.

- Sun glare (off snow and water) and eyestrain.

- Rebound from withdrawal of analgesic or vasorelaxation drugs.

- Episodes are frequently triggered by *stress*. A classic story is the onset of the headache in the let-down period immediately after an acutely stressful episode has passed. Numerous papers have described the precipitation of headache in migraine sufferers by submission to a stressful interview in which the patient has little control.

- Emotional changes and intense emotional experience. Anxiety and depression are strongly related to vascular headaches of both cluster and migraine varieties. Astute observers and researchers of migraine think there is a strong association with intense organized activity to attempt to manage feelings of anxiety, which drives the sympathetic nervous system to extremely high activity.

- Hormonal changes (menstruation, ovulation, oral contraceptives). Migraines are more common before and during a menstrual period and in women who take oral contraceptive agents. They are less common in pregnancy and postmenopausally. In migraine-prone pregnant women, headaches are much more common if pre-eclampsia is present; both conditions are related to lower levels of magnesium and are also often related to subnormal levels of progesterone.

- Studies have shown that migraine patients include a higher percentage of people with chronic candidiasis. In those with high positive candida antigen or antibody titers, a great majority enjoy marked improvement or cessation of migraines when the yeast infection is treated. (For more on candidiasis see Chapter 9.)

Holistic Prevention and Treatment

Physical Health Recommendations

Diet

Nutritional elements in prevention of migraine include decreasing fats from land animals and increasing foods that inhibit platelet aggregation (stickiness), including vegetable oils, onion, garlic, and fish oils.

Food elimination. In a number of studies of foods and migraine, a majority of migraine sufferers improve on elimination diets, and food rechallenge confirms specific food offenders. The most common offenders, in order of frequency, usually turn out to be cow's milk, wheat, orange, eggs, coffee, tea, chocolate, milk, beef, pork, corn, tomato, rye, yeast, and shellfish. If you have migraine, arbitrary total elimination of these most common offender foods from your diet may bring you great relief.

Vitamins, Minerals, and Supplements

- Since *magnesium*-deficient people are more subject to vascular headache, adequate intake (400–600 mg/day) from food or supplements is essential.

- Intravenous injection of one gram of magnesium by your physician can terminate an *acute migraine* headache within minutes—in up to nearly 100 percent of subjects in some reviews. Intravenous injection of *folic acid*, 15 mg, in one study achieved total subsidence of acute headache within one hour in 60 percent, with great improvement in another 30 percent. These two agents are strikingly successful.

- *Omega-3 oils* (EPA and DHA, average dose 1,400 mg daily) greatly reduce intensity and frequency of migraines.

- *Vitamin B-2* (riboflavin), 400 mg daily for three months, has been shown to reduce migraine frequency by two-thirds.

- *Vitamin C* (2,000 mg/day, *vitamin E* (400–600 I.U/day), *vitamin B-6* (100 mg/day), and choline (100–300 mg/day) all inhibit the tendency to high platelet in migraine.

- *Melatonin*, 10 mg each evening for two weeks, can terminate an episode of cluster headaches in three to five days.

- *5-hydroxytryptophan* (5-HTP), 300 mg twice daily, works as well as methysergide for prevention of migraine, enhanced by taking with 25 mg of vitamin B-6.

- Mixed *bioflavonoids*, 1,000 mg twice daily.

Herbs

- *Feverfew* (Tanacetum parthenium), 0.25 to 0.5 parthenolide content daily, has markedly helpful effects in migraine.

- *Dried ginger*, 500 mg four times daily, and Pueraria root also provide substantial benefit with reduction in frequency and intensity of migraine occurrences.

- Intranasal instillation of *capsaicin* has been shown to induce remissions in cluster headache.

Exercise

Appropriate regular *aerobic exercise*—brisk walking, jogging, sports activities, gardening, low impact aerobics, and water aerobics are among the options that both release tension from the system and reduce the frequency and intensity of migraine episodes.

Mental and Emotional Health Recommendations

Counseling Therapies

Counselors who understand the interrelationships of attitudes, conditioned responses, emotional state, and dis-ease, as well as the dynamics of the change process can be enormously helpful. Many people with headache and migraine feel trapped by their circumstances and the gulf between the way life is and the way it *should* be. Releasing the demands (the "shoulds") with a strong dose of forgiveness can lead to rewarding and sometimes dramatic changes.

Biofeedback and Relaxation

Learning and regularly practicing *biofeedback* or any of the systematic relaxation approaches achieves a *50 to 80 percent reduction or elimination* in both severity and frequency of migraine headache. You can achieve the same results by learning and practicing regular meditation, eliminating or reducing your need for medication. *Hypnosis*, too, has significant success with headache. Self-hypnosis has been shown to be particularly helpful in children and teenagers.

Professional Care Therapies

Manual methods. Patients treated by chiropractic adjustment report greater relief of pain compared to other manual methods.

Acupuncture in skilled hands can be very effective in migraine headache. In one study 40 percent of patients achieved a 50 to 100 percent reduction in severity and frequency of migraine episodes. Among the acupoints that can also be conveniently used for acupressure are the following:

- The ho-ku point in the soft tissue between the thumb and index finger;

- The B2 point below the inner aspect of the eyebrow;

- The GB20 and GV16 points over the spine and on both sides of the spine just below the back of the skull.

Therapeutic Touch has been shown to provide a substantial, sustained improvement in headache patterns. Other energy therapies have success as well.

MULTIPLE SCLEROSIS (MS)

Prevalence

The incidence rate of multiple sclerosis varies from 50 to 100 affected persons per one hundred thousand people in zones of higher latitude in both the Northern and Southern Hemispheres to five to ten affected persons per one hundred thousand people in the tropics; 350,000 Americans are afflicted. In Switzerland and Norway, the incidence is significantly lower in mountainous regions and higher at lower altitudes and along the seacoast. In most areas, women with MS outnumber men three to two. Onset is commonly between the ages of 20 and 40. The incidence has significantly increased since early descriptions before 1850. The disease is uncommon in emerging countries.

Anatomy and Physiology

In MS the myelin lipoprotein content of the cells that surround and insulate the nerve cells gradually breaks down and is lost. Nerve cells then lose their ability to properly conduct electrical impulses. The disease has a tendency to progress, though treatment measures can stabilize the condition for many years.

Symptoms and Diagnosis

Early diagnosis of this disease is difficult. The most frequent early symptoms in order of commonness are:

- Motor system—muscle weakness, clumsiness, dropping objects, leg-dragging
- Visual—blurring, blindness, double vision, haziness
- Sensory—numbness, tingling, "pins and needles" feelings, heaviness, tightness
- Balance—lightheadedness, vertigo, unsteadiness
- Pain—occasionally experienced

Diagnostic tests, though nonspecific, are used to confirm the suspected diagnosis. The most helpful are decreases in measures of nerve conduction and abnormalities on MRI scanning of the brain. With disease progression in severe cases, walking often becomes difficult, weakness of arm and hand movement ensues, speech may become slurred, and urinary incontinence sometimes develops. Fatigue is a frequent accompanying symptom. The disease may progress slowly and steadily or assume a relapsing/remitting pattern with long periods of stability between episodes of deterioration.

Conventional Medical Treatment

Most conventional practitioners believe that MS is inevitably progressive. Besides supportive care for complications, measures often suggested include concentrated courses of corticosteroid treatment at times of worsening of symptoms. Based on the autoimmune theory, immune suppressant drugs are also used, including Cytoxan and methotrexate. These drugs appear to have short-term benefit, but demonstration of long-term benefits is lacking. Intravenous gamma globulin, 20–30 grams daily for five days with boosters every two months, reduces relapses 70 percent in the first year of treatment. Beta-interferon is a drug that has been offered in recent years with various degrees of success in up to 30 percent of patients.

Risk Factors and Causes

The cause of multiple sclerosis is unknown. The leading theories are:

- Genetic—first-degree relatives of MS patients have up to an eightfold increased risk

- Autoimmune reactions

- Viral infection

- Nutritional—high dairy and animal sources, high saturated fat content, deficiency of omega-3 fatty acids

- Free radical damage—low glutathione peroxidase (an antioxidant enzyme)

- Environmental toxins—petrochemicals, solvents (may trigger free radical reactivity)

- Heavy metal toxicity—higher mercury levels in MS patients

- Vitamin D deficiency (higher incidence of MS at low altitudes and higher latitudes)

- Stress: some studies have found an 80 percent likelihood of a significant stressful incident within the 30 days prior to onset of the very first symptoms; many MS patients have been very busy, overactive "doers," with a distinct overly analytical tendency

- Insightful observers also frequently find a background of pervasive criticism in the family of origin

Holistic Treatment of Multiple Sclerosis

Physical Health Recommendations

Diet

The extremely low fat diet pioneered by Dr. Roy Swank of Portland, Oregon, has shown remarkable stabilizing effects in mild to moderate MS. Even including patients with advanced disease, when a low fat diet was instituted, those consuming less than 20 grams of fat daily had a 35-year mortality rate of 31 percent compared to 81 percent for those ingesting more than 20 grams of fat daily. Swank and others emphasize the extreme importance of treatment as early as possible. His regimen calls for:

- Saturated fat intake of 10 grams daily or less with 40 to 50 grams of polyunsaturated oils daily

- Complete prohibition of margarines, shortening, and hydrogenated oils
- At least one teaspoon of cod liver oil daily (high omega-3 oil content)
- Normal amounts of protein
- Emphasis on fish intake (at least three servings per week)

To hold fat intake to ten grams daily, this diet greatly restricts animal protein, which has a higher fat content. In limiting animal protein, and consequently animal fat, the diet greatly reduces the intake of pesticides, herbicides, and fungicides, which concentrate in the fat of animals. This may be one reason why the diet works well. The best approach, then, is to eat only organic foods, with a high content of live foods with a high enzyme content. The diet also reduces platelet stickiness, blunts autoimmune responses, and increases essential fatty acid levels in the bloodstream and spinal fluid. These effects probably retard the entry of toxins into brain and neural tissues.

Food sensitivities. A small study in the 1950s demonstrated positive food reactions in about 40 percent of MS patients and found that elimination of offenders led to complete or substantial remission in 10 percent and clinically significant improvement in 20 percent. Attempts to replicate this finding have been disappointing.

Vitamins, Minerals, and Supplements

- *Omega-3 oils* from fish sources are essential (3–6 one-gram capsules twice daily) and can be obtained from *flaxseed oil* as well (one tablespoonful daily).
- Daily *antioxidants,* especially *vitamin E,* 400–1,200 I.U., are important. A high dose multivitamin-mineral preparation will supply most needs.
- *Vitamin B-12* by injection in massive doses has been shown to improve nerve electrical conduction time. A reasonable dose is 1–10 mg from daily to weekly. Ask your physician if you can be taught how to do this for yourself at home.
- *Phosphatidyl choline,* 300 mg twice daily.
- *Phosphatidylserine,* 100 mg three times a day.
- *Lecithin,* 1,200 mg three times a day.

Herbs

During treatment with Padma 28, two tablets three times daily for a year, 44 percent of MS patients noted relief of symptoms and increase in strength. (Padma 28 is a combination German herbal product widely used in Switzerland for 20 years, carried in selected health food stores.)

Biomolecular Options

Autoimmune diseases are thought by many to be related to *gastrointestinal malabsorption* in failing to appropriately assimilate all the needed nutrients and prevent absorption of toxins, incompletely digested food substances, and potentially toxic organisms and chemicals that can cause abnormal responses by the immune system. Studies indicate that the gut mucosal lining in a significant portion of MS patients may leak some of these substances across the intestinal barrier. Those who adhere to this theory ask patients to undertake extensive evaluation of intestinal permeability with specimens sent to laboratories who specialize in this work. Vigorous treatment of abnormalities is undertaken to normalize the balance of organisms in the intestine and the function of the intestinal mucosal membrane. *L-glutamine*, five grams twice a day, helps restore intestinal mucosal integrity.

Preliminary experimental research with *natural alpha-interferon* derived from white blood cells has shown encouraging results with a high percentage of remission in initial two-year treatment periods. This treatment will not be generally available until further research is completed.

Bee venom therapy, administered by a small number of holistic physicians in the United States, has been researched and shown to be beneficial in reported cases. Large scale controlled trials have not been done.

Exercise

Although exercise is the last thing that fatigued MS patients think they can do, studies document improvement in upper and lower body strength and significant gains in scores on anxiety and depression tests. Holistic physicians, physical therapists, and sports medicine trainers can be helpful. If you have deterioration of function after exercise, other than 12 to 24 hours of muscle tiredness, you may be doing too much; the right balance of challenge is critical.

Mercury Toxicity

Improvement in function with removal of mercury amalgam dental fillings has been reported, but no large scale studies have been published. Removal of amalgam fillings is expensive, and the potential benefits need to be individually assessed. Significant improvement in hearing loss associated with MS was reported in 1997 in a small series of patients with removal of mercury fillings.

Mental and Emotional Health Recommendations. We have repeatedly mentioned the importance of positive attitudes and beliefs and the poisonous nature of pervasive negative emotions. In autoimmune disease, these factors are paramount. Cases of complete recovery from MS with permanent remission of all symptoms and resumption of all functions have been reported, just as cases of recovery from far-advanced cancer, intractable coma, and Lou Gehrig's disease (amyotrophic lateral sclerosis) have been reported. These possibilities are enhanced in a climate of positive attitudes and beliefs. If possible, find a health care practitioner who will support you in moving toward positivity; find positive supportive people with whom to associate; read the stories and listen to the cases of recovery. The quality of your life will be enhanced.

CONDITION

ATTENTION DEFICIT HYPERACTIVITY DISORDER (ADHD)

Prevalence

About 2 to 3 percent of the population is said to have a predisposition to hyperactivity and/or attention deficit disorder. Boys outnumber girls at least five to one.

Anatomy and Physiology

PET scans of the brain have demonstrated that the prefrontal lobes, which function to organize and sequence our thinking and behavior and maintain a mental focus, are hypoactively energized in ADHD children and adults. This phenomenon is significantly more demonstrable when scans are done following a stressful experience.

Symptoms and Diagnosis

Attention deficit disorder (ADD) encompasses a group of conditions variously termed "minimal brain dysfunction," "hyperkinetic disorder," and "minimal brain damage." Attention deficit disorder is seen with and without a component of hyperactivity. ADD and ADHD are diagnosed in about 6 percent of children in the United States but in only about 1 percent in the United Kingdom. The most common age at which the diagnosis is made is six or seven.

Children with ADHD often have converse reactions to medications, becoming "hyper" with sedatives (including antihistamines) and sedated with stimulants.

The identifying diagnostic features of ADHD are:

- *Distractibility*, inattention, short attention span, lack of perseverance, failure to finish, not listening, poor concentration
- Dysfunctional memory and thinking
- Specific learning disabilities
- Emotional instability
- Disorders of speech and hearing

- *Impulsiveness*, acting before thinking, lack of organization, abruptly shifting in activity, unable to stay in seat, settled only while participating in or watching rapid-fire activity
- Hyperactivity
- Perceptual motor impairment
- General coordination deficit
- Equivocal ("soft") neurological signs and EEG abnormalities
- PET scan abnormalities

Conventional Medical Treatment

The emphasis of conventional treatment is placed on pharmaceutical intervention. Over two million school children are currently taking the stimulant Ritalin. Other drugs which are used include Dexedrine, Cylert, SSRI antidepressants (Prozac, Zoloft), tricyclic antidepressants (desipramine), antiseizure drugs (Tegretol, Depakote) and clonidine (an antihypertensive drug with sedative properties that helps impulsiveness and aids in sleep). Associated bouts of recurring otitis media in children should be given high priority for treatment to break the cycle and eradicate underlying predisposing factors (see below).

Side effects of medications include up to one to one and a half inches of ultimate growth retardation with consistent use of the stimulants; vacation and summer drug holidays help to reduce this effect. Drug abuse is a hazard among teenagers using stimulant medications.

Risk Factors and Causes

Risk factors, based on published studies and broad experience, include:

- Genetic predisposition
- Sensitivity to food additives
- Predisposition to hypoglycemia
- Sensitivity to foods
- Standard fluorescent lighting
- Deficient essential fatty acids

Additional risk factors in ADD without hyperactivity:

- Recurrent otitis media—associated with increased risk
- Heavy metal toxicity—higher amounts of lead and aluminum have been found in ADHD children

- Specific nutrient deficits:
    1. iron deficiency is associated with decreased attentiveness and attention span, decreased persistence, and decreased voluntary activity
    2. deficiencies of vitamins C, B-1, B-3, B-5, and B-6 and bioflavonoids have all been implicated
- Hypoglycemia—occasionally found to be related
- Social and family isolation—often aggravating factors; the isolation stems from inability of family members and friends to accommodate the fact that the ADHD child is different, often disruptive, and the central focus of the family

The most common additives found to be problematic are the red, yellow, and blue FD&C dyes. Very carefully done double-blind studies show a number of children to be unequivocally sensitive to tartrazine food colorings. Over five thousand food additives are in use in the United States today: anticaking agents, synthetic antioxidants (BHA, BHT), bleaches, colorings, flavorings, emulsifiers, fillers, preservatives, thickeners, mineral salts, and vegetable gums. About ten pounds of these additives are consumed by each person in the United States each year.

Other studies find the most common food offenders to be cow's milk, wheat, corn, tomato, yeast, soy, citrus, grapes, eggs, peanuts, cane sugar, and chocolate. For reasons unclear at present, ADHD children and teenagers have been found to have significantly lower levels of essential fatty acids compared to normal children. The beginnings of this deficit may date to infancy; breast-fed children have higher levels of EFAs compared to bottle-fed children. Bottle-fed children also have higher levels of manganese, which is associated with an increased incidence of learning problems.

Holistic Treatment and Prevention
Physical and Environmental Health Recommendations

Diet
Food elimination. Elimination diets for one to two weeks followed by rechallenge with eliminated foods, one at a time, often brings to light offending foods; an appropriate elimination diet will result in substantial improvement. Most studies with positive results report 50 to 60 percent significant improvement. On a diet eliminating artificial flavors, colorings, preservatives, caffeine, monosodium glutamate, chocolate, and individually parent-suspected foods, 42 percent of hyperactive children showed nearly 60 percent significant improvement with reduced hyperactivity symptoms. Physicians who are affiliated with the American Acad-

emy of Environmental Medicine also use hyposensitization procedures, administering intradermal injections of minute quantities of antigens from the foods to which patients were sensitive, greatly reducing reactivity and all associated symptoms.

Vitamins, Minerals, and Supplements

Nutrients that have been shown to alter hyperactive and ADD behavior in up to half of hyperactive children and teenagers are:

- *Iron*—20 to 100 mg daily depending on deficits
- *Vitamin C*—one gram daily
- *Pyridoxine (B-6)*—100 mg three times daily
- *Pantothenic acid* as calcium pantothenate, 200 mg twice daily
- *Thiamin (B-1)*—100 mg three times daily
- *Niacinamide*—500 mg twice daily
- *Bioflavonoids*—500 to 1,000 mg daily of mixed bioflavonoids
- *Docasahexaenoic acid (DHA)*—100 mg three times daily
- *Pycnogenol* (oligomeric proanthocyanidin), 100 mg one to two times daily
- *L-tryptophan*, prescription-available through compounding pharmacists (one to three grams at bedtime without food for sleep; or

  5-hydroxytryptophan (5-HTP) (accompanied with 25 mg of vitamin B-6), available from health food stores and holistic practitioners; (50—250 mg at bedtime), another gentle option to help the sleep of ADHD patients whose sleep is often disrupted
- *DL-phenylalanine* (500 to 1,500 mg midmorning and midafternoon on empty stomach); helps maintain mental focus
- *L-tyrosine*, precursor of dopamine, a stimulant neurotransmitter (500 to 1,500 mg twice daily on an empty stomach)

A potent megavitamin trial in ADHD children that includes part of the suggested amounts listed here can easily be undertaken with no fear of side effects.

Herbs

- *St. John's wort*, 300 mg three times daily for the depression commonly associated with ADHD
- *Ginkgo biloba*, 80 mg twice daily, improves circulation and may enhance frontal lobe brain activity

- *Valerian* for evening and night sedative effects, tincture 1:5, 1-1½ tsp., or fluid extract 1:1, one half–1 teaspoon at bedtime

- *Mentalin*, an Ayurvedic herb containing Gotu kola (Centella asiatica) for improving memory and relieving depression (four to six tablets daily, from Metagenics in Eugene, OR)

- *Beyond Ritalin*, a specifically formulated proprietary herbal preparation (Wise Woman Herbals, Cottage Grove, OR); combining many of these elements, works well

Environment

Standard fluorescent *lighting* is related to ADHD in some studies; for patients not responding to other measures, replacement of standard tubes with full-spectrum fluorescent tubes should be tried. And for children and young adults who are not responding to dietary and food elimination protocols, lead levels should be checked. One of the least expensive tests is a hair mineral analysis, which accurately reveals heavy metal toxicities.

Biomolecular Options

Persistent antibiotic treatment for otitis media frequently changes the gastrointestinal flora, permitting overgrowth of candida. You may need to be checked and treated for candidiasis (if present), which often alters gut mucosal integrity, leading to distorted immune interactions with food antigens, and also to generalized inflammatory reactions with increased free radical activity, which may explain why antioxidants such as grape seed extract are sometimes found to be helpful.

Professional Care Therapy

Homeopathic treatment needs to be highly individualized and managed by skilled practitioners.

Mental and Emotional Health Recommendations

Biofeedback and Relaxation

Hyperactive children, though seemingly unlikely candidates for relaxation training, seem to enjoy the challenge of learning a process with a machine, much like the challenge of computer games which they also enjoy. Children learn biofeedback and relaxation skills quickly. EEG biofeedback training teaches the skills to affect a basic change in predominant brainwave function and when persistently practiced can be of substantial help. Studies have shown the benefits of biofeedback to outscore those of Ritalin. Your physicians can recommend biofeedback resources if they do not offer training themselves.

ALZHEIMER'S DISEASE (AD)

Prevalence

More than four million patients living in the United States today have been diagnosed with Alzheimer's disease (also called Alzheimer's dementia). Alzheimer's is the most common cause of senile dementia, affecting 10 percent of those over 65 and an alarming 50 percent of those over 85. Several million additional elderly have early dementia changes not yet formally diagnosed.

Anatomy and Physiology

The typical lesions found in brain tissue at autopsy of a patient who has died of the complications of Alzheimer's dementia are formations of plaque and tangles of nerve endings, particularly concentrated in the hippocampus, the center of memory and intellectual functioning in the brain. As the disease progresses, there is increasing atrophy and cellular death in many parts of the brain.

Symptoms and Diagnosis

The earliest manifestation of Alzheimer's is memory loss, particularly for recent and contemporary events. Forgetfulness, disorientation, confusion, and mood changes, including depression, are also common symptoms. The Alzheimer's process is usually progressive, often leading to paranoia, inability to manage activities of daily living, and eventual need for institutionalization where 24-hour care is available. Alzheimer's disease (AD) can easily be confused with other causes of dementia. Among them are pernicious anemia, cerebral artery insufficiency, multiple small strokes, Parkinson's disease, Huntington's chorea, drug side effects, environmental toxins, nutritional deficiencies, alcoholism, and depression. Since some of these causes are more treatable, it is important to be as specific as possible in investigation and diagnosis.

An extensive investigation includes a carefully taken history (often with a relative present), physical examination, psychological tests, and often a neurological consultation; laboratory tests, a CT scan, and an EEG are usually necessary to rule out other conditions and confirm the diagnosis.

Fingerprint patterns with increased numbers of ulnar loops (loops deviating toward the little-finger side of the hand) predominating over radial loops, whorls, and arches, were found in 75 percent of AD patients, but only 25 percent of patients without dementia, making this phenomenon a probable marker for predisposition to AD.

Right Hand Finger Prints

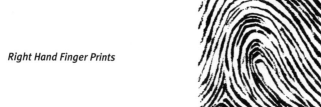
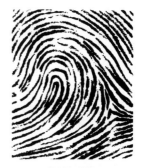

ULNAR LOOP   RADIAL LOOP

Conventional Medical Treatment

Conventional approaches have little to offer Alzheimer's patients. Among the drugs used, selegiline and cholinesterase inhibitors tacrine and donepezil may have some benefit in retarding deterioration. Diarrhea may be a side effect of cholinesterase inhibitors. Amantadine, a drug used to prevent influenza, is reported helpful in some cases and is worth trying at 300 mg twice daily.

Risk Factors and Causes

Physical Factors

Genetic

The risk for AD is three times higher if first-degree relatives have manifested Alzheimer's changes.

Nutritional

Research shows that the brain tissue of Alzheimer's patients exhibits a level of free radical activity twice that of healthy patients of the same age who have no dementia. The oxidative stress found in the degenerative process is now thought to be the primary cause. Alzheimer's patients also have lower levels of antioxidant nutrients compared to healthy elderly controls, probably because the antioxidant reserves have been exhausted by the increased free radical activity. Alzheimer's patients are deficient in vitamins B-1, B-6, and B-12, folic acid, magnesium, zinc, and selenium. Niacin (B-3) deficiency can simulate Alzheimer's disease. Functional elderly subjects with no diagnosed problems who have had lower blood levels of vitamins E and C and beta carotene in the past, as well as the present, score higher on dementia tests. Deficient body levels of docosahexaenoic acid (DHA, an essential fatty acid) are also associated with diminished cognitive function.

Toxicity

The role of *aluminum* and *mercury* in contributing to Alzheimer's disease is disputed. The amount of these minerals in brain tissue at autopsy is significantly higher in those who had Alzheimer's versus those who did not. Alzheimer's is more common in patients who have used more underarm antiperspirants containing aluminum, those who lived in districts with higher aluminum content in the water supply, and those whose aluminum blood levels were higher. Aluminum is known to be absorbed from many sources (see below). Mercury in animals accumulates to a modest extent in brain tissue and induces an anatomic appearance in the brain indistinguishable from the neurofibrillary tangles found in the brain tissue of Alzheimer's patients. Blood mercury levels in Alzheimer's patients are three times as high as in healthy controls. Studies show that mercury absorbed from silver-mercury amalgam dental fillings is the major source of the body burden of mercury in most people.

Prescription medications can cause side effects simulating Alzheimer's; the most common classes of drugs to manifest side effects of mental confusion are: tranquilizers (valium-type medications); antidepressants; antiseizure drugs; anti-Parkinson's drugs; antihypertensives; cancer chemotherapy agents; interferon; antiarrhythmic drugs; and muscle relaxants

Smoking is a risk factor in people who do not have the specific genetic marker for Alzheimer's.

Disease Associations

A recent prospective report showed that men who had elevated systolic *blood pressures* in the 1960s had detectably lower mental abilities 25 to 30 years later in 1990. Chronically high blood pressure gradually damages blood vessels, including those in the brain. Atherosclerosis and high blood pressure are major contributors to multi-infarct dementia, a deterioration of cognitive functions frequently indistinguishable from Alzheimer's. Alzheimer's is also significantly increased in those with a history of chronic *hypothyroidism*.

Biochemistry

Immune and inflammatory chemicals have been identified in brain tissue of AD patients, suggesting that a strong inflammatory component is involved in the degenerative process.

Physical Inactivity

Groups of elderly persons who lack physical activity have poorer cognitive function and slower reaction times than more active groups.

Mental and Emotional Factors. Low "idea density" in childhood and early adulthood appears to be related to increased risk of Alzheimer's. This implies that children and young people need adequate challenge and stimulation to think broadly and develop a far-ranging spectrum of mental images and ideas.

Many elderly who develop Alzheimer's have been very active and mentally and analytically focused, with little time spent in reflection, meditation, and quietness.

Social Health Factors. Medical intuitive Caroline Myss sees a significant contribution to Alzheimer's with the recent cultural shift in the social position of many elderly from being "wisdomkeepers" in society to being elderly dependents. She sees the withdrawal of contact from family and friends in AD as a reflection of the values of society which devalue the contributions of the elderly, who as a result tend to withdraw instead of engaging in the competitive fast-paced struggle for youthfulness and excitement.

Holistic Prevention and Treatment

Physical and Environmental Health Recommendations:

Special Investigations and Testing

- Evaluation for markers of free radical activity
- Functional liver detoxification testing
- Hair analysis for heavy metal contamination
- Assessment of homocysteine status

Vitamins, Minerals, and Supplements

- High antioxidant intake is important in preventing and offsetting the free radical damage associated with AD. A potent multivitamin-mineral can supply most of the needed elements, including *folic acid*. (See chapter 2 for specifics.)

- Research shows that the elderly who have higher levels of *vitamins C* (one to two grams daily), *E* (400 to 1,200 I.U. daily), *beta carotene* (10,000—25,000 I.U. daily), and *B-6* (50—100 mg daily) do best on tests of memory, recognition, and vocabulary. High doses of Vitamins C and E appear, in a recently published study, to reduce the risk of Alzheimer's.

- Supplements of *B-1* (300 to 2,000 mg/day) and *B-12* (1 mg weekly by injection or 1 mg of methylcobalamin twice daily by mouth) stabilize or improve mood and cognitive functions.

- Patients with early Alzheimer's who combine *zinc* (45 mg daily), *evening primrose oil* (three grams daily), and *selenium* (1,000 mcg daily) for four months significantly improve mood and mental function scores on testing.

- *Omega-3 fatty acids* from fish, *flaxseed oil*, or algae sources are also a feasible option (100–300 mg/day of docosahexaenoic acid content).

- *Acetyl L-carnitine*, two to three grams daily, retards deterioration and achieves moderate reversal of some of the memory, attention, and mood alterations in Alzheimer's patients.

- *Methionine*, (0.5–1.5 grams/day) and *cysteine* (one to four grams/day), sulphur-containing amino acids, enhance antioxidant enzymes.

- *NADH* (nucleotide adenine dehydrogenase), 10 mg once daily before breakfast, improves functioning in AD patients.

- *Phosphatidylserine*, another body chemical, 100 mg three times daily, also evokes noticeable improvement.

- *Reduced glutathione*, 50 mg twice daily.

- *Coenzyme Q10* (100 mg daily) has been used widely in Japan. If benefit is achieved with biosynthetic supplements, treatment needs to be continued indefinitely. An oil resin–bound form provides three times higher absorption (from Metagenics in Eugene, OR).

- It has been suggested that women taking *estrogen* for hormone replacement post-menopausally may have a lower incidence of AD. Estrogen does have antioxidant properties, which may explain these data. Not all studies concur; if you undertake hormone replacement therapy, natural hormones have less possibility for problematic side effects. (See chapter 17.)

- DHEA, if blood levels prove deficient, should be taken as a supplement (usual dose is 10–25 mg daily).

Herbs

If you are dealing with a relative with AD, *Ginkgo biloba* extract, 80 mg twice daily (standardized to 24 percent ginkgolides) is worth trying; it has a 60 percent chance of slowing the progression and even partially reversing symptoms. One study also noted improvement in electroencephalograms. A long-term trial of several months is necessary. Greater absorbability has been found in a product combining ginkgo with inositol (from Phytopharmica in Green Bay, WI.)

Exercise

For maintenance of mental function, challenging physical activities are essential. If you do not do at least 45- to 60-minutes of brisk walking or other aerobic activity two to three times each week, start working toward that goal with shorter periods of exercise (see chapter 2). Alzheimer's patients in a nursing home who participated once a week in a session in which a dozen residents seated in a circle bounced a beach ball across the circle to each other for 30 to 40 minutes became more functional and lived twice as long as a comparable group that only reminisced about old times. Physical movement is basic to every principle of health maintenance and achieving optimal health.

Environmental Options

Although the importance of aluminum and mercury in Alzheimer's dementia is still debated, since they are both identified to be toxic to the human body, excessive contact should be avoided. To reduce aluminum exposure:

- Consider using deodorants without aluminum antiperspirants (you will perspire much less if you regularly practice meditation or deep relaxation).
- Avoid aluminum cookware (use stainless steel).
- Use glass bottles rather than aluminum cans if you drink colas and beer.
- Do not use antacids containing aluminum.
- Do not store highly acid or alkaline foods in aluminum foil.
- Find salt and baking powder with no aluminum content (read the labels).
- Use pastry mixes that do not contain aluminum (again, read the labels).
- Use a water filter to remove aluminum from your drinking and cooking water (certified city water supplies can contain excessive amounts of aluminum).
- Take extra magnesium to oppose aluminum absorption.
- Avoid citric acid and citrate forms of mineral supplements, which increase aluminum absorption.

To reduce mercury exposure:

- If you are having dental cavities filled or replaced, insist that your dentist use plastic or porcelain options rather than silver-mercury amalgam material. The extra cost may well be worth it.
- Avoid high intake of coastal fish.

In a two-year research project, intramuscular injections of a chelating agent, *desferrioxamine*, significantly slowed the rate of decline in 50 patients with early Alzheimer's disease (published in *Therapeutic Drug Monitoring*, December 1993). Desferrioxamine removes heavy metals from the body.

If the onset of Alzheimer's-like symptoms in a friend or relative seems to be associated with the starting of a new prescribed medication, read the PDR (Physician's Desk Reference) in your library to find out more. Or ask the doctor about the possible relationship.

Mental and Emotional Health Recommendations. Studies have clearly shown the benefits of continued intellectual challenge in arresting the progress of Alzheimer's. New challenges including classes, reading, and playing games requiring mental skill such as board games (chess for example), card games, and crossword and jigsaw puzzles are all helpful.

Social Health Recommendations. Challenging yourself socially has also been shown to prevent or postpone the dementia-like changes of advancing age. Requiring yourself to remember names, develop new skills, interact socially and conversationally with others, and accept new challenges does make a difference.

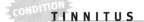

TINNITUS

Prevalence

Some ten million people have experienced sufficient tinnitus to seek medical help; it is estimated that 35 million may have symptoms at least occasionally. The symptoms are much more common in people in middle age and in the elderly.

Symptoms and Diagnosis

Tinnitus describes the persistent ringing, buzzing, hissing, or humming sounds perceived by people with this affliction. The sounds are subjective and not heard by anyone else or by your doctor. Tinnitus may be associated with hearing loss, but neither causes the other. There are no objective tests to confirm the diagnosis.

Conventional Medical Treatment

Medical textbooks frequently mention reassurance as a major therapeutic initiative for patients with tinnitus. Other suggestions commonly mentioned include removal of objects or wax from the external ear canal; potassium iodide supplements; magnesium supplements; salicylate-free diets; reduction of fat and cholesterol in the diet; vasodilators, including niacin (vitamin B-3); and the avoidance of caffeine and nicotine.

Risk Factors and Causes

Environmental Hazards. Excessive *noise* that may damage the ears includes that of firearm discharges, motorcycle riding, industrial noise, rock concerts, jackhammers, and many other consistent or loud sounds, leaving a residual tinnitus. Toxic environmental hazards include acute *lead* poisoning and leaking mercury from silver-*mercury* amalgam dental fillings, which has been reported to cause symptoms.

Pharmaceutical Side Effects. The most common *drug* causing tinnitus is aspirin (all salicylates), used daily by millions of people in the United States; moderate to high doses consistently cause ringing in the ears. In high doses some antibiotics, including erythromycin, can cause hearing loss and tinnitus. Other problematic drugs include antidepressants, antihypertensives, NSAIDs (ibuprofen, for example), atropine, chloroquine, Flexeril, ergotamines, Talwin, quinidine, quinine, and meclorethamine hydrochloride (a cancer chemotherapy drug).

Sensitivities. Tinnitus is sometimes related to inhalant or ingestant (food) sensitivities. Most likely candidates for these reactions include people with personal or family histories of allergic reactions and those who have a history of food cravings or attraction to a small number of foods that are eaten often. Great variability in tinnitus symptoms may also be a clue to the need to assess food sensitivities.

Other Causes

- Acoustic neuroma (a tumor of the auditory nerve)
- Elevated blood lipids (cholesterol and triglycerides)
- Hypertension
- Hyperthyroidism
- Meniere's disease
- Viral and bacterial ear infections
- Poorly managed stress
- Temporomandibular joint problems
- Compromised circulation
- Smoking—may aggravate tinnitus from nicotine absorption
- Coffee and caffeine—have been known to be contributing factors

Emotional Factors. Tinnitus and deafness have been energetically related to fear and negative behavior patterns. These include fears of introspection, of intellectual inadequacy, of using one's intuitive skills, of being open to the value of the ideas of others, and of using one's own power; denying elements of the truth; and unwillingness to learn from life's experiences.

Holistic Prevention and Treatment

Vitamins and Minerals which are sometimes helpful are:

- *Zinc picolinate*, up to 90 mg/day
- *Vitamin A*, 5,000 I.U. daily (vitamin A is highly concentrated in the cochlea and receptor cells in the inner ear)
- *Vitamin B-complex* ("B-50," one daily)
- Extra *vitamin B-6*, 100 mg daily (especially with fluid retention problems)
- *Quercetin*, 500 mg, two capsules three times daily as a natural antihistamine
- *Vitamin C* with mixed bioflavonoids, one gram three times a day

Sensitizer elimination. When food or inhalant sensitivities are suspected and identified, elimination of the strong offender(s) and rotation of minor and moderate food offenders is helpful. When tinnitus presents as part of a picture of progressive bilateral, sensorineural hearing loss (the hearing loss of old age) in which no specific cause is apparent, the total elimination of cow's milk is worth trying. Recovery of some hearing in this condition has recently been reported as a result of eliminating cow's milk protein antigens, which are similar to proteins in the inner ear, to which the immune system may respond by making antibodies.

Drug identification and elimination. If the timing of tinnitus is correlated with starting or taking medications, eliminate the medication if possible for about a week to see if the tinnitus subsides. Drugs shown to be related to symptoms by test elimination periods should be permanently omitted unless life-saving. Ongoing noise exposure should be eliminated. Other primary disease problems leading to tinnitus need to be handled in the best way possible to reduce symptoms.

Detoxification. The institution of a nutritional detoxification program can be helpful (see inflammatory bowel disease, chapter 11).

Herbs. Ginkgo biloba, 80 mg twice daily, has been shown to significantly reduce severity ratings in tinnitus patients; it may take up to four months to see improvement.

Biofeedback, relaxation training, and yoga have all been reported to be helpful, and upgrading of stress management skills is of great help. One study found 50 percent improvement with *biofeedback*, 30 percent with *acupuncture*, 7 percent with drug treatment, and 2 percent with placebos.

Professional Care Therapies. *Therapeutic Touch, Reiki, Zenith therapy,* and other energy therapy approaches can also be helpful. Specific *homeopathic* remedies can be helpful when carefully chosen by a well-trained professional practitioner.

Social Health Recommendations. One recent published study found significantly greater improvement in a peer-led support group, compared to those treated without group involvement.

16

Obesity

Prevalence

OBESITY IS PRESENT in women whose body makeup is over 30 percent fat, and in men whose bodies contain over 25 percent fat. Optimum body constitution is less than 24 percent body fat for women and less than 18 percent for men. Thirty to fifty percent of American adults are obese—carrying too much body fat. In the last 20 years, obesity has increased 50 percent in children and 40 percent in teenagers. The numbers of obese children and teenagers have steadily increased since 1970.

Anatomy and Physiology

Excess fat is distributed throughout the body, including increased deposition under the skin and in most of the internal organs. Two predominant patterns are seen: the "apple," or android, pattern, more common in men with extra weight predominantly carried in the chest and waist area; and the "pear," or gynecoid; pattern with fat distribution predominant in the low abdomen, buttock, and thigh areas, more common in women. The distinction is more than academic: greater risks of a number of diseases accompany the android pattern.

Symptoms and Diagnosis

Most of us fairly easily recognize our gains in weight. Our older clothes become too snug and we tend to not wear them, and our new clothes are a size bigger. Measured weight can be a distortion, however; weighing the same at 60 as we were at 20 usually means we have lost lean muscle mass and gained fat to replace it. In the United States we lose an average of 4 percent of our muscle mass each decade from age 25 to 50, and 10 percent each decade thereafter.

The associated evidences of weight gain include mild shortness of breath, decreased stamina, and increasing difficulty in managing the physical activities of daily living.

The complications of obesity include:

- Higher incidence of some cancers (liver, gall bladder, colon, rectum, prostate, uterus, urinary tract)
- High blood pressure
- Cardiovascular disease (heart attacks, strokes, sudden death events, poor leg circulation)
- Diabetes
- Gout
- Gallbladder disease
- Hernias
- Intestinal obstruction
- Arthritis of weight-bearing joints
- Poor wound healing
- Excess risk of childbirth complications
- Sleep disorders, including sleep apnea
- Excess risk of injury and falls
- Respiratory disease susceptibility
- Shortened lifespan (up to 20 percent)
- Lower metabolism

Obesity may be estimated and diagnosed by being above the norms on weight/height tables, by consulting a table for body mass index, by above normal measurements of abdominal girth, or more precisely, by measures of excess content of body fat. The latter is most simply and inexpensively done by having your external fat layers measured in three to five places by a calipers, with your percentage of body fat then calculated from standard tables. Body fat content can be determined, also, by weighing on a scale incorporating bioelectrical impedance.

Conventional Treatment

Conventional management incorporates suggestions for losing weight by reduction of caloric intake, increased exercise of an aerobic nature, and often referral to dietitians for nutritional help or to commercial diet and weight-loss programs.

Figure 1

Calculating Body
Mass Index

Draw a straight line
from your weight to
your height. Where it
crosses the middle
line is equal to your
body mass index.

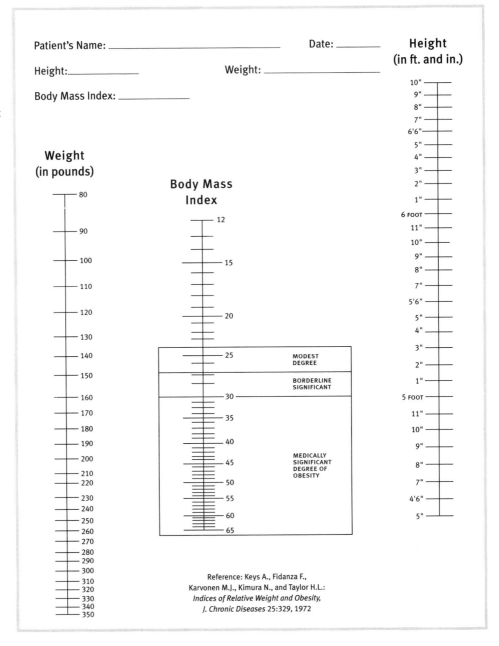

Patient's Name: _____   Date: _____

Height: _____   Weight: _____

Body Mass Index: _____

Weight
(in pounds)

Body Mass
Index

Height
(in ft. and in.)

Reference: Keys A., Fidanza F.,
Karvonen M.J., Kimura N., and Taylor H.L.:
Indices of Relative Weight and Obesity,
J. Chronic Diseases 25:329, 1972

About 70 percent of people placed on these programs lose substantial amounts of weight, but about 95 percent of the time the weight is regained, with patients sometimes winding up heavier than they were before. Appetite suppressant drugs are also used; in the 1960s and 1970s, amphetamines were prescribed but all too often were abused. Amphetamine derivatives, including fenfluramine, Bontril, and phentermine, were used in the 1980s and early 1990s. Again, problems arose from not only a tendency for habituation but also the emergence of side effects, including heart valve abnormalities and increased blood pressure in the lungs. Meridia is the latest drug approved for use in obesity. It inhibits several brain neurotransmitters. The pharmaceutical company warns against its use in patients with high blood pressure, or in combination with certain antidepressants. Orlistat, a new pancreatic lipase inhibitor, appears to assist in weight loss by inhibiting fat digestion and assimilation. Long-term results are pending. Olestra-containing foods may be suggested, to allow enjoyment of the taste of fat without the burden of assimilation and adding to caloric totals. Olestra, however, causes diarrhea in many people and inhibits absorption of vital antioxidant nutrients.

Risk Factors and Causes

The roots of obesity lie in a combination of genetic, physical, emotional, and social factors.

Genetic Factors. Carefully done studies in the 1980s showed that a significant number of obese people who adhered to a good exercise program had to decrease their food intake to at least 25 percent below the levels of lean people in order to lose weight. The reasons for this marked difference in metabolism are thought to be predominantly genetic. The hereditary causes contributing to this predisposition to obesity include:

- Low serotonin levels (hunger and craving for carbohydrate are increased by deficiency in tryptophan, serotonin's precursor amino acid), aggravated by insufficient tryptophan intake
- Insulin resistance (insensitivity), aggravated by lack of physical exercise and by diets high in sugar, refined carbohydrates, and saturated fat (increases hunger, raises set point [see under holistic treatment], decreases thermogenesis—the energy expenditure used to produce heat)
- Impaired sympathetic nervous system activity (leads to decreased thermogenesis)
- Lower percentage of brown fat (leads to 25 percent higher efficiency in producing energy and heat, leaving a net saving of calories with more calories to go into fat storage. See under holistic treatment)
- Coenzyme Q10 deficiency (in up to 50 percent of obese subjects)

Physical Factors

- Physical inactivity. The United States is a sedentary nation. In spite of a decrease in average caloric intake of 40 percent in the last 130 years, the decrease in physical exertion has been even greater, leaving more people overweight. In the majority of obese people, caloric intake habitually exceeds caloric loss from physical activity, movement, and exertion.

- Low metabolism: metabolism is deficient in many overweight people for genetic reasons and lack of physical exercise. The metabolism of stored fat in the body is considerably below that of lean tissue. So the metabolic rate of obese people is well below that of lean people, reduced by the sluggish metabolism of fat; this vicious cycle is difficult to break without vigorous physical activity.

- Certain disease states are also associated with a greater likelihood of obesity, including diabetes, hypothyroidism, hypertension, and hyperlipidemias (see chapters 14, 20).

- Food allergies and sensitivities evoke craving responses and an addiction-like pattern. Overeating in these circumstances can often be traced to intake of unusually large amounts of the foods to which there is an excessive and distorted attraction. The commonest offending foods are milk, wheat, and corn—all commonly found in snack foods.

- Men whose birth weights were over 10 pounds carry twice the risk of being overweight adults compared to those whose birth weight was under five and a half pounds. Women have a two-thirds greater risk. It is also known that there is a consistent relationship between the number of fat cells, fixed at birth, and the adult tendency to be obese. The reasons why these two factors influence adult weight are unclear.

Emotional and Mental Factors. Excessive caloric intake from unrestrained eating, including our incredible habits of snacking in the United States, is often associated with factors other than hunger. Eating may be triggered by learned responses from childhood; we all know them: "Don't waste food—children are starving in the world." "Clean your plate." "If you want dessert, you have to eat your asparagus." Childhood and adult obesity are much more common in those whose parents use or tended to use more manipulative negative and positive prompting to control their eating as children.

Emotional factors play an enormous role. Any number of emotional states can also touch off our decision to eat, such as anger, self-hatred, anxiety, and simple boredom. Overeating is also very commonplace in our society because of the tendency to use food as a source of pleasure, particularly in people—more women than men—who have experienced previous traumas in life that limit their ability to find sources of pleasure not associated with food.

Social Factors. Food is easily available in our society and is a centerpiece of social affairs of all kinds; eating can often carry a sense of social obligation. Eating is often a reason for coming together—meeting someone and/or conducting business over lunch or coffee. Extended family gatherings during holidays carry a sense of celebration and often center around large, sumptuous meals. Eating is also significantly enhanced by intense advertising. Television watching and obesity are highly associated; the more of one, the more of the other.

Holistic Prevention and Treatment

Physical Health Recommendations

Diet

High fiber intake encourages weight loss by accumulating a larger mass of food in the stomach, creating a sensation of fullness and satisfaction earlier in the eating cycle. High amounts of sugar, refined carbohydrates, and fat have the opposite effect.

Food sensitivities. If you have distinct patterns of specific food cravings, tend to eat a lot of the same foods, or have a personal or family background of allergic tendencies, a food elimination trial may well prove helpful. If you have no withdrawal symptoms whatsoever after totally omitting a specific food from your eating pattern, food sensitivity is less likely. If the thought of going a week without even a token amount of any foods that you consume in large amounts induces a sense of anxiety, then food sensitivities are more likely. If a food elimination and rechallenge trial gives significant results, proven offending foods need to be eliminated or eaten on a rotation basis (see chapter 2).

Vitamins, Minerals, and Supplements

- Specific fiber supplements have an additional dimension of effectiveness by reducing excess insulin levels and actually reducing the number of calories absorbed. Perhaps the best example is *guar gum*, a water soluble fiber derivative of the Indian cluster bean. Ten grams of guar gum twice daily before lunch and dinner achieve a weight loss of about a pound per week, while improving insulin utilization and cholesterol ratios. Start with a low dose of one to two grams before meals to avoid excessive gas. Various other fiber sources and combinations of *pectin, glucomannon* (from konjac root), beet, and barley are also effective.

- *Medium chain triglycerides* (MCTs) (fats) have been found to save 50 percent of the calories compared to a similar intake of long chain triglycerides. These triglycerides can be used as an oil in salad dressings, for instance, or taken as a supplement, one to two tablespoonfuls daily. Health food stores market products containing MCTs. To be fully effective, intake of long chain triglycerides must be kept to reasonably low—meaning a diet relatively low in animal fat.

- Overweight volunteers taking 200 mcg of *chromium picolinate* with 100 mg of **L-carnitine** daily, plus vitamins and minerals, have been shown to average a 15-pound weight loss in eight weeks. This combination was observed to increase their metabolism as well.

- *Pantothenic acid* (vitamin B-5), 2,500 mg four times daily, enabled a group of one hundred subjects to lose two and a half pounds a week over several months with no side effects.

- *Tryptophan* assimilated into the body is degraded to the amino acid *5-hydroxytryptophan*, which in turn is metabolized to serotonin. Higher serotonin levels reduce carbohydrate craving and hunger. 5-HTP is available without a prescription; doses of 300 mg three times a day in one study afforded a 12-pound weight loss in 12 weeks with almost total elimination of excessive hunger, even in the face of caloric restrictions. The only reported side effect was mild nausea in the early weeks of the study. An appropriate starting dose is 100 mg before meals, increasing after two weeks if weight loss is under one pound per week.

- Taking modest (10–20 mg) daily doses of *DHEA* in those who have low DHEA blood levels can contribute to weight loss.

- In *Coenzyme Q10*–deficient subjects, 100 mg daily achieved a weight loss of 30 pounds in nine weeks. An arbitrary trial without prior testing is reasonable.

- In animals, the combination of *ephedrine* and *caffeine* increases sympathetic nervous system activity and burning of calories by brown fat. Brown fat, located between the shoulder blades, makes up only a small percentage of total body fat. Surgical removal of the brown fat in animals leads to obesity. Severing all the nerves from the brown fat does the same thing, showing that the substantial influence on metabolic (calorie-burning) rate of this special fat is mediated through the sympathetic nervous system. In one human study, relatively low daily doses of a combination of caffeine (30 mg), ephedrine (22 mg), and theophylline, an asthma medication, (50 mg) led to an 8 percent increase in metabolism. Elevation of blood pressure, headache, heart palpitations, and headache can occur if these doses are increased beyond these minimal amounts.

Herbs

- Excellent research shows that *Yohimbine* affords a 35 percent better weight loss than placebo medication. Yohimbine is available by prescription: 15 mg daily in divided doses.

- Intake of *guggul* derivatives regularly for three months results in four times the weight loss compared to placebo (dosage: 2.25 grams twice a day).
- Botanicals (Ephedra sinica with Coffea arabica or Camellia sinensis) can also be taken in amounts to supply 30 mg of ephedrine and 100 mg of methylxanthines daily, as mentioned earlier.

Exercise

Exercise will not burn enough calories to lead to significant weight loss. For example, to lose one pound, you have to burn five hundred extra calories above maintenance levels each day for a week. That requires the equivalent of jogging for 45 minutes daily—difficult to sustain indefinitely. Exercise, however, does greatly increase thermogenic calorie burning (metabolism) not only during exercise, but also for up to four to six hours after finishing. Most people achieve about a 10 percent weight loss in six months with a well-designed aerobic exercise program alone. Aerobic exercise also reduces insulin levels by increasing insulin sensitivity and uptake in the cells of the body, as well as lowering the set point. The set point is an internally programmed weight (possibly genetically determined) below which it becomes increasingly difficult to adhere to a diet of lowered caloric intake. So *permanent weight loss is very difficult to achieve without a program of regular aerobic exercise*. Fidgeting, a manifestation of higher sympathetic nervous system energy, has been found to burn an additional five hundred to seven hundred calories daily.

Mental and Emotional Health Recommendations. If you are obese, several steps are involved in reaching nearly normal body fat constitution for the rest of your life. They include commitment to:

- Practicing a positive attitude of unconditional love and caring for your body.
- Evoking motivation to be healthy and the most attractive you that you can be. You need to do this for yourself and not because someone else wants you to.
- Changing your behavior in regard to food and eating; eating only when hungry and honoring the eating process by giving yourself enough time to eat in pleasant circumstances.
- Moving your body in ways that honor its need for physical activity.
- Forging relationships with supportive people who hold you in high esteem no matter what, and creating the circumstances that honor your need for pleasure without dependence on food.

- Becoming more aware of your eating patterns and associated emotions, gradually shifting to hunger as the major reason for eating.

You may need professional help from counselors who are thoroughly steeped in awareness of these principles. Many well-trained professionals will combine these skills with opportunities for you to learn a systematic relaxation process such as *biofeedback* and utilizing the power of *guided imagery*.

17

Women's Conditions

CONDITION

BLADDER INFECTIONS

Prevalence

TEN TO TWENTY PERCENT of all adult women in the United States have at least one bladder infection each year, triggering six to nine million physician visits annually. Two to four percent of asymptomatic women have bacteria in any random urine specimen. Women subject to recurring infections average over one episode each year, and 20 percent of women having one episode will have another. Thirty-seven percent of all women have at least one urinary tract infection in a ten-year span. The serious aspect of the recurrences is that at least one-half also involve the upper urinary tract—the kidneys. Repeated kidney infections can cause permanent and progressive degrees of kidney failure. Bladder infections in men are much less common.

Anatomy and Physiology

Urine formed in the kidneys is accumulated in the bladder for collection until eliminated at the time of urination. The bladder may accommodate up to a pint of urine before giving an elimination signal. The elimination tube, the urethra, is much shorter in women compared to men. Bacteria reach the bladder by ascending upstream from the outside through the urethra. In 90 percent of cases, the infecting organism is E. coli, a garden variety organism with permanent residence in the bowel.

Symptoms and Diagnosis

Bladder infection, medically known as cystitis, presents with urinary frequency and urgency and, particularly if the urethra is involved, a very uncomfortable burning sensation during urination. The amount of urine passed is frequently small, and the urine may be foul-smelling, cloudy, or bloody. Severe infections are accompanied by fever and chills.

The diagnosis is confirmed by examination of a urine specimen, which may be cultured in the laboratory for identification of the offending bacterium to guide antibiotic treatment.

Symptoms of a bladder infection may be present with no bacteria found in the urine. In fact, some studies show that this happens about 25 to 40 percent of the time. When this occurs, you and your doctor will need to search for other pelvic and nervous system causes for your symptoms.

Conventional Medical Treatment

Conventional precautions to prevent episodes and recurrences emphasize adequate hydration. It is helpful to achieve the goal of six to eight glasses of water daily, sufficient to keep the urine a pale yellow. If you have a history of bladder infections, it will reduce your risks if you urinate more frequently, avoiding any tendency to ignore the bladder's signals of being full when you are overly busy. What Mother taught you, to wipe from the front to the back after urinating, is probably also important. Although some authorities disagree, most think that urinating after sexual intercourse makes real sense and recommend it for those with susceptibility to recurrent infections. Cranberry juice reduces the frequency of infections; it has been documented to make it more difficult for bacteria to attach to the bladder wall.

The first line of medical treatment usually involves the prescribing of antibiotics. The most common ones used include sulfa drugs, broad spectrum penicillins, fluoroquinolones (Cipro, Noroxin), and nitrofurantoins (Macrodantin). The previous standard was a ten-day prescription; three to five days has been found to work just as well most of the time in uncomplicated infections. For frequently recurring episodes, some physicians recommend low antibiotic dosage daily for several weeks or months.

A common hazard with any antibiotic treatment is the destruction of normal friendly bacteria in the intestine and overgrowth of other organisms, including candida (see chapter 9).

Occasionally when a tight urethral opening is a contributing factor in recurring infections, urological dilation and gentle stretching of the urethral opening may help the emptying process.

Risk Factors and Causes

The propensity for women to have a bladder infection on becoming sexually active is well known. Bladder infection is likewise common in pregnancy. Women in menopause and approaching menopause are more susceptible to infections as well, apparently due to some weakening of pelvic structures with decreases in estrogen. Diaphragms used for contraception also increase risk for infection. Spermicidal creams containing nonoxynol-9 alter the vaginal bacterial flora and encourage the proliferation of E. coli. Feminine hygiene sprays and frequent douching are also hazards. Recurring or persistent vaginal infections (see below) also predispose to bladder infections.

Resistance to infection depends on the flushing action of urine moving from the kidneys to the bladder and then to the outside of the body. If this flushing activity becomes sluggish, the hazard of infection taking hold increases. Contributors to this problem are diseases that interfere with regular urination (spinal cord injury, for instance), partial obstruction by spasm or tightness of the urethra, or underhydration, all contributing to the stagnation effect. Compromised immune resistance to any infection is present in hypothyroidism.

Some foods tend to be bladder irritants or to adversely affect the bladder's natural rhythms, including caffeine in coffee, tea, and colas; alcohol on occasion; and specific sensitizing foods in susceptible people.

Excessive sympathetic nervous system activity due to the tension of unmanaged stress predisposes to spasm and incomplete emptying of the bladder.

Holistic Prevention and Treatment

Physical Health Recommendations

Diet

- Sugar inhibits bacterial destruction and should be avoided.

- Blueberry juice, although harder to find than cranberry juice, also contains the inhibitor that prevents adherence of bacteria to the bladder wall. Since most cranberry juices on the market are sweetened with sugar (which inhibits bacterial destruction) and unsweetened cranberry juice is not very palatable, blueberry juice is probably preferable: a reasonable intake is eight ounces a day.

- Alkalinizing the urine also is beneficial; one study showed 80 percent relief from bladder symptoms after four grams of sodium citrate three times daily for two days. The best agents are *calcium*, *magnesium*, or *potassium citrate*; the amounts of the elemental minerals should be 250 mg four times a day.

Vitamins and Supplements

- *Vitamin C* is also effective in bladder and urethral infections. Vitamin C has distinct antimicrobial properties and taken in large doses (one to two grams three to four times daily) is quickly hyperconcentrated in the urine. Calcium, magnesium, and potassium ascorbate will alkalinize the urine at the same time.

- *Vitamin A*, which helps with many infections, can be taken in large doses of 50,000 I.U. daily for up to a week in adults and for two days in a row in children and infants. Do not take if pregnancy is a possibility.

- *Acidophilus* and *bifidus* supplements correct imbalances in the vaginal flora, which, when seriously damaged, tend to lead to both vaginal and bladder infections.

Food Sensitivities

The urine specimens of up to 40 percent of women with typical symptoms of bladder or urethral infection have no detectable bacteria. Chronic interstitial cystitis is a chronic bladder irritation without bacterial infection. Food sensitivities can cause urinary frequency and urgency and may be a cause of interstitial cystitis. If you have recurring or chronic irritative bladder symptoms and examinations find no bacterial infections, a food elimination trial and rechallenge is well worth doing.

Herbs

- *Uva ursi* (bearberry) is an herb with a long history of use in preventing and treating bladder infections with recent research documentation of effectiveness; dosage in 1:5 tincture form: 1–1½ teaspoons three times daily (standardized extract).

- *Goldenseal*, taken as a 1:5 tincture, 1–1½ teaspoons three times daily, is also efficacious against many of the bacteria commonly involved.

- *Gotu kola* (centella asiatica) has been used with success in interstitial cystitis; take an extract supplying 60 mg daily of the active ingredients—triterpenic acids.

- *Juniper berry* and *cornsilk* teas have therapeutic benefits.

Biomolecular Options

Capitalizing on the known increase in recurrent infections in menopausal women, astute observers found in one study that use of one of the three natural human estrogens, *estriol*, in an intravaginal cream used nightly for two weeks each month, reduced the frequency of infection recurrences *92 percent*. And oral supplementation with low doses of estriol (2 mg daily) has been shown to reduce bladder and vaginal reinfection rates *16-fold*. Your doctor can prescribe oral or intravaginal estriol (0.5 mg daily) to be obtained from a compounding pharmacist.

Professional Care Therapies

Homeopathy. Classic homeopathic diagnosis and treatment may be curative for recurrent cystitis. Symptomatic homeopathic remedies to use for treatment include Apis Mel or Cantharis. *Acupuncture* also can be of help with recurrent infections.

Mental and Emotional Treatment Options. If you have a high level of stress and tension in your life, incorporating some measure of regular relaxation practice will tend to improve bladder emptying and reduce the frequency of recurrences. Meditation, biofeedback, and other techniques all decrease sympathetic nervous system activity, reducing the contribution made by urethral spasm and poor bladder emptying. Immune responses also improve with the practice of these skills.

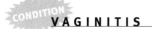

VAGINITIS

Prevalence

Thirty-five to fifty percent of American women have dealt with a vaginal infection at some time in their lives. In a recent study, three out of four young sexually ac-

---

A CASE HISTORY

On noticing that my patient Carol, age 42, looked very tired, I inquired why. She volunteered that she had not been sleeping well, and she had not slept really well for at least 20 years. The major problem, urinary frequency, which she said roused her from bed six times each night to empty her bladder, had been constant since high school. During the day she emptied her bladder at least once an hour. Her urgency during the day and at night was such that she felt in danger of wetting her underclothing if she procrastinated. Her problem had been thoroughly investigated years before, but no pathology was ever found.

Carol had hay fever and allergy to milk as a child and had colic as an infant. She was very willing to undertake a food elimination program, intending to avoid milk, corn, wheat, sugar, citrus fruit, nuts, eggs, chocolate, and food dyes and preservatives for a week.

Three days later she talked ecstatically with my staff, reporting that she had gotten up only twice the previous night and that she was voiding at about two-hour intervals during the day. By the end of the week, she was passing large quantities of urine at each voiding. She then systematically rechallenged herself with each of the eliminated foods, one at a time in pure form. When she reintroduced milk, and later pure chocolate, within hours she returned to the urgent every 45 minutes schedule, with nighttime frequency returning to almost hourly. Following her discovery, she had no further urgency and urinary frequency except after an occasional episode of bingeing on chocolate.

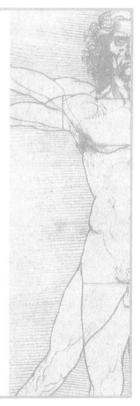

tive women had one or more types of infection; vaginal infections have now been shown to be six times more common than bladder infections. The incidence of vaginitis, particularly the variety caused by yeast organisms, is extremely common and is on the increase. About 1.3 million women are treated or treat themselves for vaginal yeast (candida) infections each year; the number of yearly antifungal prescriptions has risen over 50 percent in the last decade. Antibody studies indicate that between 30 and 100 percent of adults have been infected with both varieties of herpes organisms, which can cause infections in the vagina as well as elsewhere. Chlamydia infection is found in 5 to 10 percent of young sexually active women.

Anatomy and Physiology

Vaginal infections may be limited to superficial invasion of the outer layer of the vaginal mucosal surface, may be part of a more serious generalized infection, including the cervix of the uterus, or may be a total pelvic inflammatory disease process involving the uterus and Fallopian tubes as well. The pH of the vagina is normally mildly acidic.

Symptoms and Diagnosis

Three organisms—Trichomonas vaginalis, Candida albicans, and Gardnerella vaginalis—cause 90 percent of vaginal infections. Other invading organisms include Chlamydia trachomatis, Neisseria gonorrhea, and Herpes simplex.

- Trichomoniasis is caused by a single-celled parasite transmitted by sexual intercourse and manifests as a foul-smelling greenish discharge, with itching and burning. The diagnosis is made by finding the organism in a microscopic examination of the vaginal secretions, the pH of which is usually between 5.5 and 5.8 (mildly acidic).

- Candida albicans (yeast) is a normal fungal resident of the vaginal flora and may overgrow (due to factors mentioned under causes), causing intense itching and a white cottage-cheesy discharge.

- Gardnerella vaginalis (formerly Hemophilus vaginalis) is found in over 90 percent of nontrichomonas, nonyeast infections, usually called nonspecific vaginitis (NSV). Minimal itching and a more profuse odorous discharge are clues to this infection. Gardnerella is an opportunistic invader that is found in 40 percent of women with no symptoms and contributes to nonspecific infection when the vaginal medium is compromised. Other anaerobic bacteria are more probably the key causative organisms in NSV.

- Chlamydia trachomatis, a sexually transmitted parasitic disease, is a major cause of deep pelvic infection and consequent infertility. It is a serious infection leading to many complications and needs to be handled as such.

- Gonorrhea, a sexually transmitted, bacterial disease, commonly called the clap, is cultured in 50 percent of serious deep pelvic inflammatory infections and often manifests as a bloody, pus-containing discharge.

- Herpes simplex infection is the most common sexually transmitted infection in the United States today. Both herpes type 1 and type 2 viruses may be involved. Vulvo-vaginal herpes manifests as localized, blistery sores that usually ulcerate, becoming painful (sometimes excruciatingly so), and taking about two or more weeks to completely heal. Vaginal herpetic infections are most commonly transmitted by genital, manual, or oral contact.

Conventional Medical Treatment

Standard advice includes avoiding routine douching, not using scented toilet paper or tampons, and removing tampons after no more than eight hours.

Trichomoniasis is treated with Flagyl, an antiparasitic agent, prescribed in a large single dose or in smaller amounts over five to seven days. Sexual partners need to be treated at the same time as well. Nausea affects 12 percent of users, metallic taste is common, and seizures and persistent neuropathy have been reliably reported.

Candida infection is treated by intravaginal prescription and OTC creams and suppositories; the most popular are Gyne-Lotrimin and Monistat; generic OTC preparations are also available. For herpetic outbreaks, acyclovir (Zovirax) and similar drugs are used effectively in ointment form, orally (200 mg every 4 hours, five doses daily), and even intravenously, injected over an hour, three times daily for two to five days. It should not be given intravenously in those who are pregnant or who have any degree of kidney failure; it can produce nausea, headache, and malaise. Long term daily prophylactic use is also prescribed for patients with a history of frequent recurrences.

Nonspecific vaginitis, gonorrhea, and chlamydia infections are all treated with antibiotics. Some strains of Neisseria gonorrhea are now resistant to the usual treatment with penicillin and common broad-spectrum antibiotics. Antibacterial prescription creams (Cleomycin, Metrogel) are also used for bacterial vaginitis. *As mentioned previously, antibiotics do not alter the circumstances predisposing to the infections in the first place.*

Risk Factors and Causes

Vaginitis involves the invasion of infecting organisms from the reservoir of organisms in the colon and rectum or transmitted through sexual contact. Infection can also arise from multiplication of normal organisms resident in the vagina that proliferate or overgrow due to changes in the vaginal medium—including the pH (acid-alkaline balance), the presence of blood at the time of the menses, the population and balance of normal organisms, the level of sugar in the blood and vaginal tissues, the adequacy of the natural flushing action of vaginal fluids, and the presence of immunity-determined resistance factors.

Predisposing factors contributing to these imbalances include:

- Diabetes—elevated blood and tissue sugar levels encourage growth of yeast (candida) and diminish immune resistance.

- Pregnancy and oral contraceptive agents change the hormone balance, encouraging yeast growth and imbalances in intestinal flora as well.

- Treatment with immune suppressants, chemotherapeutic anticancer agents, or cortisone drugs compromises immune resistance.

- Poor nutritional habits—high sugar and low antioxidant intake—compromise immune resistance.

- Antibiotic treatment severely reduces the population of normal organisms (L. acidophilus), promoting yeast proliferation.

- Wearing panty hose made of synthetic materials triples the incidence of yeast infections compared to the wearing of cotton underclothing.

- Multiple sex partners increases the risk of sexually transmitted organisms, including Trichomonas and Herpes.

- Failure to use barrier contraceptive methods (which reduce transmission of organisms) increases risk.

- Stress that is not managed well results in tension, high levels of which compromise immunity and resistance to infection in the vagina as well as elsewhere.

- Semen has a pH of about 9 (alkaline); it takes about eight hours for the normally mildly acidic vagina to return to normal. Sexual intercourse several times in 24 hours alters the normally acidic pH, tending to support abnormal organisms.

- Scented and perfumed toilet paper and tampons containing deodorants are often irritating and predispose to invasion by infecting organisms.

Studies have shown that in women with recurrent vaginal candida infections, 75 percent have the same yeast strains in the gastrointestinal tract. As most women know, yeast infections of the vagina (as well as the gastrointestinal tract), are highly associated with the use of broad spectrum antibiotics. Candida infections tend to aggravate or evoke more frequent generalized allergic reactions.

The onset of vaginitis may have a psychosocial implication as well. In *Women's Bodies, Women's Wisdom,* Dr. Christiane Northrup says: "Chronic vaginitis is a socially acceptable way for a woman to say no to sex."

Holistic Prevention and Treatment
Candida

Diet
- Avoid sugar.
- Avoid milk and milk products including cheese.
- Avoid foods with high yeast or mold content: nuts, melons, dried fruits, alcohol.
- Avoid fermented foods: vinegar, pickles, tempeh.
- Augment your water intake. Women subject to candidiasis have a 25 percent higher rate of loss of water through the skin.
- Omit any known food allergens.

Vitamins, Minerals, and Supplements
- Take a high potency multivitamin-mineral supplement with megadose *antioxidants.*
- Orally ingested *acidophilus* reestablishes normal intestinal populations.
- When vaginal yeast overgrowth is present, overgrowth in the intestine is also likely, since the predisposing factors favoring yeast multiplication affect the entire body. Nutritional agents that address the concurrent treatment of intestinal candidiasis with vaginal treatment include *garlic* and *short chain fatty acids* (*caprylic acid*) and herbs containing berberine.
- *Grapefruit seed extract,* 2 capsules before meals.

Simultaneous Treatment of Intestinal Candidiasis
There is evidence that treating the intestinal candidiasis at the same time as the vaginal infection reduces the rate of recurrences. The mechanism by which intestinal infection affects the vaginal manifestations is not completely clear but may occur through an allergic phenomenon or by transmission of organisms from the anorectal area. Conventional treatment of the intestinal infection utilizes nys-

tatin, one 500,000-unit tablet four times daily, or more potent systemic medications such as Diflucan and Nizoral.

Local Treatment

- Reestablish normal vaginal organisms by douching daily with a solution of Lactobacillus acidophillus, prepared from a high quality supplement with live organisms, or an active-culture yogurt (most live organism preparations have to be refrigerated). Use an amount supplying one billion organisms and mix with one-third ounce of water and inject into the vagina with a syringe once or twice daily. A vast majority of women using yogurt instilled into the vagina in one half-ounce amounts twice daily become asymptomatic within 1–3 months.

- Boric acid capsules or suppositories (600 mg twice daily) have a higher treatment success rate than antifungal prescription creams and suppositories. Persistent treatment for several months achieves the greatest success in reestablishing totally normal vaginal flora. Side effects of minor burning sensations are usually not severe enough to think about discontinuing treatment.

- Positive results have also been reported with insertion of a *gentian violet*–soaked tampon into the vagina daily for 7–14 days. The only hazard of this approach is that gentian violet is an intensely potent dye and needs to be handled with great care to avoid irrevocable staining of clothing.

- Betadine, available in pharmacies, contains iodine, which has wide antibacterial, antifungal, and antiparasitic activity. Iodine is, after all, used to treat water to make it potable. A solution of one part Betadine to 100 parts water can be used as a douche on a daily basis for two weeks. Studies have shown *100 percent effectiveness* in vaginal candidiasis.

Homeopathy
Yeast-gard is a well tolerated homeopathic remedy.

Trichomonas. Iodine douche is 80 percent successful.

Nonspecific Vaginitis. Iodine douche is 93 percent effective in mixed infections.

Herpes. Treatment options in herpes vaginalis include the following.

Diet
- Low arginine intake (avoid chocolate, peanuts, seeds, almonds, nuts)
- Increase in *lysine* foods (most vegetables, legumes, fish, turkey, chicken)

Vitamins and Minerals

- Oral *vitamin C*, two grams daily
- *Zinc*, 50–75 mg daily
- *Lysine*, 1,000 mg three times daily
- Mixed *bioflavonoids*, 1,000 mg daily

These oral supplements help assist with healing lesions as well as being highly effective in prevention of recurrences.

Topical (Local) Nutrients

- *Vitamin C* solution (Ascoxal) significantly accelerates the rate of healing.
- *Zinc sulfate* solution, 0.025 percent, accelerates healing and prevents outbreaks. A prescription your physician could write for topical zinc is as follows: "$ZnSO_4$ 0.25% in sat. sol. camphor water; apply one-half–2 hours at outbreak. Disp 30 cc." The solution can be daubed on and allowed to dry each time. When the solution is applied immediately at the outset of the tingly prodrome that tells you an outbreak is imminent, it will abort the outbreak up to 90 percent of the time. If an outbreak does occur, it is attended with much less pain and greatly accelerated healing.

Herbs

- Topical application of 70:1 concentrated extract of lemon balm (Melissa officinalis) two–four times daily in cream form has been shown in a German study to prevent recurrences 100 percent of the time when used continuously.
- Licorice root (glycyrrhetinic acid) applied topically twice daily speeds healing and reduces pain; Licrogel (Scientific Botanicals in Seattle, WA) cream supplies appropriate amounts of licorice root.

Biomolecular Agents

Bovine thymus extracts improve cellular immunity. Take 500 mg of crude polypeptide fraction daily (or 120 mg of purified polypeptides).

Additional Recommendations for Treatment of All Vaginal Infections

Mental and Emotional Health Recommendations. Regular practice of *meditation* and *relaxation skills* improves immunity. Outbreaks and recurrences of herpes, candida, and other chronic infections follow times of acute stress a strikingly high portion of the time.

Social Health Recommendations. Keen observers discern symbolic significance relating immune strength, a clear sense of one's internal sense of power, and clarity in sexual relationships. If ambivalence in regards to sexual relationships is present; if you sense that you cannot state what you want, say, in not having sexual relations at a given time and need to have an excuse, such as a vaginal infection, you will probably benefit from brief counseling. Greater self-esteem will enable you to be clear about your wants and feel okay about negotiating comfortable solutions about issues regarding sexual relations. The psychological and spiritual growth that ensues will enhance your psychospiritual energy and benefit your body and your immune system.

FIBROCYSTIC BREAST DISEASE (FBD)

Prevalence

Estimates of the portion of women who have a degree of fibrocystic breast disease (FBD) go as high as 80 percent. The disease disappears at menopause as strong hormonal influences disappear.

Anatomy and Physiology

The fibrocystic masses that cause noticeable, palpable breast lumpiness in this disease are most commonly cystic and may contain up to two ounces of fluid and be two inches or more in diameter. The involved areas are often tender, due to the inflammatory factor, and may at times be confusing enough that a biopsy is undertaken to rule out cancer. The more you are able to minimize the fibrocystic changes with the options mentioned here, the less likely it is that you will be in the position of needing a biopsy.

Conventional Medical Treatment

Conventional physicians accept major responsibility for monitoring breast masses, which if persistent, may need to be biopsied. Medications for pain are usually made available.

Risk Factors and Causes

Genetic. There is evidence that women with cystic breast disease have a hereditary predisposition to greater sensitivity to methylxanthines (caffeine-like compounds).

Diet factors

Consistently low iodine levels are found in animals with fibrocystic breast disease. This is thought to render the breast tissues more sensitive to estrogen effects.

Consumption of coffee is strongly associated with PMS symptoms. The incidence and severity of symptoms was seven times greater in those drinking eight to ten cups of coffee daily compared to non–coffee drinkers. Caffeine and methyl xanthines have been shown to contribute to cystic breast disease in a number of studies. In those that have not come to this conclusion, total elimination of all caffeine was apparently not achieved during treatment.

Deficiencies of vitamin E may also contribute to increased risk.

Habit Factors. Cystic breast changes are associated with constipation; women having less than three bowel movements per week have a four to five times greater incidence of fibrocystic changes than women with a daily bowel habit. This association is probably due to reabsorption of estrogenic steroids or absorption of toxic metabolites of estrogenic steroids formed by bacteria in the large bowel.

Hormonal Factors. Since cystic breast disease regresses permanently at menopause, hormone factors loom large in the list of potential causes. FBD appears to be related to a higher than normal estrogen to progesterone ratio. Higher levels of prolactin have also been shown to be present in FBD, probably secondary to the higher estrogen levels.

Holistic Prevention and Treatment
Physical Health Recommendations

Diet
- *Avoid* chocolate, caffeinated beverages, and OTC caffeine medicines. Elimination of caffeine must be 100 percent, since even small amounts of caffeine can be problematic, such as the 3 percent caffeine content in decaffeinated coffee. Significant improvement in over 95 percent of patients who totally eliminate caffeine has been reported.

- *High fiber intake* is associated with a 50 percent lower incidence of FBD, as well as a lower rate of breast cancer. Greater amounts of fiber are excreted in the colon of women on high fiber, mostly vegetarian diets. Your nutritional intake should minimize animal meat, dairy products, and processed sugars.

  The daily intake of seaweed sources high in iodine (kelp, dulse) is thought to be associated with the much lower incidence of cystic breast disease in many oriental and southeast Asian cultures.

Vitamins, Minerals, and Supplements
- *Vitamin E* has a clearly researched record for reducing symptoms and findings in two-thirds of patients with FBD (600 I.U. daily). A few studies have found it less

useful. Vitamin E appears to lower pituitary LH and FSH hormones, reducing estrogen stimulation.

- *Vitamin A*, although less researched, brought about partial or full disease remission in 50 percent of those treated in one study (150,000 I.U. daily). This is a high dose and needs to be used when other measures fail; monitoring by a physician is essential; it should not be used if you have any possibility of becoming pregnant.

- In the liver, estrogen breaks down to glucuronic acid for elimination into the intestine. Adequate *B-complex vitamins* are necessary to accomplish the task ("B-50," one daily).

- Other antioxidant elements should include *vitamin C*, one to two grams daily, *beta carotene*, 25,000 I.U. daily, *zinc*, 30 mg daily, and *selenium*, 200 mcg daily.

- Because of its effect on equilibrating inflammatory factors in the body, *flaxseed oil* (high in omega-3 oils), one tablespoon daily, or *fish oil*, two 1,000-mg capsules twice a day, are important.

- *Evening primrose* and *borage oils*, high in gamma linolenic acid, are also helpful in doses of two capsules three times daily.

- In a study of 140 women with painful fibrocystic breast disease, 72 percent became totally asymptomatic after treatment with *iodized casein*. Lugol's solution or elemental iodine, two to eight drops daily, can be used but should be supervised by a physician; excess doses can alter thyroid function and lead to a toxic condition called iodism. Five to twelve drops per day of SSKI, a prescription expectorant, will also suffice. After the cystic changes have largely subsided, recurrence can be controlled with increased iodine intake from kelp tablets, four to six daily.

- Probiotics L. *acidophilus* and *bifidus* also appear to increase estrogen excretion and are worth at least a six-month trial. Take a preparation supplying one to five billion live organisms in a day's dose.

Biomolecular Options

A 1981 study achieved partial or total relief in three of every four FBD patients by using Synthroid, 0.1 mg daily for two months, in spite of the fact that the thyroid blood tests were normal in all but one patient.

Mental and Emotional Health Recommendations. Consistent observers of women with fibrocystic breast disease see clear patterns of exacerbation during times of stress. Regular practice of *biofeedback*, *deep relaxation*, or *meditation* techniques are of considerable help in bringing together healing energies. *Imagery* and repetition of positive *affirmations* regarding the health of your body and breasts also helps.

Psychotherapy. The pain of cystic breast disease may be intertwined with residual blocked energy from past painful experiences involving the breasts. Recalling repressed memories of childhood and early adulthood experiences and psychological traumas, especially those with a sexual connotation, may be part of the psychotherapy of resolving pain manifestations in the breast or genital organs. It is important to be gentle and forgiving of yourself in letting past issues be acknowledged, resolved, and then dispatched to the past where they belong. As mentioned in chapters 3 and 4, we are whole beings with bodies, feelings, thoughts, and spiritual beliefs. All aspects need to be integrated to provide the best opportunity to experience optimal health.

CONDITION PREMENSTRUAL SYNDROME (PMS)

Prevalence

An estimated 30 to 60 percent of women experience bothersome premenstrual symptoms. Ten percent of women experience severe degrees of disturbance which interfere with activities of daily living. The greatest incidence occurs in women in their thirties and forties.

Anatomy and Physiology

Endocrine (hormonal), reproductive, gastrointestinal, and psychological systems of the body are involved in PMS.

Symptoms and Diagnosis

Premenstrual syndrome describes the collection of distressing symptoms occurring in the one to two weeks before the onset of the menses in many women. The array of symptoms includes tension, anxiety, irritability, insomnia, depression, mood swings, food cravings, depleted energy, headache, backache, abdominal bloating, edema of hands and feet, altered sex drive, and tenderness and swelling of the breasts.

The diagnosis is strongly suspected on the basis of the history, and hormone abnormalities can be confirmed by blood tests, including thyroid profile and progesterone, estrogen, and prolactin levels.

Conventional Medical Treatment

Some conventional physicians believe that premenstrual symptoms are a variant of depression, and patients are too often still told: "It's all in your head." This may stem from the fact that there is not a simple, definitive laboratory test. Suggestions are often made to suppress ovulation with oral contraceptive medication (birth control pills). This temporarily relieves the symptoms, but underlying problems remain. Antidepressant prescriptions are common; severe water retention has been treated with diuretics.

Risk Factors and Causes

The most important contributing factors in PMS appear to be:

- Stress, endorphin deficiency
- Depression—low brain neurotransmitter levels (serotonin and gamma butyric acid)
- Decreased vitamin B-6 levels
- Obesity—body fat manufactures estrone, an estrogen
- Deficient exposure to natural light, with a predisposition to seasonal affective depression
- History of growing up in an alcoholic family system in which women are scripted to take care of every situation. Dr. Christiane Northrup, in *Women's Bodies, Women's Wisdom*, describes this as a "relationship addiction."
- PMS complaints are significantly more common in those with mercury amalgam dental fillings compared to women without mercury fillings.
- Hypothyroidism—a high percentage of PMS patients exhibit overt or subtle laboratory evidence of low thyroid function. Several studies have found a 70–90 percent incidence of low thyroid status in women with PMS versus 0–20 percent in controls without PMS.
- Elevated prolactin (a pituitary hormone that stimulates milk production after childbirth)—contributes to breast tenderness
- Excess estrogen
- Deficient progesterone; an increased estrogen/progesterone ratio is common

An increased estrogen/progesterone ratio tends to lead to:

- Decreased serotonin production (leads to anxiety, depression, sleeplessness)
- Mildly increased aldosterone secretion (contributes to water retention)
- Increased prolactin production (causes breast tenderness and swelling)
- Diminished liver function with decreased bile flow
- Apparently, depleted vitamin B-6 levels (impairs neurotransmitter and prostaglandin synthesis)

Precipitating events associated with onset of PMS, as listed by Dr. Northrup are:

- Onset of menses with puberty
- The one to two year period before menopause
- After stopping oral contraceptives
- After a pregnancy complicated by toxemia
- After a time of amenorrhea (no periods)
- After tubal ligation for contraception
- Following intense stressful psychological trauma

Compared to women without PMS, women with PMS have:

- Up to fivefold greater consumption of dairy products
- Greater intake of caffeine (soft drinks, coffee, tea, chocolate)
- Up to two and a half times as much sugar consumption
- Excess amounts of fat in their diets
- Noticeable deficiency of micronutrients: vitamins C, E and B6, magnesium, and selenium

Holistic Prevention and Treatment

Physical Health Recommendations

Diet

The following choices are therapeutic.

- Move toward a more whole foods, vegetarian diet.
- Reduce intake of fat.
- Remove as much of the sugar as possible from your diet.
- Deemphasize foods contaminated with estrogen-mimicking pesticides (DDE, PCB, dieldrin, chlordane)—higher in animal meats, eggs, and milk products.
- Increase phytoestrogen-containing foods (soy, seeds, nuts, apples, parsley, alfalfa).
- Omitting beverages and food with caffeine diminishes anxiety and reduces breast sensitivity.
- Limit salt intake to less than two grams/day.
- Maintain good body hydration.

Vitamins, Minerals, and Supplements
Helpful daily amounts include:

- *Vitamin B-6*—100 mg; accompany this with a B-complex preparation containing 25 mg of each of the B vitamins
- *Vitamin E*—400–800 I.U.
- *Calcium*—one gram
- *Magnesium*—800 mg
- *Manganese*—5 mg
- *Flaxseed oil*—one tablespoon
- *Evening primrose* or *borage oil* capsules
- *Tryptophan*—two grams, available from compounding pharmacists by prescription; or 5-HTP (5-hydroxy tryptophan), 200–400 mg
- *Taurine*—1,500 mg in last half of menstrual cycle for antidepressant effect
- *L. acidophilus* and *bifidus* reduce excess estrogen assimilation from nutrient sources

A high potency multivitamin-mineral supplement will supply many of these elements and reduce the number of pills you have to take. Check the content on the labels.

Herbs
(For dosages see menopause.)

- *Black cohosh*
- *Chasteberry*
- *Dong Quai*
- *Licorice root*

Biomolecular Options.
High dose treatment with progesterone vaginal suppositories in the last half of the menstrual cycle is also used, with mild to moderate benefit reported (dosage 200–800 mg daily, available by prescription). Other prescription natural progesterone options are oral doses of 100 mg daily or cream form for topical use on the skin, one-quarter teaspoon twice daily, also in the last half of the menstrual cycle.

A report in 1982 detailed the highly successful treatment of PMS with the subdermal injection of tiny, subpharmacological, desensitizing doses of dilute aqueous progesterone, which gives substantial and sometimes dramatic relief in 85 percent of cases. You could give this reference to your physician: *OB Gyn* May 1982; 59(5):560–64.

If you have not obtained substantial relief with other initiatives, you may wish to consider the possibility that yeast infection might be playing a causative role. In a published study, improvement in PMS was observed in two-thirds of women who had not responded to standard treatment when they were given Nystatin (specific treatment for candida) and placed on a sugar-free diet; this success in treatment implies the frequent presence of candida in PMS. Empirically trying a low sugar diet and getting a prescription for Nystatin (one tablet, or one-quarter teaspoon of the powder if available, four times daily for one to two months) is an option based on this research.

With demonstration of hypothyroidism, shown by either sophisticated thyrotropin releasing hormone (TRH) tests or the finding of low basal body temperatures (see chapter 20), a trial of small amounts of thyroxin or Armour whole thyroid will often bring great or complete relief (See *New England Journal of Medicine*, December 1986). Small doses of thyroid supplements even in women who had normal thyroid tests gave prompt relief, "sometimes dramatic," in three out of four women treated.

If you tend to have lowered moods in the winter in northern latitudes and do not get significant daily outdoor exposure to winter sun or at least cloudy weather, arrange to be exposed to full spectrum bright light for at least two hours daily (light boxes or full spectrum lighting).

Exercise

Aerobic workouts 30 to 45 minutes three times weekly have been shown to greatly reduce breast tenderness, water retention, tension, and depression compared to those of nonexercising women. Consistent exercise also markedly improves mood and reduces irritability symptoms.

Professional Care Treatments

Weekly ear, hand and foot *reflexology* treatments of 30 minutes each has been shown in a controlled study to reduce physical and emotional symptoms by 40 percent. *Cranial osteopathy* in PMS also has particularly good results. *Homeopathy* also deals frequently with PMS problems; an individualized, constitutional prescription is complicated and requires a knowledgeable practitioner.

Mental and Emotional Health Recommendations. Negative patterns of coping with stress and PMS symptoms need to be acknowledged and steps taken to move them in a positive direction. Self-destructive responses that worsen the cycle of symptoms include overeating, becoming sedentary, becoming an observer (e.g., television) instead of a participator, and lapsing into habits of overspending and depending on prescription and illicit drugs. You can work at greater self-acceptance, letting go toxic emotions, and evoking a determination to be a participant in life rather than a bystander. It may be very helpful for you to enlist short-term assistance from a skilled *counselor*. Be discerning in choosing one who himself or herself is optimistic, enthusiastic, and active rather than depressed and passive. *Biofeedback* and relaxation practice are also therapeutic and empowering options.

MENOPAUSE

Prevalence

The numbers of women experiencing menopausal symptoms vary considerably from culture to culture. Research shows that Mayan Indian women experience neither osteoporosis nor any menopausal symptoms. In the American culture, however, between 65 and 85 percent of women experience symptoms during onset of menopause.

Anatomy and Physiology

Menopause is the phenomenon in women experienced with cessation of menses. Menopause is thought to occur as the ovaries run out of ova (eggs) and can no longer participate in the hormone cycles involving ovulation. Some one million ova are present at birth, with an estimated four hundred thousand present at puberty; about four hundred ova mature during menstrual years, with the remainder involuting by the time of menopause. The cessation of normal hormonal reproductive cycles occurs between the ages of 45 and 55 in American women, with an average of 52 years.

As the ovaries become unable to respond, the pituitary gland secretes large amounts of the ovarian stimulating hormones FSH and LH. The ovaries respond with androgenic hormone secretion, which is converted into estrogen in the fat cells of the hips and thighs. This converted estrogen, present in levels far below those during reproductive years, makes up the majority of the low levels of circulating estrogen in menopausal women. The decrease in estrogen levels is responsible for the hot flashes and other associated symptoms experienced by a great majority of women.

Symptoms and Diagnosis

The concept of menopause as a disease rather than a simple natural life phenomenon arose in the 1960s. Conventional medicine authorities began to regard menopause as a treatable illness in which estrogen replacement therapy was emphasized. As indicated earlier, the symptoms of this change in hormonal and reproductive status in women vary tremendously from culture to culture. The symptoms most commonly experienced by women in America are:

- Hot flashes with or without heavy soaking perspiration (especially at night), fast heart rate, headaches, and dizziness
- Weight gain
- Sleeplessness
- Fatigue
- Atrophic vaginitis with drying and thinning of the vaginal mucosa
- Increased coldness of hands and feet
- Moodiness
- Mental fogginess with forgetfulness and inability to concentrate

Libido may be decreased, and increased urinary frequency with susceptibility to bladder infections is often encountered (the outer third of the urethra is estrogen sensitive). Menopause is often heralded by missed periods or a change in menstrual flow in the prior two to three years. Other accompanying phenomena include an increase in coronary heart disease and osteoporosis following menopause.

Premature menopause occurs if a hysterectomy for any reason is accompanied by removal of both ovaries. Hormone replacement (see below) is a very important consideration in this circumstance.

The diagnosis of menopause is made with an identification of a typical history of symptoms. Confirmation may be sought with laboratory evidence of an increased FSH blood level.

Conventional Medical Treatment

Menopause is an occasion for a health reevaluation, including examination of the genital organs and breasts, assessment of blood chemistry, cholesterol, and the status of thyroid and adrenal function, determination of bone density, and arrangement for breast mammography follow-up.

Recommendations for estrogen replacement after menopause are standard. Estrogen vaginal cream can be obtained on prescription when vaginal symptoms predominate. Oral estrogen is prescribed for perimenopausal and menopausal women for its properties of relieving hot flashes and vaginal dryness and retarding the progression of osteoporosis and for its apparent benefits in reducing risks of heart disease. However, recent studies have carefully separated out other confusing variables and have shown no significant benefits for heart disease prevention. Hazards of hormone replacement therapy (HRT) include:

- Estrogen-only replacement is associated with a marked increase in the incidence of uterine cancer and a modest increase in breast cancer. If you have high risk factors for uterine or breast cancer, you need to weigh the benefits and risks of this therapy very carefully. Smaller doses of 0.6 mg/day of Premarin, the most commonly prescribed drug, appear to be as sufficient as higher doses. Estrogen patches are also satisfactory.

- Conventional prescriptions for estrogen are often accompanied by a prescription for the progestin drug Provera, which reduces the risks for uterine cancer from estrogen but does not affect the breast cancer risk.

- The incidence of adult-onset asthma in postmenopausal women using HRT is double that of nonusers.

- Clotting problems and phlebitis incidence increase in HRT users.

- The incidence of gallstones and gallbladder inflammation increases noticeably in users.

- Complaints of breast tenderness, water retention, headaches, and depression are bothersome to many users, leading to a decision to quit hormone therapy by some women.

- Liver abnormalities, exaggeration of blood sugar variations, and enlargement of uterine fibroids are also a problem for some women.

Estrogen replacement therapy is considered by most to be contraindicated in uterine and breast cancer, clotting disorders, obesity, diabetes, acute liver disease, and not-yet-diagnosed vaginal bleeding.

Risk Factors and Causes

The direct cause of menopausal symptoms is the cessation of high levels of estrogen production from the ovaries. Women who smoke double the likelihood of an early menopause before the age of 50. Caffeine and alcohol consumption tend to aggravate hot flashes.

Japanese women, who have far less severe menopausal symptoms compared to American women, also have much higher levels of phytoestrogens in their bodies. Soy is a major source of these compounds.

Holistic Treatment

Physical Health Recommendations

Diet

Phytoestrogens from food have weak but detectable estrogenic activity. Phyto-estrogens occupy the same estrogen receptor sites as pharmaceutical estrogens, preventing occupation by these more powerful hormones and therefore reducing total estrogenic influence in the body; this may explain the lower incidence of es-trogen dependent cancers such as breast cancer in women who consume high amounts of phytoestrogens from soy, flaxseed and its oil, nuts, whole grains, ap-ples, parsley, and alfalfa. The consumption of phytoestrogens by Japanese women, who enjoy one of the lowest incidence rates of hot flashes, hormone-related can-cers, and osteoporosis in the world, is estimated to be 200 mg daily. Reduction and avoidance of coffee and alcohol is usually helpful.

Vitamins, Minerals, and Supplements

- *Gamma-oryzanol*, a substance derived from rice bran oil, in doses of 300 mg/day totally or partially relieves hot flashes and other menopausal symptoms in over 85 percent of users.

- A combination of *vitamin C* (1,200 mg) and *hesperidin* (a citrus bioflavonoid, 900 mg), daily has been shown to give nearly total relief from hot flashes in over 55 percent and partial relief in 35 percent of users.

- *Vitamin E*, 400–800 I.U. daily, totally relieves distressing menopausal symptoms in over 25 percent of menopausal women and affords partial relief in another 25 percent.

- Women with higher calcium intake experienced a later menopause.

- A high dose multivitamin-mineral combination is good insurance for meeting all micronutrient needs in aging women, whose intestinal assimilation tends to de-cline each decade.

- *Para-amino benzoic acid* (PABA), two to four grams/day, equilibrates conversion of estrogenic compounds.

Herbs

- *Black cohosh* (Cimicifuga racemosa) enjoys wide use in relieving hot flashes, de-pression, and vaginal atrophy, modulating symptoms in 80 percent of users in six to eight weeks (tincture 1:5, 1–1½ tsp., or fluid extract 1:1, one tsp., three times/day)

- *Dong Quai* (Angelica sinensis) is broadly used in Asian cultures for menopausal symptoms and other problems, including painful and heavy menses. It has demonstrable estrogenic properties (tincture 1:5, one tsp., or fluid extract 1:1, ¼ tsp., three times/day).

- *Licorice* (Glycyrrhiza glabra), tending to raise progesterone levels, is also helpful in premenstrual syndrome (fluid extract 1:1, one tsp. three times/day).

- *Chasteberry* (Vitex agnus castus) has effects on pituitary hormone function (40 drops each morning of a tincture standardized to contain nine grams of the fruit per 100 ml of solution).

- *Ginkgo biloba* improves circulation, giving relief to cold hands and feet and improving memory (40 mg three times/day).

- *Korean ginseng* (Panax ginseng), 500 mg two times/day, contributes to homeostasis and neutralizing fatigue symptoms.

Biomolecular Options

Estriol in doses of eight mg daily improved hot flashes and improved vaginal lubrication 90 percent within six months without detectable endometrial build-up. Natural forms of estrogen can be prescribed for menopausal symptoms with less risk and fewer side effects. A formula pioneered by Dr. Jonathan Wright of Kent, Washington, consisting of estriol, estrone, and estradiol in an 80:10:10 ratio can be obtained through compounding pharmacists on prescription. These three estrogens roughly approximate the ratio of the same estrogens secreted by the ovary during a woman's menstrual years. The cancer risks stem mainly from the estrone and estradiol fractions; this formula therefore reduces the risk of cancerous stimulation. Appropriate doses of this "tri-est" formula are two and a half to five mg daily.

Estriol vaginal cream prepared by a compounding pharmacist (0.5 mg per gm) can be used in doses of one-quarter teaspoon daily for a week followed by one dose three times a week for maintenance. This improves vaginal dryness and prevents thinning and atrophy. It is also helpful in breaking the cycle of recurrent bladder infections (see above).

Progesterone derived from natural sources can be readily absorbed through the skin when applied regularly or taken by mouth. Appropriate doses of the progesterone cream are one-quarter to one-half level measuring teaspoon daily, rotated over seven different sites of the body, avoiding thicker skin—one site for each day of the week. Oral micronized progesterone capsules need to supply 10 to 15 mg in a daily dose. Both can be formulated by a compounding pharmacist. Progesterone has a potent effect in promoting the rebuilding of osteoporotic bones. Osteoporosis is a major consideration and is discussed in chapter 8. Progesterone carries no known hazard of stimulating either uterine or breast cancer. In fact, women with higher levels of progesterone at the time of biopsy for breast cancer have a better prognosis. A pharmaceutical pure progesterone product, Prometrium, has been on the prescription market since 1998.

If laboratory tests have shown low thyroid function, or if basal temperatures are low (see chapter 20), you should discuss thyroid hormone replacement with your physician. If adrenal function is low, replacement doses of DHEA, 15 to 25 mg daily, are reasonable.

If diminished libido is a problem, consideration should be given to cautious supplementation with testosterone. Testosterone can be prescribed as a skin cream or as a capsule. The usual beginning test dose is 10 mg/day.

Habits
Maintaining regular sexual activity, with or without a partner, promotes the healthy condition of the vagina. Smoking abatement is also on the recommendation list.

Exercise
Women spending half an hour daily in vigorous exercise have significantly fewer hot flashes and much less mood distortion. Most exercising women in one study were able to negotiate the menopausal time without hormone replacement treatment. For many other reasons as well, regular exercise fosters health.

Professional Care Therapies
Homeopathic physicians frequently work with women to evolve a satisfactory remedy for relief. The most common remedies used are Lachesis, Pulsatilla, Bryonia, and Sepia.

Mental and Emotional Health Recommendations. If depression is a persisting problem, give consideration to the benefits of exercise and botanical approaches, or, if necessary, pharmaceutical prescriptions.

It is extremely helpful to focus on menopause as the opportunity for the beginning of a creative, expressive, freer time of life rather than the end the reproductive years. The less menopause is seen as a problem, the better. Medical intuitive Caroline Myss associates the frequently seen depression with blocked energy of sexual expression and sexual pleasure. Menopause may be a time to "finish up" old business linked to these energy distortions. It is also a time to affirm your trust that your body's ability to remain healthy in this natural change is intact.

Relaxation and mental imagery. The vasomotor blood vessel instability of hot flashes improves with regular practice of relaxation and meditation. Helpful images would be of the vaginal walls as healthy, pink, and lubricated. Affirmations, such as "My genital organs are normal and healthy," can be incorporated.

ENDOMETRIOSIS

Prevalence

It is estimated that 10 to 20 percent of all women of child-bearing age in the United States have some degree of endometriosis. The incidence is highest in women in their twenties and thirties and into the mid-forties. Some 40 to 50 percent of all women who undergo laparoscopy for infertility are found to have endometriosis. Many authorities believe the incidence is increasing.

Anatomy and Physiology

The endometrium, the tissue lining the uterine cavity, is ordinarily confined to the uterus itself. In endometriosis, endometrial tissue is found within the uterine musculature, on the outside of the uterus, ovaries, fallopian tubes, and side walls of the pelvis and sometimes on the outside surface of the intestines as far away as the liver. Some of the collections of tissue may be as small as a pinhead.

Symptoms and Diagnosis

Diagnosis of endometriosis is not always easy, and many patients see a number of doctors before the problem is pinpointed. The presence of endometriosis is suspected in women who have unusual pelvic pain, abnormal menstrual cycles, and infertility. The pain, sometimes debilitating, tends to crescendo at the time of the menstrual period. In women who have endometriosis, fibroids are frequently found as well. The diagnosis is ultimately made by observing the presence of endometrial tissue outside the uterus at the time of pelvic laparoscopy.

Conventional Medical Treatment

The most common avenues of treatment include oral contraceptive pills to suppress ovulation, synthetic progestinal agents (Provera), danocrine (Danazol), and synthetic gonadotropin-releasing hormones (Synarel and Lupron). All these hormonal approaches reduce the amount of estrogen present, inactivating the disease but taking no steps toward a cure.

Danazol can have masculinizing effects, including deepening of the voice, excessive hair growth, and weight gain. Gonadotropin-releasing hormone can cause hot flashes, thinning of the vaginal lining, and bone loss.

Lupron and Synarel cause the pituitary to terminate ovarian hormone secretion and an artificial menopause is created. Fibroids, if present, shrink, and the cycles of pain stop. These drugs are not recommended for longer than six months of consecutive use.

Since many of the medical treatments are not totally satisfactory, surgery is also a possibility. In extreme cases, especially if you are not wanting to be pregnant or be pregnant again, a hysterectomy is performed, terminating the menstrual cycle and the disease. Hysterectomies are frequently done for this disease. Meticulous pelviscopic surgery crafted to remove absolutely all the errant endometrial tissue meets with a high degree of success, with residual pain in only 10 percent of patients. A surgeon with wide experience with the disease is required.

Risk Factors and Causes

The cause is unknown. The classic theory is that endometriosis results from retrograde menstrual flow, moving from the uterine cavity up the fallopian tubes with endometrial cells being transplanted into the pelvis. Another possibility is that primitive cells that develop into endometrial tissue in embryonic life do not all migrate to the uterus and are present outside the uterus at birth. Some studies have shown that women with endometriosis have antiendometrial antibodies, potentially marking the condition as an autoimmune disease like rheumatoid arthritis.

Some authorities connect the increasing incidence of endometriosis to the earlier onset of menstruation in teenagers and longer times until first pregnancy. Other research has shown that many with this problem have an ambivalence about becoming pregnant and indeed, in vitro ("test tube") fertilization for infertility has less success if endometriosis is present. At any rate, endometriosis is clearly a hormonally related condition, with symptoms peaking at the time of highest estrogen levels in the menstrual cycle.

Uterine fibroids, which may accompany endometriosis, are benign uterine tumors that are also estrogen sensitive. Infertility problems, which are greater in women with endometriosis, have been shown to be significantly worse with increasing amounts of alcohol intake.

Medical intuitive Caroline Myss relates endometriosis and other female pelvic organ dysfunctions to: patterns of fear and insecurity, including a sense of powerlessness regarding sexual relationships; feelings of sexual inadequacy and childbirth; fear of never having enough (even poverty); resentment over the authority of a sexual partner and manipulation by other people; feelings of powerlessness so great that a tendency to manipulate others is adopted in order to gain some sense of control; and dealing dishonestly in sexual and interpersonal relationships.

Dr. Myss also sees endometriosis as a disorder of competition. In this sense, the affected woman is conflicted between what the world is demanding of her and the meeting of her innermost emotional needs. Women with endometriosis are often in a home or business situation in which they feel unsupported.

Holistic Prevention and Treatment

Physical Health Recommendations

Diet

A low fat, high fiber diet will decrease estrogen levels and tend toward some lessening of pain. Fibroids also tend to shrink on a diet that eliminates red meats, chicken, and refined sugar. Phytoestrogen food sources (soybeans are high in plant estrogens daidzein, genistein, equol, and kaeonpferol) also lower estrogen levels by blocking estrogen receptor sites with weaker estrogen forms.

Vitamins, Minerals, and Supplements

- *Inositol* (a B-complex vitamin)—up to 4 gm/day
- *Choline* (a B-complex vitamin) —one to two grams/day
- *Methionine* (an amino acid)—one to two grams/day
- A potent *B-complex vitamin*—one "B-50"/day (50 mg of each major B-complex element)
- *Magnesium*—400–800 mg/day
- A well-formulated megadose multivitamin-mineral high in antioxidants is desirable
- *Vitamin E*, 800 I.U. daily
- Proinflammatory prostaglandins participating in the pain cycle can be reduced by adding anti-inflammatory precursors, including *omega-3 oils* (two to four grams twice daily) or *flaxseed oil* (one tablespoon daily)
- *Gamma linolenic acid* from *borage oil*—one to two capsules three times daily (supplying 500 mg/day of gamma linolenic acid)
- *Quercetin*, a potent flavonoid in many fruits and other plants, has an anti-inflammatory effect, and doses of 400 mg three times a day before meals are helpful

Herbs
- *Dong Quai* (one and a half grams three times daily)
- *Licorice root extract* (one-fourth–one-half teaspoon in hot water twice daily)
- Solid extract of *alfalfa* (one-fourth–one-half teaspoon dissolved in hot water twice daily)

Biomolecular Options

Natural progesterone from plant sources is commonly tried. It is available in cream form for application to the skin, from where it is absorbed into the system; the usual dose is one-half level teaspoon daily from days 10 to 28 of the menstrual cycle. The sites for application are rotated to seven different areas to complete the cycle in a week. Natural progesterone capsules for oral use are available from compounding pharmacists as prescribed by your doctor in doses of 50 to 200 mg daily from days 10 to 28 of the cycle.

Professional Care Therapies

Homeopathic remedies, carefully chosen, can be quite beneficial. *Acupuncture* also addresses problems of pain and endometrial dysfunction. *Massage therapy* has been used to great benefit by many women with this problem.

Mental and Emotional Health Recommendations. If you have endometriosis, a *counselor* who understands the issues listed under the risk factors listed above will be a valuable resource. Formal counseling to help shift the beliefs, attitudes, and feeling states toward empowerment and equanimity can be enhanced by training and practice in *biofeedback* or the practice of *meditation.*

The use of *imagery* in this disease, which has such a distinct anatomical presentation, can be very powerful. The repetition of *affirmations,* too, has an important place in recovery from this affliction. Use an affirmation such as: "I am a worthy self-assured human being." Or: "I am fully in charge of my sexuality and sexual functioning."

18

Vision Problems

MACULAR DEGENERATION

Prevalence

MACULAR DEGENERATION is the cause of blindness for over 150,000 Americans. It is the second most common reason for loss of vision in older people. Thirty percent of people over age 75 are affected by some macular degenerative change. About 20,000 new cases of macular degenerative blindness occur each year.

Anatomy and Physiology

The macula is the center of retinal vision for fine detail. The yellowish color of the macula arises from its high concentration of cells containing the yellow carotenoid pigments called lutein and zeaxanthin. Macular degeneration results from free radical damage to these pigmented cells. As damage to the central retina develops, debris called lipofucsin accumulates from damaged cells, causing extrusions (called drusen) in the macula, which distort the visual field.

Symptoms and Diagnosis

There are no early subjective symptoms of macular degeneration. The diagnosis is made by ophthalmoscopic examination of the eye, usually at the time of a checkup by an ophthalmologist or optometrist for visual complaints or perceived need for adjustment of lens correction. Macular degeneration symptoms begin with the subtle onset of slight blurring in fine vision required for reading. Minute visual details are frequently overlooked, and there is often a distortion of images or a dark spot in the center of the visual field.

Conventional Medical Treatment

There is no standard recognized treatment for the atrophic form of macular degeneration, which comprises 95 percent of all cases. Five percent of the problem presents as a neovascular or "wet" form, which is treated very effectively by laser photocoagulation, especially when caught in the earlier stages.

Risk Factors and Causes

Major contributing causes include:

- Smoking
- Arteriosclerosis
- Advanced age
- Excessive ultraviolet light exposure
- High saturated fat diet
- Deficient intake of lutein and zeaxanthin (increases risk over 40 percent)
- Deficient intake of the carotenoid lycopene (increases risk over 50 percent)
- Higher intake of alcohol (weak evidence)

Holistic Prevention and Treatment

Diet

The essential nutrients that are known to delay, halt, or reverse the process are those that increase antioxidant levels. The carotene-containing foods rank high in importance. The best food sources for the essential carotenoids are:

- *Lutein:* kale, collard greens, spinach, Swiss chard, mustard greens, red peppers, okra, romaine lettuce, parsley, dill, celery, carrots, corn, tomatoes, potatoes, fruits
- *Zeaxanthin:* kale, collard greens, spinach, Swiss chard, mustard greens, red peppers, paprika, corn, okra, romaine lettuce, parsley, dill, celery, fruits
- *Lycopene:* tomatoes, tomato juice, tomato catsup, watermelon, guava, pink grapefruit, dried apricots, green peppers, carrots

Fruit and vegetable intake is inversely correlated with the degree of macular degeneration. Fruits with intense red, blue, and purple coloring, containing high amounts of anthocyanidin bioflavonoids, are especially helpful (see Herbs, below). Foods recommended are blackberries, raspberries, blueberries, huckleberries, cherries, tomatoes, and plums.

Vitamins, Minerals, and Supplements

The most important vitamins and minerals are:

- *Carotenoids*—mixed carotenoids, 50,000 I.U./day (lutein, zeaxanthin, lycopene, beta carotene); supplements of lutein (30 mg daily) derived from palm oil are better absorbed than synthetic forms and should be used if available
- *Riboflavin*—10–25 mg/day
- *Vitamin C*—500–2,500 mg/day
- *Vitamin E*—400–1,200 I.U./day
- *Selenium*—200–400 mg/day
- *Manganese*—5–10 mg/day
- *Zinc*—in patients who took 80 mg of zinc or a placebo daily for 12–24 months, the zinc group preserved their vision 42 percent better than those on placebo, whose vision steadily deteriorated; zinc actually improved vision in a small percentage of the subjects.
- *Copper*—2–3 mg/day

In one study, daily intake of a combination of vitamin C, 500 mg, Vitamin E, 400 mg, beta carotene, 45,000 I.U., and selenium, 250 mcg, halted or reversed the vision decline in 60 percent of macular degeneration patients.

Herbs

- *Ginkgo biloba.* Significant improvement in distance vision occurs in macular degeneration patients taking ginkgo biloba extract, 80 mg twice daily for six months. Ginkgo improves circulation to the eye and brain.
- *Bilberry* (Vaccinium myrtillus), 80 mg three times daily (25 percent anthocyanidin content), also substantially slows, halts, and sometimes reverses the degeneration. Its key flavonoid, anthocyanidin, has potent antioxidant qualities and healing action in the retina.
- *Grapeseed* extract (Vitis vinifera), 150 to 300 mg daily (95 percent procyanidolic content), also restrains progression of the degeneration.

Nonspecific General Management Options

In addition to the specific biochemical, nutritional, and botanical options in preventing and delaying macular degeneration, all generic measures for restraining free radical proliferation mentioned in chapters 2, 3, and 4 are helpful, including avoidance of toxins from the environment, exercise, and adequate management of stress.

Smoking abatement (and avoidance of passive exposure) and control of blood pressure are important measures. Protection from excessively long hours of bright sunlight should be undertaken, particularly for those exposed to light reflection off snow and water and those living in climates with long hours of bright sunlight for great portions of the year. In these situations, sunglasses that filter out 98 percent or more of the ultraviolet spectrum may be necessary.

CONDITION

CATARACTS

Prevalence

Cataracts are the leading cause of loss of vision in the United States. Four million Americans have a degree of visual impairment from cataracts, and 40,000 are legally blind as a result. The largest single item in the Medicare budget is the cost for surgical lens replacement, at a price of three billion dollars per year.

Anatomy and Physiology

Cataracts describe the cloudy, opaque degenerative changes that may occur in the crystalline lens of the eye. Ordinarily clear, the lens deteriorates as a result of dehydration and synthesis of polyols by an enzyme called aldose reductase.

Symptoms and Diagnosis

The very earliest cataract changes are usually not subjectively perceivable and are discovered only during routine eye examinations being done for modification of lens corrections.

Conventional Medical Treatment

The development of lens replacement surgery has been a highly successful advance in professional eye care, resulting in preservation of vision for millions of people. Surgery achieves restoration of totally normal vision in over 98 percent of cases.

Risk Factors and Causes

The clouding of the lens of the eye is, in great part, the result of degeneration secondary to damage by free radical proliferation.

Contributing factors are:

- Diabetes
- Toxic exposures
- Excessive ultraviolet and near-ultraviolet light exposure

- Smoking (two to three times higher risk)
- Deficiency of antioxidants—carotenoids, vitamins A and E, and selenium (levels of selenium in the aqueous humor of the eye, part of the refracting medium, are 60 percent lower in people with cataracts)
- Low levels of superoxide dismutase (SOD), a major antioxidant enzyme of the body
- Depleted zinc—90 percent lower in cataracts compared to healthy lenses
- Depleted copper—90 percent lower in cataracts compared to healthy lenses
- Depleted manganese—50 percent lower in cataracts compared to normal lenses
- High levels of the heavy metal cadmium (two to three times higher in cataracts compared to normal lenses); smoking is a major source of cadmium
- Side effects of medications; long-term use of cortisone-like drugs contributes to the risk of cataract formation

Holistic Prevention and Treatment

Diet
Fruits and vegetables with high antioxidant nutrient content top the list of important foods, and higher intakes are correlated with greater protection against cataracts. Avoiding sugar, alcohol, and salt is indicated. Important on the list of high antioxidant foods are the carotenes. High carotene foods include leafy greens, yams, carrots, broccoli, and other highly colored yellow vegetables. Spinach intake is a more efficient source of antioxidants than carrots for prevention of cataracts.

Vitamins, Minerals, and Supplements
A host of studies documents a 25 percent lower risk of cataracts in people who take multivitamins and minerals. The reduction in risk with antioxidant vitamins and minerals is even greater in smokers. Validated case reports have documented the partial regression of cataracts in five months of treatment with a high dose combination of antioxidants.

Documented benefits have been shown with daily doses of:

- *Vitamin C*, 2.5 gm, will reduce your risk of cataracts 75–85 percent compared to people taking no supplements
- *Vitamin A* and *carotenoids*—those with highest intakes are 40 percent less likely to have cataracts (25,000 I.U. of mixed carotenoids)
- *Beta carotene*—may act as a filter against light-induced damage to the fibrous part of the lens, functioning in a manner similar to its action in the skin

- *Vitamin E*—1,200 mg
- *Riboflavin*—limit doses to 15 mg/day; higher riboflavin doses have a contradictory effect
- *Pyridoxine*—80–100 mg
- *Selenium*—600 mcg
- *Calcium*—500 to 1,000 mg—protective action demonstrated
- *Folic acid*—protection demonstrated; may be important in maintaining high levels of tetrahydrobiopterin, a protein which has been found to be low in senile cataracts
- *Quercetin*, a bioflavonoid; contains pentahydroxyflavone, which opposes aldose reductase induced damage to the lens (400 mg three times daily before meals)
- *Methionine*, an amino acid; a component in methionine sulfoxide reductase, an essential antioxidant enzyme in the lens (500 mg twice daily).
- *Cysteine*, an amino acid metabolized from methionine; also beneficial in cataract treatment (500 mg three times daily)
- *EPA/DHA* (omega-3 oils), three grams/day

Herbs

- *Bilberry*—80 mg three times daily (25 percent anthocyanidin content); combined with vitamin E blocked progression of cataracts in 48 of 50 patients in a European study
- *Grape seed* extract—150 to 300 mg daily (95 percent procyanidolic content)
- *Pine bark* extract (pycnogenol)—30 mg four times daily or 85 mg twice daily
- *Curcumin* (Curcuma longa, or turmeric)—200–400 mg three times/day between meals
- *Ba-wei-wan* (hachimijiogan), a traditional Chinese herb that has been used in Asia for hundreds of years for treating cataracts; a mixture of Rehamia glutinosa and seven other herbs, in a study published in 1985 was demonstrated to halt progression of cataracts in 20 percent of patients and partially reverse the deterioration in vision in 60 percent; increases antioxidant levels within the lens.

Biomolecular Options

Melatonin, a pineal gland hormone, is a powerful antioxidant that inhibits cataract development in animals. The development of cataracts increases with age, parallel to the decrease in melatonin levels with increasing age.

All the measures to restrain free radical proliferation previously mentioned in chapter 2 are valid additions to a cataract prevention and treatment program.

CONDITION

GLAUCOMA

Prevalence

About two million people in the United States are estimated to have glaucoma. The increased intraocular pressure of glaucoma in about a quarter of this group has not been recognized, diagnosed, or treated. Glaucoma is the third leading cause for vision loss in aging people after macular degeneration and cataracts. The incidence rate in the elderly population is thought to be about 3 percent.

Anatomy and Physiology

The cornea and lens of the eye have no blood supply. Nutrients are provided to these structures through the aqueous humor, a thick, clear liquid that is secreted into the central chamber of the eye. As it slowly circulates, the aqueous humor supplies nutrients and removes waste products, exiting through a spongelike connective tissue network of collagen around the margin of the eye, to then be absorbed into the bloodstream. Damage to the collagen, the most abundant protein in the body, clogs the egress of aqueous humor from the eye, increasing the pressure within the globe of the eye—the central problem in glaucoma.

Symptoms and Diagnosis

In early stages, glaucoma is usually totally asymptomatic. With the passage of time and increased pressures, chronic open-angle glaucoma manifests in gradually compromised peripheral vision, marked by blind spots. It usually affects both eyes.

A more rare condition, acute or closed-angle glaucoma, is heralded by severe pain, nausea, vomiting, one-sided presentation, blurring of vision, the impression of a halo effect around images, cloudiness of the cornea, redness of the eye, and intraocular pressures over 40 mmHg. Acute glaucoma threatens sudden loss of vision and constitutes an emergency.

The diagnosis of glaucoma is usually made during a routine eye examination occasioned by the need for new prescription lenses. The pressure is measured by sophisticated equipment that gauges the degree of indentation of the eye globe from a quick puff of a tiny jet of air. The eye pressure can also be measured by a tenometer, a small instrument placed on the eye after the corneal surface has been made numb by a topical anesthetic. Early diagnosis is important, since early treatment forestalls visual deterioration. All too few primary care physicians, however, make testing for eye pressure a regular part of an interval examination. People at high risk should have a routine screening examination every two years after age 65, or after age 40 for African Americans.

Conventional Medical Treatment

Medications to control ocular pressure are of two varieties: sterile topical drops to be instilled in the eyes; and pills to be taken by mouth. Local agents for use in the eye include Betopic and Timoptic. Significant amounts of the local drugs are absorbed into the system, and the drug literature warns of possible respiratory and heart reactions, especially in those with asthma and abnormal heart rhythms. These medications are beta-blockers (see heart disease, chapter 14) and should be withdrawn slowly before any general anesthetic is given. Systemic agents to be taken by mouth include beta-blockers, carbonic anhydrase inhibitors (Diamox), and vasoconstrictors, the latter for use in acute closed-angle glaucoma.

Risk Factors and Causes

The immediate cause of increased intraocular pressure is the free radical–mediated deterioration of the spongelike connective tissue network of collagen, which gradually obstructs the egress of aqueous humor from the eye. The obstruction results in an increase of pressure within the eye, leading to a subtle distortion of the eye globe itself, in which visual images fail to focus on the retina, causing blurred vision. The increased pressure also damages the functional parts of the visual apparatus. Normal intraocular pressures are 10 to 21 mmHg; with onset of chronic glaucoma, pressures can be up to 40 mmHg.

Contributing to the risk for glaucoma are:

- Genetic factors, if you have family members with a history of glaucoma
- Side effects of medications: antihistamine, anti-inflammatory (cortisone), and antihypertensive drugs can increase intraocular pressure
- Hereditary influences with certain diseases involving errors of collagen metabolism (Marfan's syndrome, osteogenesis imperfecta)
- Diabetes and high blood sugar
- Food sensitivities
- Being African American
- Being over 65
- Severe nearsightedness
- Stress—rises in intraocular pressure are correlated with periods of increased stress and emotional reactions; marked rises in pressures can be induced by initiating a discussion of a glaucoma patient's significant personal conflicts

Holistic Prevention and Treatment

Physical Health Recommendations

Diet

A variety of fresh fruits and vegetables is in order, with an emphasis on foods containing vitamin C and bioflavonoids. Fish meals supply a high amount of omega-3 fatty acids.

Food allergens. Elimination of food allergens accomplished through elimination and rechallenge trials has successfully lowered pressures in selected patients. In susceptible people, rise in pressure of up to 20 mmHg has been demonstrated following exposure to known allergenic foods.

Vitamins, Minerals, and Supplements

- One published study from the 1960s documented an average fall of 16 mmHg in eye pressures after treatment with megadoses of *vitamin C*. A recent study reaffirmed the same effect: addition of vitamin C or ascorbate with mixed bioflavenoids to bowel tolerance levels (two to nine grams daily) reduced pressures an average of 5.6 mmHg (28 percent).

- A multivitamin-mineral with B-complex elements at 50 mg each is recommended.

- Addition of a *magnesium* supplement, 240 mg daily, reduced intraocular pressures in glaucoma subjects 10 percent, while improving the visual field.

- *Chromium* as well as vitamin C deficiencies have been correlated with increased pressures. Addition of chromium (200 mcg/day) improves blood sugar management.

- In laboratory animals, intraocular pressures are cut in half with the addition of fish oil to food intake. Reasonable human dosages are: *omega-3 oils*, two grams twice daily, or *flaxseed oil*, one tablespoon daily.

Herbs

Herbs and food bioflavonoids containing anthocyanidins maintain capillary integrity and stabilize the strength of collagen tissues by preventing free radical damage and forming more cross-linked bonds within the protein matrix. *Bilberry* is outstanding in this regard. *Rutin*, a citrus bioflavonoid, has been shown to lower pressures in patients unresponsive to medications alone. *Grapeseed extract*, or *pycnogenol*, 100 mg three times a day, supplies similar essential agents. *Ginkgo biloba* extract (24 percent ginkgolides) has improved pressures in doses of 80 mg twice daily for a month with 40 mg three times daily thereafter. *Amla* (50 mg daily) is an

Ayurvedic herb (Indian gooseberry) with the highest vitamin C concentration of all known plants.

Biomolecular Options

Melatonin in small doses (0.2 to 0.5 mg) in the evening decreases intraocular pressures about 10 percent through the rest of the night. Intraocular pressures are 25 percent higher in people with hypothyroidism; they fall to normal when an appropriate dose of replacement *thyroid* or synthetic thyroxin is reached.

Exercise

In one study, the average intraocular pressure in sedentary glaucoma subjects dropped from 23 to 19 mmHg after 12 weeks of regular aerobic exercise.

Mental and Emotional Health Recommendations. In management of stress, the benefits of regular relaxation practice and meditation, as well as regular aerobic exercise, apply here as in most diseases. Acknowledging and releasing the demands of stressful situations will insulate you from the intense emotional and nervous system responses which raise ocular pressure. Falls in intraocular pressures following disciplined practices of relaxation, biofeedback, and meditation are frequently great enough to be able to reduce medication or stop it altogether. The lower the necessary dose of medication, the greater the likelihood for the disappearance of side effects.

19

Food Allergies and Sensitivities

Prevalence

THE INCIDENCE RATE of allergic responses in Americans may be as high as 60 percent. Allergies and reactions to food are seen in 25 percent of young children. And the incidence of allergic diseases is increasing.

Anatomy and Physiology

Allergy is the overresponsiveness of the immune system to foreign inhalant molecules or ingested food molecules. The common target organs in classical allergy are the nose and sinuses (hay fever or allergic rhinitis), the lungs (asthma), and the skin (hives and eczema). A less accepted but well-researched holistic medical principle embraces the concept that all organs of the body can be the targets of the allergic response.

Allergic responses to foods include:

- Respiratory tract: allergic rhinitis, asthma (see chapter 6)
- Skin: eczema, hives (see chapter 21)
- Joints: rheumatoid arthritis (see chapter 8)
- Connective tissues: lupus erythematosus, scleroderma, dermatomyositis
- Brain: ADHD (see chapter 15), memory problems, epilepsy
- Veins: phlebitis
- Stomach: gastritis, ulcers (see chapter 11)
- Intestines: ulcers, Crohn's disease, ulcerative colitis (see chapter 11)
- Kidney: nephrosis
- Bladder: enuresis, urinary urgency
- Heart: arrhythmias, atherosclerosis, hypertension (see chapter 14)

- Ears: otitis media (see chapter 6), hearing loss
- Metabolic system: fatigue (see chapter 9)

Symptoms and Diagnosis

The diagnosis of food allergy disease is made on the basis of:

- History of appropriate target organ symptoms not otherwise explained
- Consistent relation of symptoms to food exposures
- Evidence on examination:
  - Dark circles and puffiness under the eyes (allergic shiners)
  - Horizontal creases in the lower eyelid
  - Horizontal crease across the front of the lower nose
  - Chronic water retention without other identified cause
  - Chronically or recurrently swollen glands (lymph nodes)
  - Inflammation, swelling, tenderness in affected organ or tissue
- Positive results with improvement in symptoms while on a food elimination-rechallenge testing diet
- Confirmation with positive blood tests

The most commonly used testing procedure is called *food elimination and rechallenge*. The three approaches for clinical testing to demonstrate food reactivity require five to seven days of:

- A (five-day) water fast; or
- Elimination of a limited number of foods (omitting the *most* likely offenders—cow's milk, wheat, sugar, corn, eggs, nuts, chocolate, citrus, soy, yeast, and additives); or
- An oligoantigenic food diet (allowing *only* the *least* likely offenders: lamb, rice, pears, banana, and a cruciferous vegetable—cabbage, broccoli)

If food sensitivities are ultimately found to be present, symptoms will initially get worse in the first three to four days of the testing period as the sensitizing food is eliminated from the system; on the fourth or fifth day, the symptoms will usually have totally abated, leaving the patient feeling enormously better.

If symptoms improve during the test period, foods are then reintroduced one at a time, in a pure form, with careful recording of results. Reexposure to an offending food typically precipitates symptoms that are often far worse than they were before testing. Objective evidence of reactivity may also be gauged by a significant increase in the pulse rate in the first hour after the test meal.

There are some limitations to be mentioned. A five-day fast should be undertaken only by those who are physically and mentally disposed to undertake this rigorous approach. None of the three approaches should be undertaken in someone whose asthma is precariously controlled or those who are subject to life-threatening anaphylactic reactions. It is very helpful to work with an experienced practitioner who can guide you through this process. You can also do much of the work yourself by reading books, including *The Five-day Allergy Relief System* (by Marshall Mandel) and *Allergies and the Hyperactive Child* (by Doris Rapp).

Conventional Medical Treatment

Conventional allergists tend to recognize food allergies only in children. Parents are often told that the food reactions will be outgrown. Some allergists do skin tests for foods, but reliability of skin tests for food reactions is very low. The RAST or ELISA blood tests occasionally used by conventional doctors are subject to up to 50 percent error with many false positives and false negatives.

Risk Factors and Causes

Allergic reactions occur when the body reacts adversely to the ingestion of food molecules. Using a limited definition, allergic reactions are mediated by the immune system. Food sensitivity reactions may also occur in other nonimmunological reactions involving histamine, prostaglandins, serotonin, and other body chemical systems. Food proteins, starches, and contaminants (colorings and other additives) can all cause reactions. The reactions in the case of classic allergy involve the formation of antibodies that bind to the antigenic food molecules. The terms *food sensitivity* and *food intolerance* are encompassed by these mechanisms.

Predisposing factors:

- Genetic: a 70 percent chance of problems if both parents are food reactive.

- Frequent consumption of high amounts of a small number of foods.

- A surprising number of people have a deficiency in acid production in the stomach. Gastric acid content in allergic children also tends to be lower than in nonallergic children. The resulting incomplete digestion of food elements may lead to assimilation of molecules to which the immune system reacts adversely.

- Deficiency in pancreatic digestive enzyme secretion can be contributory to incomplete digestion as well.

- The presence of intestinal candida overgrowth can likewise derange immune function and will often aggravate allergic reactions.

- Stress: food reactions develop or become aggravated during times of high stress, particularly if it is not well managed (may be due to decreased secretory IgA, which ordinarily protects the intestinal mucosa and prevents assimilation of foreign substances into the bloodstream).

- Low levels of DHEA predispose to greater risk of allergies. If DHEA levels are determined and found to be low, taking replacement doses will improve food allergy symptoms.

Holistic Prevention and Treatment

Diet

If food elimination and rechallenge tests prove positive, the offensive foods can be handled in two ways:

- Total elimination may be necessary for the foods to which you are most sensitive. This is, of course, difficult when traveling and eating away from home.

- Rotation of mildly and moderately offensive foods. Rotating of offending foods by consuming them on a regular basis every fourth, fifth, or sixth day has a high degree of success. Many allergic people find that this approach, followed for a number of months, actually results in a loss of intolerance for some of their offending foods.

Vitamins, Minerals, and Supplements

Daily dosages of micronutrients that reduce allergic reactions include:

- *Vitamin C* (1,000–3,000 mg)
- *Vitamin E* (400–800 I.U.)
- *Beta carotene* (15,000–25,000 I.U.)
- *Vitamin B-6* (50–100 mg)
- *Calcium* (400–1,000 mg)
- *Zinc* (30–60 mg of zinc picolinate)
- *Magnesium* (300–600 mg)
- *Selenium* (200 mcg)

Herbs

Nettles have antihistaminic and anti-inflammatory activity; one-half teaspoon of the tincture four times daily, or preparations of nettle tea can be helpful.

Biomolecular Options

A complete evaluation of intestinal function may be necessary to evaluate these possibilities, with specimens sent to laboratories skilled in analysis of stool chemistry and microbiology.

The use of a prescription blocking agent is sometimes helpful. Gastrocrom (cromolyn sodium) taken two capsules four times daily before meals and at bedtime blocks the release of inflammatory chemicals from sensitized pro-allergy mast cells in the intestinal tract.

Professional Care Therapies

Biofeedback and *relaxation training* substantially benefit patients with asthma related to food allergies, sometimes dramatically. People with food allergic reactions often experience great reduction in their symptoms when they learn and practice regular *meditation*. A helpful addition involves *imagery* in which the patient visualizes the ingestion of offending foods with no reaction.

You might also choose to utilize *hypnosis,* using a good hypnotherapist or learning self-hypnosis from a qualified teacher. A percentage of asthmatics seem to lose their asthmatic tendency completely, while the majority experience benefit that needs to be reinforced by periodic repeat hypnosis sessions. The importance of the mind in allergy has been underscored by the demonstration of the ability of certain subjects under controlled conditions to turn their skin tests from positive to negative with hypnosis, and by the simultaneous disappearance of an acute allergic reaction on the spontaneous shifting from one personality state to another in subjects with multiple personality disorder.

Positive results with elimination of allergies are reported with the use of *N.A.E.T.* (Nambudripad's Allergy Elimination Technique) by practitioners skilled in the use of this energy technique.

Numerous placebo studies have confirmed the importance of *beliefs* in regard to allergic phenomena. You may want to seek the help of appropriate *psychotherapists* or *spiritual counselors* to help in shifting your beliefs toward a more positive worldview. Numerous placebo studies have demonstrated the relapse into an acute allergic state when a patient is exposed to a placebo believed to be an antigen.

Acupuncture has been used with success. *Spa hydrotherapy* and *cranial manipulation techniques* can also be helpful, sometimes dramatically so.

Homeopathy. Remedies more commonly used include Apis mel, Allium cepa, and Histaminum.

A CASE HISTORY

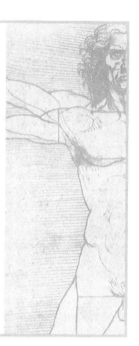

Sally, in her early 40s, had been a friend for some time. I was aware that she had been struggling with fatigue for several years with little success. She decided to seek a second opinion with me after a complete workup in a university medical center failed to identify the cause of her fatigue and ringing in the ears.

Respecting her previous, rather complete evaluation, I elicited a history of childhood allergy, as well as the fact that she occasionally experienced great remission from her fatigue symptoms for two to three days at a time. I suggested that she might find it worthwhile to investigate the possibility of an allergic basis for her fatigue.

Sally went on a five-day water fast, becoming so exhausted on the third day that she missed work and could barely crawl from her bed to the bathroom. On the fifth day, however, she awakened "feeling more energetic than I had in ten years." On pursuing food rechallenge, she became incredibly fatigued two hours after eating wheat, and a few days later after eating chocolate. Her energy, on eliminating these two foods, returned to a level she had not experienced in several years.

20

Endocrinological Disease

Hypothyroidism

Diabetes

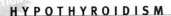 **HYPOTHYROIDISM**

Prevalence

More than five million people in the United States suffer from thyroid problems; the vast majority are women with hypothyroidism. Hypothyroidism is a condition of insufficient thyroid hormone.

Anatomy and Physiology

The thyroid gland straddles both sides of the trachea (windpipe) at the base of your neck, below the Adam's apple. The gland secretes a hormone that is responsible for controlling the rate of metabolism of the whole body. When thyroid hormone blood levels are low, all physiological functions of the body slow down. The secretion of thyroid hormone is controlled by another endocrine gland—the pituitary. This "master gland," located at the base of the brain, secretes the thyroid-stimulating hormone (TSH) to stimulate the thyroid gland to increase its production of thyroid hormone if the blood level is too low.

The primary form of thyroid hormone produced within the thyroid gland is called thyroxine, or T4. However, we usually require the more active thyroid hormone, triiodothyronine, or T3, to stimulate every one of the trillion cells in our bodies; T4 is normally converted to T3 outside of the thyroid gland through the interaction of enzymes that are capable of converting one form to the other as needed. It is T3 that stimulates nearly every organ and system in the body and triggers all physiological functions.

Symptoms and Diagnosis

Hypothyroidism can cause a myriad of symptoms affecting nearly every system of the body. The most prominent symptoms are usually:

- Fatigue

- Weight gain

- Constipation

- Cold intolerance

- Dry, flaky skin

- Hair loss

- Brittle nails

- Recurrent infections/decreased immune function

- Menstrual problems—heavy flow or painful menstruation, PMS

- Depression

The most reliable blood test to diagnose hypothyroidism is for *TSH*. If TSH is normal it means that the pituitary gland is satisfied with the blood levels of thyroid hormone. If TSH is high, then the circulating level of thyroid hormone is usually too low. The test is highly sensitive, and in some instances where TSH is elevated (indicating low thyroid hormone), the blood test for thyroid hormone may be normal. That's why the test for TSH has recently replaced that for T3 and T4 as the best means of diagnosing hypothyroidism. With the use of thyroid hormone blood tests many cases of hypothyroidism that went undetected are now being diagnosed. Some individuals have "tissue resistance" to thyroid hormone, and their body needs more hormone, even though the amount in their blood is normal.

Although TSH is currently the recommended blood test, one of the oldest but less reliable methods of evaluating thyroid function is *basal body temperature measurement*. If you suspect hypothyroidism you can perform this test on yourself by following these instructions:

1. Use any mercury oral or rectal thermometer. Do not use a digital or electronic thermometer. Shake it down before going to bed to 96 degrees or less and put it by your bedside.

2. In the morning, as soon as you wake up, put the thermometer deep in your left armpit and close your arm on it firmly for ten minutes, then record the temperature. Do this before you get out of bed, have anything to eat or drink, or engage in any activity. This will measure your lowest temperature of the day, which correlates with thyroid gland function. The normal underarm temperature averages 97.8—98.2 degrees F. The temperature should be taken for five days. The lower

the temperature (especially 97.0 or less), the more suspicious you should be of hypothyroidism. Oral or mouth temperature does not correlate closely with thyroid function.

3. For women, the temperature should be taken starting the second day of menstruation. This is because a considerable temperature rise may occur around the time of ovulation and give incorrect results. If you miss a day, that is okay, but be sure to finish the testing before ovulation. For men and postmenopausal women, it makes no difference when the temperatures are taken. However, do not do the test when you have an infection or any other condition that would raise your temperature.

Conventional Medical Treatment

Conventional treatment of hypothyroidism with *thyroid replacement therapy* is usually quite effective in correcting this hormonal imbalance. An appropriately prescribed dose of thyroid hormone can enable sufferers of this condition to regain full health without unpleasant side effects. The standard form of thyroid hormone supplement is synthetic thyroid. Synthroid, which is pure T4, is probably the most often prescribed form of synthetic thyroid. However, some people are not able to convert T4 to T3, and the body requires both to function normally. For this reason, a more natural form of thyroid called *Armour thyroid*, containing both forms of thyroid hormone, T4 and T3, is the best first choice for thyroid supplementation. Armour, extracted from cows and pigs, has only one significant drawback. Because T3 is absorbed so erratically through the digestive system, people who are taking it can experience dramatic fluctuations of their thyroid blood level. Close clinical and blood test monitoring initially help to establish the correct dose for any form of thyroid supplement. Once the proper dose is established, this treatment is safe and effective, but because it is long-term, even life-long, periodic monitoring by your doctor is essential.

Risk Factors and Causes

Physical Factors. Hypothyroidism is caused by failure of the thyroid gland to produce an adequate amount of thyroid hormone to maintain good health. Factors that might contribute to thyroid failure are:

- Heredity—usually a parent or grandparent with hypothyroidism
- Nutrient deficiencies—iodine (rare), zinc, copper, iron, selenium, tyrosine, niacinamide, and thiamine; some of these nutrients are involved in T4 production or in converting T4 to T3
- Stress—excessive cortisol levels can block the conversion of T4 to T3

- Hashimoto's disease—an autoimmune disorder (the body becomes allergic to itself) that destroys the thyroid gland

- Pituitary gland dysfunction—inadequate production of TSH

- Heavy metal toxicity from mercury, lead, cadmium, and chemical contamination—may be important resistance factors disrupting the thyroid hormone's effect on the cells

Mental and Emotional Factors. Emotional issues most often associated with hypothyroidism are:

- Reticence in speaking one's truth and being assertively expressive

- Suboptimal self-motivation

- Missing opportunities to experience gratitude about life's opportunities

Holistic Medical Treatment

Physical Health Recommendations. For almost everyone afflicted with hypothyroidism, the *primary treatment is thyroid hormone supplementation.* However, there are foods, supplements, and herbs that can strengthen thyroid function.

Diet
The following foods can nourish and enhance the thyroid:

- *Iodine*: from fish; sea vegetables like kelp, dulse, arame, hijiki, nori, wakame, kombu; root vegetables such as potatoes; and sea salt. Iodized salt can be used but usually contains aluminum

- *Zinc*: from beef, oatmeal, chicken, seafood (especially oysters), liver, dried beans, bran, seeds (especially pumpkin seeds), nuts, and tuna

- *Copper*: from liver and other organ meats, eggs, yeast, legumes, nuts, and raisins

- *Tyrosine* (from phenylalanine): found in soy products, beef, chicken, and fish

- *Water*—maintain hydration with high intake

Foods that naturally slow down the functioning of the thyroid should be *avoided:* broccoli, spinach, cabbage, Brussels sprouts, mustard greens, turnips, kale, peanuts, pine nuts, millet, peaches, and pears. Both antihistamines and sulfa drugs can also affect the thyroid in this way.

Vitamins, Minerals, and Supplements

- *Iodine*—225 to 1000 mcg/day (available in the foods suggested earlier or in liquid or tablet form)
- *Vitamin B*-complex—25 to 50 mg/day
- *Vitamin A* or *beta carotene*—10 to 25,000 I.U./day
- *Zinc*—15 to 30 mg/day
- *Magnesium*—400 to 500 mg/day
- *Copper*—2 or 3 mg/day
- *Selenium*—200 to 250 mcg/day
- *Tyrosine*—300 to 1000 mg/day
- *Iron*—18 mg/day (especially for menstruating females and anemia)

Herbs

Take *kelp* (rich in iodine), 10 drops, one or two times/day; or in capsules (10 to 30 grains), one or two times/day.

Exercise

Yoga, and specifically the shoulder stand and plough positions, can be beneficial to the thyroid. People with hypothyroidism often derive significant benefit from *aerobic exercise*, probably as a result of enhanced circulation and greater cellular uptake of thyroid hormone. Exercise should be performed for at least 30 minutes three times per week.

Professional Care Therapies

Both *homeopathy* and *acupuncture* are effective complements to the treatment of hypothyroidism. The treatment of candidiasis (see chapter 9) and of heavy metal toxicity can also enhance the effect of thyroid hormone supplementation.

Mental and Emotional Health Recommendations. Taking steps to be appropriately more assertive, encouraging yourself to learn the art of self-motivation, and permitting yourself to become more expressive of gratitude for life's gifts will all tend to improve the energy function of the thyroid gland. Cultivating the art of joyful singing can be a specific practice embodying these principles.

DIABETES

Prevalence

Diabetes incidence in the United States is about 4 percent of the population; it is the seventh leading cause of death. It does not occur to any extent in emerging nations but is a phenomenon of advanced societies. About 90 percent of patients have type II disease, so-called adult onset diabetes. The remainder, 10 percent, have juvenile onset diabetes, type I. The incidence of diabetes in the American people is increasing a little over 5 percent each year.

Anatomy and Physiology

Diabetes mellitus is a chronic disorder of carbohydrate, protein, and fat metabolism. It results either from a lack of insulin production in the specialized beta-cells in the islets of the pancreas or from resistance to proper utilization of insulin at the receptor sites on the cell surfaces. When insulin is deficient or not properly utilizable, the cells of the body begin to be fuel-depleted, while the level of sugar in the bloodstream rises to very high levels.

Insulin is attracted to insulin-receptor sites on the membrane surfaces of the cells in the body, where it facilitates the passage of molecules of sugar into the body of each cell to be used as the major source of fuel.

Symptoms and Diagnosis

The classical signs of diabetes are:

- Excessive thirst
- Excessive appetite
- Frequent urination
- Weight loss.

The diagnosis of diabetes depends on the finding of a morning fasting blood sugar level of 140 mg per dl or greater on at least two occasions or a blood sugar concentration of 200 mg per dl or more at two hours after the ingestion of 75 grams of sugar. When the diagnosis is in doubt, a six-hour test measuring blood glucose and insulin levels at hourly intervals after ingestion of 75 grams of glucose in 10 ounces of water may be undertaken. At least 50 percent of patients whose glucose tolerance test was normal (no insulin determinations) have an abnormal glucose-insulin tolerance test.

In juvenile onset (type I) diabetics, extreme deprivation of sugar availability in the cells of the brain can cause unconsciousness (diabetic coma), and the excess burning of fat for fuel can create a serious condition called diabetic ketoacidosis. In adult onset diabetics, stress combined with dehydration can lead to a life-threatening condition called hyperosmolar nonketogenic coma. Ketoacidosis and hyperosmolar nonketogenic coma are life-threatening emergency situations requiring urgent hospitalization.

Long-term complications of diabetes include damage to the kidneys, peripheral nerves, blood vessels, and the retina and lens of the eye. Diabetics tend to have premature onset of arteriosclerosis, heart attacks, strokes, and poor circulation. Compromised circulation to the legs can lead to skin deterioration and pre-gangrenous changes in the feet. A majority of these complications are associated with the accumulation of sorbitol (an alcohol) in body cells. Diabetics with high sugars cannot perform the normal conversion of sorbitol to fructose; accumulated high sorbitol levels are destructive to cells in a variety of ways. Thyroid function is also impaired in uncontrolled diabetics.

Conventional Medical Treatment

Upon proper diagnosis, management of diabetes begins with proper nutritional control, reducing simple sugars, decreasing fat, and increasing starch consumption to 60–70 percent of caloric intake. In juvenile diabetics, insulin becomes required, sometimes after a "honeymoon" period during which sugar is temporarily easier to control. Proper insulin adjustment based on blood sugar readings is imperative. In "brittle" diabetics, a device known as an insulin pump may be used.

In adult-onset diabetics, properly constituted diet is equally important. Appropriate exercise is prescribed. Ninety percent of type II diabetics are overweight, and weight loss for these obese persons becomes very important. Prescription of oral antidiabetic agents is common. Frequently prescribed agents include the sulfonylureas (Diabeta, Diabinese, Glucotrol) and newer agents including the biguanides (Glucophage or metformin), the thiazolidinediones (Troglitizone), and the glucosidases (Precose). Sulfonylurea drugs can cause hypoglycemia; death from heart attack or stroke is also significantly higher compared to patients controlled by diet, weight loss and exercise alone. The biguanide drugs can lead to acidosis and increased cardiovascular mortality in susceptible patients. The thiazolidinediones can cause liver damage and fatalities have been reported. The glucosidases inhibit carbohydrate absorption from the intestine, lowering peak sugar levels. When diet and oral drugs do not sufficiently control glucose levels, insulin treatment is undertaken.

Conventional management includes careful attention to the monitoring of patients for diabetic complications, including nerve pain and numbness (neuropathy), accelerated arteriosclerosis, kidney deterioration, (nephropathy), eye damage (retinopathy), sexual dysfunction, and neurogenic loss of bladder control.

Risk Factors and Causes

Diabetes presents in two forms. The characteristics of type I are:

- Onset in infancy, childhood, and young adulthood up to about age 35
- Results from total destruction of the beta-cells of the islets of the pancreas, the site of insulin production
- Inevitably insulin dependent
- May be linked to cows' milk exposure early in life (see below)
- Nitrates degraded to N-nitroso compounds are capable of producing beta-cell damage and may be problematic; foods such as cured meats (ham, bacon, smoked meats) and drinking water may contain significant amounts of nitrates.
- Diet and stress management very important in disease control
- Exercise plays a modest role in disease control

The characteristics of type II diabetes mellitus are:

- Onset at any time from early adulthood on
- May or may not become insulin dependent
- Hereditary factors play a major role
- Sufficient insulin combined with insulin resistance
- Availability of insulin receptor sites on cell surfaces decreases with increasing sugar intake and lack of exercise
- Highly associated with obesity
- Lack of antioxidant nutrients plays a role; insulin facilitates vitamin C passage into body cells; white blood cell vitamin C is 33 percent below levels in nondiabetics even though oral intake is the same
- Insufficiency of vitamins B-6 and biotin increase risk
- Magnesium, calcium, and potassium deficiency increase risk
- Manganese deficiency compromises glucose tolerance
- Smoking: risk of developing type II disease for those smoking more than 25 cigarettes/day is twice as great as for nonsmokers
- Sedentary lifestyle greatly accelerates onset
- Suppressed anger plays some role in onset

Taking certain drugs increases risks for induction of diabetes; these include:

- Corticosteroids (cortisone, prednisone)
- Estrogens, including oral contraceptive agents
- Thyroid medications
- Catecholamines (adrenaline-like drugs)
- Diuretics
- Antidepressants and other psychotropic medicines
- Chemotherapy drugs
- Isoniazid (a tuberculosis drug)

Energy diagnosticians, medical intuitives, and astute counselors aware of energy fields sense diabetes as a disorder related to personal maturation and self-responsibility, with:

- Resentment or fear on having to take responsibility for another person or for one-self
- Anger at being neglected or ignored while constantly giving to others
- Discomfort with and codependent excuse-making for irresponsible behavior or attitudes of others
- Intense efforts to prevent others from maturing into self-responsibility with less need for one's presence and help
- Resentment in children when parents, out of ineptitude or immaturity, demand to be parented by the children; for example, a significant number of diabetics are children of alcoholics

Holistic Prevention

Physical Health Recommendations

Diet

Vegetarians (meat or poultry less than once a week) have a 38 percent lower risk of developing diabetes than nonvegetarians, probably because of high fiber intake.

Food sensitivities. Cow's milk. Children breast-fed exclusively for their first 90 days have a 35 percent lower risk of developing type I diabetes compared to those not breast-fed. Those fed cow's milk formula in their first 90 days of life are 50 percent more likely to develop diabetes than those not given cow's milk. Cow's milk contains a protein closely resembling a surface molecule in pancreatic beta-cells, which produce insulin. *Antibodies to this unique 17–amino acid protein found in cow's milk were present in 100 percent of newly diagnosed Finnish diabetic children but not found at all in nondiabetic healthy children or adults.* Immune cells reacting to the milk also attack the beta-cells in a free radical–mediated process, gradually destroying them. The implication of cow's milk as an early sensitizing agent in susceptible populations is very clear. Studies also confirm an 88 percent correlation between the amount of milk drunk by children and the risk of diabetes. *Preventing juvenile diabetes begins with the promotion of exclusive breast-feeding for infants for at least three to six months and the sparing use of cow's milk in early childhood.* If breast-feeding is not possible, alternative milk sources (goat, rice bran, soy) should be used.

Vitamins

Long-term treatment in prediabetic patients with doses of nicotinamide (*niacin*) of one gram/day may be helpful. The implication of benefit from increasing *antioxidant* and *vitamin C* intake to remedy deficiencies is quite apparent (one to two grams/day).

Habits

- *Obesity* is a highly significant predictor of adult-onset diabetes, particularly in those with a genetic family predisposition. In one research study, maintenance of normal weight decreased the likelihood of type II diabetes 75 percent compared to those who became obese. Obesity is a more specific predictor of diabetes than lack of exercise.

- *Smoking:* in persons who have abated smoking, the risk of developing type II diabetes drops 20 percent in only two years. Kidney damage, a consequence of chronic diabetes, progresses four and one-half times as rapidly in smokers as non-smokers. If you are diabetic and smoke, attempts to stop are paramount.

Exercise

Exercise more than once a week reduces the risk of developing adult-onset diabetes 35 percent; a 35-year study placed the risk reduction at 42 percent. Those exercising five or more times a week reduced the risk of developing diabetes 50 percent in a study from Harvard. In those with a family diabetic history, regular aerobic exercise postpones the onset of diabetes by 10–12 years. Dr. Steven Blair, of the Cooper Aerobics Institute in Dallas, Texas, presents evidence showing that those among the most active 20 percent of aerobic exercisers have essentially no chance of developing Type II diabetes.

Mental and Emotional Health Recommendations. *Stress management* is unequivocally related to both prevention and control. The stress of marital or personal separation is linked to onset of diabetic symptoms. In a study of children aged five to nine, loss or threatened loss of parent relationships increased the risk of developing type I diabetes 80 percent compared to a group with low loss experiences. Poorly managed stress increases cortisone, increasing insulin requirements. In experiments with dietary intake and exercise held constant, episodes of elevated blood sugar, diabetic acidosis, and near-coma can be induced by intentional exposure to stress. Learning and applying stress management skills help prevent diabetic crises.

Holistic Treatment

Physical Health Recommendations

Diet

The best standard diet omits simple sugars and processed grains, and emphasizes increased intake of high complex carbohydrate, fiber, fruit, and vegetable intake with modest protein, and low fat consumption. Cultures with high cold-water fish consumption have significantly lower incidence of diabetes. Starchy foods vary significantly in the degree to which they raise blood sugar levels. The rate at which they digest is a major variant. Potentially useful foods that have a lower glycemic index (raise blood sugar less) than white bread include:

- Legumes (beans, peas, peanuts, soybeans)
- Vegetables such as carrots and beets
- Pasta, especially whole grain
- Grains, including parboiled rice and bulgur (cracked wheat) and bran cereals
- Fruit (apples, oranges)
- Fructose
- Dairy milks (unless lactose intolerant)
- Nuts
- Whole grain breads such as pumpernickel

Vegetarians who also adhere to very little or no sucrose in their diet are known to control blood sugars well. Neuropathic pain of diabetic neuropathy was completely alleviated or partially relieved in diabetics who adhered to a program of exercise and a vegan diet of unrefined foods; numbness, although persisting, noticeably improved within 25 days.

Low protein, low phosphorus diet. In a revealing dietary study, type I patients with clinical nephropathy (compromised kidney function) were treated with a low protein (less than 0.6 gm protein per Kg of ideal body weight per day, a little over an ounce for most people), low phosphorus diet (less than 1 gm phosphorus per day). After three years, kidney function had deteriorated 67 percent more slowly in those on the low protein, low phosphorus diet compared to patients on a standard American Diabetic Association diet.

Fiber. High fiber foods (whole grains, vegetables, and fruits) lower blood sugar and insulin levels and decrease insulin requirements.

Vitamins, Minerals, and Supplements

- *Vitamins C and E.* Diabetics given vitamin C, one gram per day for three months, had an 18 percent reduction in HbA_1c; high HbA_1c is an indicator of poor long-term blood sugar control. Elderly diabetics significantly improve glucose control after receiving vitamin E, 900 mg/day for 4 months.

- *Vitamin B-6.* In diabetics whose vitamin B-6 status is normal, double-blind studies show that the addition of 50 mg/day of B-6 as a vitamin supplement improves long-term blood sugar control 6 percent. A form of B-6 called pyridoxine alphaglutarate given 600 mg three times daily for four weeks to insulin-dependent juvenile diabetics achieved a 30 percent fall in fasting blood sugars and a 32 percent improvement in long-term blood sugar control (decreased HbA_1c). Type II diabetics experienced a 24 percent decrease in fasting blood sugars and a 24 percent decrease in HbA_1c. After stopping the pyridoxine alphaglutarate, all values returned to previous levels within three weeks.

- *Vitamin B-12/folate*, particularly by injection, have shown benefits.

- *Biotin.* Average blood biotin levels are significantly lower in type II diabetic patients compared to healthy controls. Raising plasma biotin decreases fasting blood sugars in diabetics. The blood sugars of type II diabetics taken off insulin and treated with 16 mg/day of biotin for *one week* have been shown to *decrease* significantly.

- *Inositol*, given 500 mg twice daily to diabetics with peripheral neuropathy, has been reported to significantly improve nerve sensation. Not all reports confirm this finding.

- *Chromium* aids insulin action and assists in losing weight. A reasonable dose is 200 mcg/day.

- *Zinc* tends to be utilized in higher amounts in diabetics, and zinc supplementation is a wise precaution (30 mg/day).

- *Magnesium* levels are lower in diabetic patients compared to healthy people. And levels in diabetics with heart complications were significantly lower than those without heart involvement. Magnesium levels in elderly persons are significantly lower than those of younger persons. Insulin production and insulin utilization improves greatly in magnesium-supplemented type II diabetics (400–800 mg/day).

- *Manganese* is commonly low in diabetics; 5–15 mg per day is a reasonable supplemental intake.

- *Iron* stores are elevated in 50 percent of poorly controlled type II diabetics. The most accurate index of iron stores is a blood ferritin test. In order to reduce iron content, patients with elevated ferritin have been treated with intravenous desferrioxamine (an iron chelating agent that removes iron), 10 mg per Kg twice weekly for 5–13 weeks. In 90 percent of those treated, *in spite of the discontinuance of oral antidiabetic drugs, significant improvement occurred in blood sugars* and triglycerides. Iron stores can be decreased by blood donations and avoiding iron in supplements.

- *Omega-3 fatty acids.* Supplementation with omega-3 fatty acids enhances insulin binding to cells. Eicosapentaenoic acid given to diabetics results in significant inhibition of platelet aggregation (i.e., platelets were made less likely to enhance blood clots). Doses should be limited to 2.5 grams per day. Diabetic patients with neuropathy (nerve damage) given four grams per day of evening primrose oil, high in gamma-linolenic acid, improve their pain and numbness symptoms. Red blood cell membrane flexibility (decreased in diabetics) improves to normal with sardine oil and other marine oils (omega-3 oils, two to four grams per day) after only four weeks. Increased red blood cell membrane flexibility improves circulation.

- *Onion and garlic* have both been shown to have blood sugar lowering effects and can be used liberally with benefit.

- *Alpha lipoic acid*, 200 mg twice daily, adds a new helpful dimension in treatment, with especial benefits in diabetic neuropathy.

Herbs

- Two bioflavonoids, *catechin* (one gram daily) and *quercetin* (400 mg twice daily) have been shown to stimulate the action of insulin and to scavenge free radicals. They are frequently helpful in control symptoms of diabetic neuropathy. Aloe, one-half teaspoon daily for 4–14 weeks in Type II patients, has been shown to reduce fasting blood glucose from levels in the high two hundreds to 150 mg per dl.

- Type II patients given 100 or 200 mg per day of *ginseng* for eight weeks improved fasting glucose levels and resulted in weight loss. Those receiving 200 mg daily demonstrated improvement in HbA_1c (better long-term sugar control). Normalization of fasting blood sugars was achieved in four times as many patients treated with ginseng compared to those treated with placebo.

- Momordica charantia (*bitter melon*), prepared as a juice of the unripe tropical Asian fruit, lowers blood sugar (25-50 gm three times a day).

- *Gymnema sylvestre* is an Ayurvedic blood sugar–lowering botanical contained in a product called Bio Gymnema, taken up to three capsules three times daily. It also contains other antidiabetic agents, including Pterocarpus marsupium (see page 465), chromium, and biotin.

- In patients with type II disease due to liver cirrhosis, 600 mg of *silymarin* daily significantly reduces average fasting blood sugar, HbA_1c, daily insulin need, fasting insulin levels, and blood free radical levels.

- *Fenugreek*, defatted, 100 gm daily, is recommended. Compared to baseline control values, non-insulin-dependent patients given 100 grams per day of defatted fenugreek seed powder for 10 days decreased their fasting blood sugars 30–65 percent.

Biomolecular Options

Levels of DHEA an adrenal hormone, are consistently significantly lower in diabetics compared to levels in healthy persons. In animals, DHEA improves diabetic control. Current research will shed light on the possibilities for human use.

Exercise

In studies of type I diabetics, the mortality rate of those regularly doing moderate or strenuous exercise is *70 percent lower* than the mortality of those exercising minimally or not at all. Dr. Steven Blair, with the Cooper Institute for Aerobic Exercise in Dallas, Texas, recently stated that those in the upper quintile (top one-fifth) for exercise frequency and intensity *do not get type II diabetes. After only one week* of exercising on a treadmill 60 minutes daily at 60 percent of maximal heart rate, men with type II diabetes dropped their average blood sugar two hours after a sugar load from 227 to 170 mg per dl and blood insulin from 172 to 106 mcU per ml; 80 percent had *normal* glucose and insulin tolerance tests at the end of the week. Exercise markedly increases availability of insulin receptor sites and efficiency of insulin utilization and diminishes insulin resistance. Resistance exercise training programs also improve blood sugar readings.

Mental and Emotional Treatment. Stress. Diabetics who learn to incorporate stress management techniques have far better diabetic control. *Relaxation practices* (below), *exercise*, and *attitudinal shifts* are all helpful skills upgrading the management of stress.

Biofeedback and relaxation. Learning these practices is a major part of managing stress and reducing its damaging effects. Three diabetic subjects with non-healing diabetic ulcers of the toe, ankle, and leg participated in 20 sessions of biofeedback training over 15 weeks with thermal biofeedback at the ulcer site plus hand-warming training and home practice. Two of the three showed significant healing. Practicing *biofeedback*, *meditation*, and *autogenic training* all decrease circulating cortisone levels, improving diabetic control.

Counseling. Control of blood sugar is known to deteriorate during periods of depression. It is important that depression and other negative feeling states be recognized and treated. Psychotherapy approaches for depression have been shown to work better than the use of drugs, many of which actually tend to make blood sugar control worse.

Yoga. In a recent study, type II diabetic patients learned and practiced yoga visceral cleansing procedures, body postures, and breathing exercises for 90 minutes in the morning and 60 minutes in the evening for 40 days. There were significant improvements in oral glucose tolerance and decreases in the amount of oral hypoglycemic drugs required. Average fasting blood sugar decreased from 135 to 100 mg per dl. Seventy percent showed good to fair response to therapy.

Quitting smoking. The elimination of smoking needs to be a major goal.

Responsibility issues. Based on energy diagnoses linking diabetes with issues of responsibility, related conflicts over this issue may need professional counseling help for resolution.

Proactive education. Diabetic subjects participating in a 45-minute interactive session regarding information-seeking and medical decision-making and completing a home followup guide showed significantly fewer physical limitations in activities of daily living and significantly better sugar control than controls four months later. In every disease process, patient involvement—being informed and participating in decisions—predicts a better outcome.

Holistic Reversal of Diabetes

Case history reports in juvenile-onset type I diabetics have shown reversal of diabetic retinopathy when excellent blood sugar control is achieved. High doses of niacinamide in newly diagnosed juvenile diabetics have been reported to reverse the glucose handling problems and prevent the onset of full-fledged disease. The children's doses used in successful trials were 100–200 mg daily. Not all studies have confirmed this phenomenon.

Many type II diabetics who have required oral antidiabetic drugs and/or less than 20 units of insulin daily, after assuming a lifestyle incorporating optimum weight, diet, supplements, and exercise, are frequently found on retesting to be nondiabetic and requiring no insulin or medications. At a minimum, improvement in lifestyle factors may eliminate or reduce insulin requirements in adult-onset diabetics while improving sugar control.

The arteriosclerotic complications of diabetes can likewise be controlled and at least modestly reversed with good blood sugar control and adoption of the measures discussed under coronary heart disease.

Epicatechin, a flavonoid extracted from the bark of Pterocarpus marsupium, long used in Ayurvedic medicine, has shown promise in pancreatic beta-cell regeneration in animals. It is not yet available in the United States.

21

Dermatological Conditions

Acne

Dermatitis

ACNE

Prevalence

Acne vulgaris, or acne, affects millions of teenagers, but also persists or recurs in later life in about 6 percent of men and 8 percent of women. The incidence is much greater in adolescent males, beginning at puberty. Acne is uncommon to rare in tribal cultures and emerging societies.

Anatomy and Physiology

Acne is a derangement in the function of the sebaceous glands of the hair follicle that produce oils and waxes to lubricate the skin. These constitute a substance called sebum, which reaches the surface by way of the pore through which the hair shaft passes. The greatest concentration of sebaceous glands is on the face, upper back, and upper chest, the sites of the greatest concentration of acneiform lesions when they occur.

The cells lining the pore of the hair shaft are activated by testosterone to produce keratin, the principal protein of the hair, nails, and outer layer of skin. This probably explains the predominant incidence in teenage boys rather than girls. Exudation of excessive amounts of keratin tends to clog the skin pores. When the blockage is complete, the sebum collects beneath the surface as a whitehead; when the blockage is partial, some sebum reaches the opening of the pore, turning dark on becoming oxidized to form the notorious blackhead. Clogging of the pore also leads to overgrowth of the normal resident bacterium, Propionibacterium acnes, which causes inflammation and swelling of the lesion, later leading to formation of cysts and nodules.

Symptoms and Diagnosis

Acne presents as a collection of skin disruptions, including blackheads, whiteheads, inflamed nodules with pus collections, and pockmarks and scarring in burned-out lesions that have healed. The diagnosis is made by identification of these typical lesions.

Conventional Medical Treatment

Topical agents such as benzoyl peroxide gel or cream (5–10 percent concentration, OTC) dry the skin and loosen keratin plugs. Conventional advice also includes encouragement of adequate rest, avoiding oil-based makeup, using water-based "nonacnegenic" products, avoiding overwashing, and judiciously using a comedone extractor.

Tretinoin (Retin-A, retinoic acid), a vitamin A derivative, is prescribed if benzoyl peroxide has not produced good results. Tretinoin reddens the skin and can cause marked irritation if used too often. It must not be used in any women who might become pregnant.

Topical antibiotic creams including clindamycin, erythromycin, and tetracycline are prescribed for control of infection. Systemically acting oral antibiotics are still often prescribed (tetracycline, erythromycin, clindamycin) for oral use if other approaches fail to bring about improvement. All too often, low dose antibiotics are prescribed for weeks, months, and even years. The well-known complication of severe depletion of normal bacteria in the intestine occurs here, with attendant overgrowth of candida organisms and the emergence of resistant pathogenic bacteria.

Accutane is an oral form of tretinoin and is a last resort option in severely disfiguring acne. The PDR lists contraindications and complications of use, including total prohibition in women who might become pregnant (causes severe life-threatening fetal anomalies), decreased night vision, formation of cataracts, evoking of inflammatory bowel disease, elevation of triglycerides and fall in HDL cholesterol, liver toxicity, excessive hardening of bones, cracking of the skin around the mouth, eye irritation, joint pains, and peeling of the skin of the soles and palms.

Risk Factors and Causes

Contributing factors include:

- Heredity
- Pharmaceuticals

  Cortisone family medications

  Dilantin (an epilepsy drug)

  Lithium (a bipolar depression drug)

- Local irritation—overwashing, scrubbing

- Chemicals—coal tar derivatives, chlorinated hydrocarbons
- Toxins absorbed from the intestines have higher blood levels in acne patients
- Higher levels of 5-alpha-reductase, the hormone converting testosterone to dihydrotestosterone
- High carbohydrate diet—accelerates testosterone to dihydrotestosterone conversion
- Deficiency in zinc—lower levels in 13–14-year-old males than in any other subgroup
- Stress—clearly related
- Foods high in iodine—highly salted foods (most salt is iodized), sea vegetables like kombu
- Selenium and vitamin E deficiency
- Hypothyroidism
- Higher incidence of intestinal candidiasis secondary to long-term antibiotic treatment in many patients

Holistic Prevention and Treatment

Diet

A 45 percent protein diet appears to restrict the conversion of testosterone to the more potent dihydrotestosterone and is helpful. Sugar is contraindicated, if for no other reason than its tendency to compromise immune resistance to infection; dairy products may also be problematic. The inclusion of more whole foods, including grains, fruits, vegetables, nuts, and seeds and the reduction of highly refined grains and other foods are indicated. Additional fiber and water discourage constipation, which is probably a contributing factor based on research cited earlier. If antibiotics have been used in treatment and candidiasis is likely, the anticandida diet is important (see chapter 9).

Vitamins, Minerals, and Supplements

- *Pyridoxine* (B-6) supplements (50–200 mg daily) benefit premenstrual acne flare-ups in women, probably decreasing sensitivity to testosterone.
- *Pantothenic acid*—a Chinese study found marked improvement in one hundred acne patients using 2.5 grams of pantothenic acid four times daily with application of a 20 percent pantothenic acid cream to acneiform lesions four to six times daily.
- *Vitamin C*, 1–2 grams daily, is recommended.
- *Vitamin A* supplementation in high doses (200,000–400,000 I.U. daily) elicits improvement but requires medical supervision and must not be used by women who

could become pregnant. Use of 25,000 I.U. daily (unsupervised) is somewhat beneficial. Again, use in sexually active women should be limited to 5,000 I.U. daily.

- *Vitamin E* and *selenium*—E acts to facilitate the full biochemical effectiveness of vitamin A and interacts synergistically with selenium to enhance production of the essential body-synthesized antioxidant enzyme glutathione peroxidase, which tends to be deficient in acne patients (vitamin E, 400–800 I.U., and selenium, 200 mcg daily). A highly absorbable combination of vitamins A and E is available in liquid form from Metagenics (Eugene, OR).

- *Zinc* is very successful. Zinc-sulfate-hydrate, 10 ml three times a day initially, followed by 50–80 mg daily of zinc picolinate are often required for up to 12 weeks to achieve improvement. One study found 75 percent of zinc-treated subjects improving compared to 25 percent of a placebo treated group. In many Scandinavian dermatology clinics, zinc is thought to bring about improvement comparable to oral antibiotics.

- *Copper*, 2–3 mg daily, will compensate for losses due to long-term zinc therapy.

- *Chromium* supplementation (200–500 mcg daily) improves acne.

- Four percent *niacinamide gel*, applied twice daily, exceeds the success of topical clindamycin antibiotic gel.

Herbs

- *Tea tree oil* from Melaleuca alternifolia (an Australian tree) has antibacterial activity, and a 5 percent solution is as effective as a 5 percent solution of benzoyl peroxide, with substantially fewer side effects; 10 to 15 percent solutions are required for more severe acne and may occasionally induce a contact dermatitis.

- *Azelaic acid* from Pityrosporum ovale (a fungus), applied as a 20 percent cream, has been shown to be as effective as benzoyl peroxide, retinoic acid, and tetracycline, with significantly less inflammation compared to the other two topical agents. It was not as effective as the prescription drug Accutane.

- Natural antimicrobials: *goldenseal/berberine*, 250–500 mg three times daily; or *Uva ursi*, 250–500 mg three times daily; neither are recommended during pregnancy.

Biomolecular Options

- Hypothyroidism, if present, needs treatment.

- Three to ten percent sulfur lotions and creams are also effective, with few side effects (Enzymatic Therapy in Green Bay, WI, Nature Derm cream, OTC, and others).

- Persistent modest exposure to sunlight is also therapeutic.

- Imbalances of intestinal bacteria and candida development resulting from antibiotic treatment need to be addressed by your physician.

- One hundred percent of antibiotic-resistant acne patients improved up to 70 percent in two months on an oral dose of 1 mg per day of colchicine (a gout medicine available on prescription) in a very recent report.

Biofeedback, Relaxation

Any technique that reduces sympathetic nervous system responsiveness at rest and under stress is helpful in skin problems. Regular relaxation practice and/or meditation both bring substantial results, but incorporation into a daily routine is often difficult for most American adolescents.

Professional Care Therapies

Homeopathic constitutional prescribing has long-term benefits; some of the more common remedies ultimately chosen include Kali bromatum, sulphur 6c, Calcarea sulphur 6c, Hepar sulphur 6c, and Antimonium tartaricum 6c.

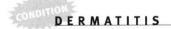

DERMATITIS

Prevalence

Eczema, the most common dermatitis, affects 5 to 15 percent of the population. It is most common in infants, disappearing in about 50 percent of children by 18 months of age, but does occur in all age groups.

Hives, another form of dermatitis, are experienced by 20 percent of the population at one time or another.

Anatomy, Physiology, Symptoms, and Diagnosis

Dermatitis describes an acute and often recurring chronic inflammation of the skin in infants, children, adolescents, and adults, characterized by redness, swelling, itching, and the appearance of tiny blister-like papules. Blisters may develop and weep small amounts of fluid, become scaly and crusting, and are often associated with and/or lead to a drying and thickening of the skin.

Many varieties of dermatitis have been classified. The most common, with their most common causes, are as follows.

Contact dermatitis. In this situation the skin reacts allergenically to physical contact with a variety of substances.

Atopic dermatitis, or *eczema*, occurs at any age, more commonly affecting the face, neck, wrists, hands, and inner aspect of the elbows and knees.

Neurodermatitis is a term sometimes applied to eczematoid rashes that seem to have a major stress-related component. Increased nerve stimulation during times of tension releases excess amounts of a neurotransmitter chemical (acetyl choline) in the skin itself. Copious amounts of acetyl choline cause irritation and severe itching.

Hives, or *urticaria*, presents with the appearance of extremely itchy, raised welts (wheals) that appear in response to either pressure contact with the skin or allergic response to inhalants or foods. The welts result from the release of histamine within the skin. A deeper variety of swellings, *angioedema*, involves the subcutaneous tissues as well. In many patients there is a heightened swelling response to mechanical pressure , stroking, or scratching of the skin.

Conventional Medical Treatment

Conventional treatment of contact dermatitis includes application of cortisone-containing topical creams and ointments, the prescription of antihistamines, and of course avoidance of the offending substance if known.

Conventional treatment of atopic dermatitis, after identification of known inhalant and ingestant triggers, begins with avoidance, including dietary restructuring. Oral antihistamines have been widely used. For children, many of these drugs have sedative properties, reducing the symptoms of itching. Other drugs used to control itching include Atarax, Temaril, and Vistaril.

Topical hydrocortisone in cream or ointment form is commonly used to control eczema symptoms; OTC forms are available. Solar treatments with UVA exposure are used in severe cases.

Treatment of hives includes many some of these same measures. In emergency situations, hives may be a part of a life-threatening state called anaphylactic shock, requiring injection of adrenalin and cortisone.

Risk Factors and Causes

Contact Dermatitis. Substances known to trigger contact dermatitis responses include metals (e.g., nickel, chrome, and gold), petrochemicals, plastics, leather, and cologne. Items of clothing, whether treated with dyes and chemicals or not, are potential causes; wool and wool fat (lanolin) are perhaps the most common. Contact with poison ivy, oak, and sumac plants is a common cause; even contact with the smoke from the burning of these plants can cause a reaction.

Atopic Eczema. *Heredity.* Family members frequently have a history of allergies as well.

Allergy. Eczema is a skin response to an allergic challenge from inhalant substances or ingested foods. Other manifestations of allergy, including hay fever (allergic rhinitis) and asthma often appear later as the eczema disappears. Predisposing skin characteristics include unusual dryness, decreased itching threshold, and increased susceptibility for superficial infections. Elevated immunoglobulin E (a class of immune antibodies) is found in 80 percent of patients. Skin allergy tests are very frequently positive.

The most common *food triggers* include milk, eggs, peanuts, chocolate, and other nuts. The most common inhalants include molds, yeasts, dust mites, and pollens.

Inflammatory prostaglandins. The diseased skin of patients with atopic dermatitis has significantly higher levels of LTB4, a strongly proinflammatory prostaglandin, compared to the content in the skin of normal healthy volunteers. The reason for this disparity is unknown.

Unmanaged stress, tension, and anxiety are contributing and aggravating factors. Emotionally disturbing events are quite commonly associated with recurrences of eczema. Itching increases as subjects discuss stressful events.

Hives or Urticaria.

Foods. Food triggers include alcohol and almost any food, most commonly chocolate, milk, egg, chicken, peanuts, cinnamon, and, in season, strawberries, melons, and tomatoes. In children, food additives, including flavorings, preservatives, colorings, and stabilizers can be the culprits, as well as natural salicylates in food. Foods on the list of those containing vasoactive amines are more likely to be problematic and include cured meats, alcohol, cheese, chocolate, citrus fruits, and shellfish.

Infections. In patients with simultaneous hives and peptic ulcers, 20 percent have been shown to be due to the presence of a bacterium in the stomach, Helicobacter pylori, which is associated with peptic ulcers. Hives were eliminated in all 20 percent when H. pylori was eliminated by drug treatment. Hepatitis viruses and other viral infections can cause hives. Hives may also occur secondary to candida (yeast) infections.

Stress is an extremely frequent primary cause, as well as secondarily lowering the threshold to reactions to drugs, other ingestants and inhalants. Some studies have found stress is *the most frequent* causal factor.

Other causes. Contributing causes to hives include overheating of the skin, from physical exercise, saunas, hot tubs, and excessively spicy foods, and excessive response to cold stimuli. *The most common cause in adults is the intake of drugs.* A wide variety of medications can lead to hives, but the most common are aspirin, penicillin and other antibiotics, and sedatives. Other causes include a secondary response to microorganisms, yeast, and fungal infections, for example.

Holistic Prevention and Treatment
Physical Health Recommendations

Contact Dermatitis

- *Elimination* of known sensitizing contact substances, if possible, is a first order of business.

- *Nutritional changes.* The incidence of dermatitis in carefully studied subjects exposed to poison oak when pretreated and concurrently treated with oral vitamin C and 600 mg of vitamin C given intravenously was found to be only 4 percent compared to 87 percent in subjects not given any supplements. Vitamin C has antihistaminic activity.

Atopic Eczema

Again, elimination of known sensitizing inhalant and ingestant substances, if possible, is paramount.

- *Breast-feeding.* Infants exclusively breast-fed, even though they have a positive family history, have a lower risk of atopic eczema development and develop symptoms at a later age. This may reflect later contact with cow's milk, a common sensitizer. Infants who are being breast-fed may react allergenically to molecules of food ingested by the mother and passed through the breast milk. Consequently, the breast-feeding mother of an infant with a recalcitrant eczema should avoid the same high profile foods listed on page 472.

- *Elimination diets* may be needed to identify specific offenders. The most extreme approach is a total water fast for five days to see if symptoms get better. Less extreme is a diet eliminating all but the least allergenic foods, including pears, rice, lamb, and vegetables, again to see if symptoms improve. Less rigorous still is a diet incorporating avoidance of cow's milk, corn, wheat, sugar, chocolate, eggs, peanuts, citrus fruits, and fish for a week, which will eliminate about 85 percent of the probable food offenders. In adults shellfish needs to be added to this list. Offensive food additives are found most often in cured meats, alcoholic beverages, cheese, and chocolate-containing foods.

Vitamins, Minerals, and Supplements

- *Essential fatty acids.* Atopic eczema patients randomly assigned to take 360 mg of gamma linolenic acid per day (as *evening primrose oil*) for three months had significantly greater improvement in inflammation, dryness, itching, and percentage of body surface involved compared to those taking a placebo, and the use of cortisone cream was two-thirds reduced. *Omega-3 fish oils*, 10 grams daily, greatly reduces scaling, itching, and total symptom scores compared to placebo. Unrefined *flaxseed oil* (1–2 tsp. daily; 1 tablespoon for adults) also supplies significant amounts of alpha-linolenic acid

- *Vitamin E*, 400 I.U. daily
- *Vitamin A*, 25,000 I.U. daily; highly absorbable forms of vitamins A and E available from Metagenics, Eugene, Oregon
- *Zinc*, 60 mg/day
- *Quercetin*, 400–1,000 mg three times daily before meals (antihistaminic properties)
- *Green tea extract*, 200–300 mg three times a day (three to four cups of green tea daily is also an option)
- *Vitamin C* or ascorbate with bioflavonoids, 1 gram three times daily
- *Pantothenic acid* (vitamin B-5), 500 mg twice daily

Herbs

- *Licorice*, solid extract 4:1, 250–500 mg three times daily.
- *Topical calendula* cream

Mental and Emotional Treatment. Relaxation techniques. Because part of the pathology of dermatitis is related to excessive generation of neurotransmitter chemicals in the skin, the acquisition of relaxation skills through *biofeedback, progressive relaxation,* or *meditation* techniques is often markedly helpful. Imagery combined with relaxation techniques is often successful, partially because the skin is such a visible organ to the observing eye, as opposed to internal organs, which cannot be as accurately pictured.

Hypnosis is known to profoundly affect the immune responses to challenge antigens. Numerous allergic subjects have been shown to change strongly positive skin test reactions from as much as 72 mm^2 of reaction to 0 after hypnosis. Energies of the mind profoundly influence skin reactivity to antigens, including cases of hives and eczema. Entrée into the utilization of these energies for clinical benefit occurs in hypnosis, imagery and meditation/relaxation training.

Hives

Nutritional options. Vitamin C has antihistaminic activity; reasonable doses can go up to 8–10 grams/day if tolerated by the bowel. *Magnesium* in daily doses is helpful (400–800 mg daily) with more in an acute situation, again, as tolerated by the bowel. Diarrhea may result from too much C or magnesium. *Quercetin*, a bioflavonoid, may also be helpful (1,000 mg three times daily). Food preservatives should be noted and avoided; these include BHT and BHA, sulfites, and benzoic acid (used in fish).

Relaxation techniques. Biofeedback, progressive relaxation, and meditation techniques are frequently successful in managing hives. Imagery is also an extremely valuable tool.

Hypnosis has also been shown to be of significant benefit in a very high percentage of patients with hives who participated.

Beliefs. Our beliefs about body organ functions are a major determinant of outcomes. The skin is one of the better examples of this phenomenon. In the 1950s, experiments were done on volunteers susceptible to hives, in which a small paddle was used to strike the forearm a sharp blow. The site of the blow immediately reddened and swelled into a welt, as blood vessels dilated to deliver nutrient chemicals and white blood cells to repair the damage done by the blow. Much later, after the arms of volunteers had returned to normal, a sham blow was delivered toward the arm without contacting the skin. The area of skin reddened just as before, as if the skin had been struck. After returning to normal, the procedure was repeated yet a third time, except that the subject was told in advance that a sham blow was to be delivered. No reddening of the skin occurred after the subject was forewarned.

A second experiment was done on a subject predisposed to hives. The patient was struck a sharp blow on the skin of the forearm, following which a typical reddening reaction developed, followed quickly by the development of a welt at the site of the blow. After the reddening and the welt had totally subsided, a very painful family-of-origin situation was brought into the discussion. When the subject was asked about his attitude, he replied that he "was just thinking about the things they did to me." At that point, the hive immediately recurred at the site of the previous blow to the forearm. So stressful psychological blows and even their recall can lead to the hive response in the skin just as a physical blow can.

Appendix
Health Care Therapies Commonly
Practiced by Holistic Physicians

THE ART AND SCIENCE of holistic medicine is inclusive and comprehensive, employing both conventional western, or allopathic, medicine, and all of the more common therapies that most people think of as *alternative* or *complementary* medicine. *Alternative medicine* is a popular but ambiguous term that is loosely used to refer to any health care approach that is not commonly taught in conventional Western medical schools. (It's only since the mid-1990s that allopathic medical schools have begun including one or more alternative therapies as part of their curriculum.) The growing popularity of alternative medicine is due at least in part to an equally growing dissatisfaction with conventional medical care. Ironically, however, what many of its adherents fail to recognize is that alternative medicine, like conventional medicine, is primarily focused on treating disease, while not necessarily caring for people from the holistic perspective of body, mind, and spirit. The primary difference is that, instead of employing drugs and/or surgery as the chief therapeutic options, alternative practitioners may use herbs, acupuncture, or a number of other complementary therapies. But unless the practitioner, either alone or as part of a therapeutic team, is treating the whole person—body, mind, and spirit—he or she is not truly practicing holistic medicine. A strong emphasis on optimal health also distinguishes holistic physicians from their alternative and conventional brethren.

Recognizing the need for a standard of excellence and competence in the emerging field of holistic medicine, in 1996 physician members of the American Holistic Medical Association created the American Board of Holistic Medicine (ABHM), with coauthor Bob Anderson, M.D., serving as ABHM's current president; ABHM's mission is to firmly establish holistic medicine as medicine's newest, and most comprehensive, specialty. The organization is accomplishing this mission by certifying physicians (M.D.s and D.O.s) in holistic medicine. This will provide an improved quality of standardized health care and a new breed of well-trained physicians who are skilled in both the use of conventional therapies, such as drugs and surgery, and complementary therapies that both the public and insurance companies are seeking. In addition, it will help establish a leadership position for holistic medicine as it becomes the standard-bearer for health care in the twenty-first century.

The principal therapies that are most commonly employed by holistic physicians are the following:

Allopathic or Western medicine (practiced by M.D.s and many D.O.s). The primary system of medicine practiced in the United States, allopathic medicine believes that the cause of disease is physical and ultimately visible. Treatment is generally restricted to surgery and pharmaceutical medications. The technology developed within the field of allopathic medicine makes it well suited for trauma care, and it is unrivalled when it comes to treating acute, life-threatening illness.

Ayurvedic medicine (Ayurveda). This branch of traditional Indian medicine is, along with traditional Chinese medicine, one of the oldest and most complete medical systems ever devised. Recognizing the integral relationship between body, mind, and spirit, Ayurvedic physicians view disease primarily as an imbalance in a person's life force (known as *prana*) and his or her predominant *dosha*, or basic metabolic condition. The three primary doshas are *pitta*, *vata*, and *kapha*. Restoring balance to the doshas and a person's pranic energy is the goal of Ayurveda. This is accomplished using diet, medicinal herbs, *pancha karma* (detoxification), *pranayama* (breathing exercises), and the most well-known components of Ayurveda in the West, meditation and yoga.

Behavioral medicine. This emerging therapeutic modality is based on the recognition that behavior, including attitudes and feelings, is a fundamental factor in both health and disease. Much of the research on behavioral medicine stems from the new understanding of health and disease that has been an outgrowth of psychoneuroimmunology (PNI), especially the role played by emotional stress. Behavioral therapists employ a variety of stress-reduction techniques to treat people with intractable pain, heart disease, cancer, stroke, and other chronic and "terminal" conditions.

Bodywork and massage therapy. The various therapies within the category of bodywork and massage therapy all focus on relieving physical tension and stress and improving posture and structural deficiencies in order to enhance health. Many of these therapies are also highly effective for rehabilitating physical injuries and improving recovery from illness. Some approaches also result in greater self-awareness and can help people learn to improve the way they sit, stand, and walk, thereby reducing stress and musculoskeletal tension. Others can also help heal repressed emotional pain related to muscular "armoring" and diminished breathing patterns. Shiatsu, reflexology, Rolfing, deep and Swedish massage, manual lymph drainage, the Alexander technique, Trager, Feldenkrais, Hellerwork, and polarity therapy are some of the more common forms of bodywork and massage therapies.

Botanical medicine (herbology). Botanical medicine employs the flowers, leaves, stems, bark, and roots of a wide range of plants to both treat specific health conditions and rejuvenate physiological systems. Perhaps the oldest form of medicine, botanical medicine has been a part of every culture throughout history, and is also a vital component in Ayurveda, traditional Chinese medicine, and naturopathic medicine. Botanicals are typically classed as food-grade (including food seasonings) and medical, and can be either self-prescribed or administered under professional supervision. Subsets of botanical medicine include aromatherapy and flower essence therapy.

Chelation therapy. Chelation therapy is the practice of injecting EDTA (*ethylene diamine tetracetic acid*, also called *edetic acid*) into the veins, where it attaches itself to harmful plaque, lead, and other heavy metals, enabling them to be excreted from the body via the urine. At the physician's discretion, vitamins and other supplements can also be included in the EDTA solution. Chelation therapy originally was found to be effective in treating heavy-metal poisoning in the mid-1900s, but in recent decades, growing numbers of physicians have recommended it as an effective option in place of bypass surgery and angioplasty in treating coronary artery disease. It should be pointed out, however, that chelation therapy is controversial and at best still a form of symptom care that does not address the causes of coronary heart disease. It only relieves their symptoms. If you are considering chelation therapy, contact the American College for Advancement in Medicine (ACAM), 23121 Verdugo Drive, Suite 204, Laguna Hills, CA 92653, (800) 532-3688, or the American Board of Chelation Therapy, 1407-B North Wells Street, Chicago, IL 60610, (800) 356–2228 to locate a physician who has been properly trained in its application.

Chinese medicine. Traditional Chinese medicine (TCM), along with Ayurveda, represents one of the oldest and most complete medical systems ever developed.

Dating back at least five thousand years, TCM views disease as an imbalance between the body's nutritive substances, known as *yin*, and the functional activity of the body, or *yang*. This imbalance causes a disruption in the flow of vital energy (*qi*) that circulates through the body's energetic pathways, known in TCM as *meridians*. Traditional Chinese medicine also recognizes the role played by thoughts and emotions in creating or destroying health, as well as seasonal changes and the properties of the Five Elements (wood, water, metal, earth, and fire). Instead of treating disease, the goal of TCM is to maintain or restore the proper balance between the yin and yang energies, thus enabling the patient to regain and maintain a state of equilibrium. The most widely known modality of TCM in the West is acupuncture, which rebalances the body's vital energy through stimulation of specific meridian points. Acupressure, Chinese herbology, t'ai chi and qigong, moxibustion, meditation, diet, and exercise are other aspects of TCM.

Chiropractic.   Developed over one hundred years ago by David Daniel Palmer, the goal of chiropractic (Greek for "done by hand") is to maintain the health of the nervous system through the adjustment of bones and joints. Chiropractic theory holds that spinal misalignment (called *subluxation*) interferes with the flow of vital energy, or what Palmer described as the body's "innate intelligence." Since the nervous system's primary pathway is along the spine, when any part of the spine is subluxated, nerve impulses can be impeded and eventually result in dis-ease in the body's various organs. Chiropractors (or D.C.s) restore spinal alignment with a variety of adjustment and manipulation techniques and comprise a large portion of the alternative practitioners in the United States. Many chiropractors also employ kinesiology (muscle testing) and provide nutritional counseling in their practices.

Energy medicine.   Including a wide range of subtle bioenergetic techniques and the use of both conventional and experimental microcurrent and magnetic energy devices, energy medicine may well become one of the most important aspects of holistic medicine in the twenty-first century, due to its ability to diagnose and treat disease in the human bioenergy field, often before it manifests physically in the body. Bioenergetic therapies within the field of energy medicine include Therapeutic Touch, healing touch, Reiki, and jin shin jyutsu. Distance healing, prayer, and meditation are other aspects of energy medicine, as are light, color, sound, and music therapies. Magnetic therapy, t'ai chi and qigong, and microcurrent therapies (using devices such as the Acuscope and cranial electrical stimulation tools) also fall under the heading of energy medicine.

Environmental medicine. Concerned with both environmental hazards and the growing incidence of food allergy, environmental medicine seeks to preserve and enhance the quality of human environments (both social and work-related) and prevent the harmful effects of environmental toxins, including chemicals, air and water pollution, radiation, sensitizing substances, and communicable disease. It includes occupational, climatological, and social environmental concerns. In addition to addressing individual aspects of these experiences, group, community, and societal concerns fall under this specialty's purview, with an emphasis on improving the environment in which people live in order to enhance health.

Homeopathy. Since its discovery and development in the late 1700s by German physician Samuel Hahnemann, homeopathy has grown to become one of the primary medical systems in much of the world today and was a major force in American medicine at the early part of the twentieth century. (The establishment of allopathic medicine, with its emphasis on pharmaceutical drugs, was the primary reason for homeopathy's decline in the United States, but in recent years homeopathy has experienced a resurgence in popularity.) The two primary tenets that inform homeopathy are "like cures like," known as the Law of Similars, and "healing occurs from the inside out," or Hering's Law. Homeopaths identify substances that cause symptoms of a particular disease when taken in large doses by healthy people. Persons suffering from that disease are then given an extremely dilute solution of the same substance in order to assist the body's natural healing capacity. Recognizing that there is a unique vital force in each individual that strives for health, and that disease occurs when this force is disrupted, homeopathy is the art and science of properly administering the specific homeopathic formulas, or remedies, that are best suited to each patient's particular needs.

Mind/body medicine. Mind/body medicine deals with the relationship between thoughts, attitudes, beliefs, and emotions and how they affect the body's nervous system, hormone production, and organ health. While the majority of the alternative therapies used by holistic physicians have long recognized the interconnectedness between the mind and body in creating both health and disease, it was not until the 1970s that Western medicine also began to consider this dynamic. Now, however, Western researchers are in the forefront of those who are scientifically quantifying the physiological effects produced by our thoughts and emotions. Based on this research, it is now estimated that at least 80 percent of all disease conditions have a "psychosomatic" component to them. The goal of the mind/body practitioner is to help patients better manage the way they think and feel by replacing limited or negative beliefs with more positive attitudes that are more "present-oriented" and free of worries, fears, upsets, and regrets about the past and future. This, in turn, helps patients to feel more empowered and better able to cope with stress, which plays a primary role in most disease conditions. Examples of mind/body therapies include meditation, visualization and guided imagery, breathwork, hypnotherapy, NLP, humor therapy, and biofeedback. From the perspective of holistic medicine, mind/body medicine is often considered a subset of behavioral medicine.

Naturopathic medicine. Along with osteopathic medicine, naturopathic medicine (also known as naturopathy) represents one of the first truly holistic systems of medicine to be developed in the United States. Naturopathic physicians, or naturopaths (N.D.s), operate on the basis of six healing principles: *the healing power of nature; find the cause; first do no harm; treat the whole person; the physician is a teacher;* and *prevention*. Incorporating many healing traditions (including diet, nutrition, herbology, TCM, homeopathy, exercise therapy, and hydrotherapy), naturopaths seek to restore and maintain overall health rather than simply providing symptom relief. They accomplish this by enhancing the body's own natural healing responses through noninvasive measures and health promotion. Naturopathic medicine is capable of treating both acute and chronic diseases and is making great contributions to the healing arts in the fields of immunology, clinical nutrition, and botanical medicine.

Nutritional medicine. Due to a variety of modern-day factors, a healthy diet alone is often not enough to meet the body's daily nutritional requirements. Nutritional medicine addresses this fact through preventive and therapeutic nutritional supplementation and dietary intervention. Basic aspects of nutritional medicine include the use of whole, unprocessed foods; identification of food allergies; and appropriate supplementation with vitamins, minerals, amino acids, fatty acids, accessory food factors, metabolic intermediaries, and natural hormone therapy. In some cases, supplementation can be in a pharmaceutical dosage range that is far in excess of the normal recommended daily intake (RDI). The use of supplements in such dosage levels is known as *orthomolecular medicine* and requires professional supervision in order to safeguard against unwanted side effects.

Osteopathic medicine. Developed by M.D. Andrew Taylor Still in 1874, osteopathic medicine can rightly be called the predecessor of holistic medicine. Still taught that physicians needed to study prevention as well as cure, and should treat *patients*, not *symptoms*. Osteopathic medicine (also known as osteopathy) is based on a body, mind, and spirit approach to evaluating and treating patients. Osteopathic manipulative treatment (OMT) is its primary hands-on approach to diagnosis and treatment and is based on the interrelationship of body structure and function. OMT, in addition to its holistic philosophy, is a major characteristic distinguishing osteopathic medicine from allopathic medicine. However, today in most other aspects of training and practice, osteopathic medicine differs very little from conventional medicine. Osteopathic physicians (D.O.s), like M.D.s, are licensed to prescribe drugs, perform surgery, and in many instances receive their specialty training in M.D.-residencies and certification by the M.D. specialty board.

Recommended Reading

THE FOLLOWING BOOKS can help you further understand the principles and information contained in this book.

General Reference

Anderson, Robert A. *Wellness Medicine.* New Canaan, CT: Keats Publishing, 1990.

Ballentine, Rudolph. *Radical Healing: Integrating the World's Great Therapeutic Traditions to Create a New Transformative Medicine.* New York: Harmony Books, 1999.

Gaby, Alan. *The Patient's Book of Natural Healing.* Rocklin, CA: Prima Publishing, 1999.

Golan, Ralph. *Optimal Wellness.* New York: Ballantine Books, 1995.

Goldberg Group, Burton, edited by Larry Trivieri Jr. *Alternative Medicine: The Definitive Guide.* Tiburon, CA: Future Medicine Publishing, 1993.

Gordon, James S. *Manifesto for a New Medicine: Your Guide to Healing Partnerships and the Wise Use of Alternative Therapies.* New York: Addison-Wesley, 1996.

Heimlich, Jane. *What Your Doctor Won't Tell You.* New York: HarperCollins, 1990.

Pizzorno, Joseph. *Total Wellness.* Rocklin, CA: Prima Publishing, 1996.

Shealy, C. Norman, editor. *The Complete Family Guide to Alternative Medicine.* Boston: Element Books, 1996.

———. *The Illustrated Encyclopedia of Natural Remedies.* Boston: Element Books, 1998.

Weil, Andrew. *Natural Health, Natural Medicine.* Boston: Houghton-Mifflin, 1990.

PART ONE

Anand, Margo. *The Art of Sexual Ecstasy.* Los Angeles: J. P. Tarcher, 1989.

Andreas, Connie, and Steve Andreas. *Heart of the Mind.* Moab, UT: Real People Press, 1989.

Benson, Herbert, with Marg Stark. *Timeless Healing: The Power and Biology of Belief.* New York: Scribner, 1996.

Borysenko, Joan, *Minding the Body, Mending the Mind.* NY: Bantam Books, 1987.

Brigham, Diedre Davis. *Imagery for Getting Well: Clinical Applications of Behavioral Medicine.* New York: W. W. Norton, 1994.

Campbell, Don. *The Mozart Effect.* New York: Avon Books, 1997.

Chopra, Deepak, *Ageless Body, Timeless Mind.* New York: Harmony Books, 1993.

———. *Quantum Healing: Exploring the Frontiers of Mind/Body Medicine.* New York: Bantam, 1989.

Cooper, Robert K. *Health and Fitness Excellence.* New York: Houghton Mifflin, 1989.

Cousens, Gabriel. *Conscious Eating.* Santa Rosa, CA: Vision Books International, 1992.

Danielou, Alain, translator. *The Complete Kama Sutra.* Rochester, VT: Park Street Press, 1994.

Dienstfrey, Harris. *Where the Mind Meets the Body: The Search for the Mind's Effects on the Body.* New York: HarperCollins, 1991.

Dispenza, Joseph. *Live Better Longer: The Parcells Center Seven-Step Plan for Health and Longevity.* San Francisco: HarperSanFrancisco, 1997.

Dossey, Larry. *Healing Words: The Power of Prayer and the Practice of Medicine.* San Francisco: HarperCollins, 1993.

———. *Prayer Is Good Medicine: How to Reap the Healing Benefits of Prayer.* San Francisco: HarperCollins, 1996.

Douillard, John. *Body, Mind, and Sport.* New York: Harmony Books, 1994.

Epstein, Gerald. *Healing Visualizations: Creating Health through Imagery.* New York: Bantam Books, 1989.

Fulford, Robert C., with Gene Stone. *Dr. Fulford's Touch of Life: The Healing Power of the Natural Life Force.* New York: Pocket Books, 1996.

Gawain, Shakti. *Creative Visualization.* San Rafael, CA: Whatever Publishing, Inc., 1978.

Gerber, Richard. *Vibrational Medicine: New Choices for Healing Ourselves.* Santa Fe: Bear, 1988.

Goleman, Daniel. *Emotional Intelligence.* New York: Bantam Books, 1995.

———. *Working with Emotional Intelligence.* New York: Bantam Books, 1998.

Graham-Pole, John. *Illness and the Art of Creative Self-Expression.* Oakland, CA: New Harbinger Publications, 2000.

Grimes, Carl E. *Starting Points for a Healthy Habitat.* Denver: GMC Media, 1999.

Haas, Elson M. *Staying Healthy with Nutrition: The Complete Guide to Diet and Nutritional Medicine.* Berkeley: Celestial Arts, 1992.

Hay, Louise L. *You Can Heal Your Life.* Carlsbad, CA: Hay House, 1984.

Hendrix, Harville. *Getting the Love You Want: A Guide for Couples.* New York: Harper and Row, 1988.

Holmes, Ernest. *The Science of Mind, Fiftieth Anniversary Edition.* New York: Tarcher/Putnam, 1997.

Jampolsky, Gerald. *Love Is Letting Go of Fear.* New York: Bantam Books, 1979.

Jahnke, Roger. *The Healer Within.* San Francisco: HarperCollins, 1997.

Joy, Brugh. *Joy's Way.* Los Angeles: J. P. Tarcher, 1979.

Justice, Blair. *Who Gets Sick: How Beliefs, Moods, and Thoughts Affect Your Health.* New York: Putnam, 1987.

Kabat-Zinn, Jon. *Full Catastrophe Living.* New York: Delacorte Press, 1990.

Kaptchuk, Ted. *The Web That Has No Weaver.* Chicago: Congdon and Weed, 1983.

Kreiger, Dolores. *Accepting Your Power to Heal.* Santa Fe: Bear, 1993.

Krippner, Stanley, with Patrick Welch. *The Spiritual Dimensions of Healing*. New York: Irvington, 1992.

Laskow, Leonard. *Healing with Love*. San Francisco: HarperSanFrancisco, 1992.

Levine, Stephen. *Healing unto Life and Death*. New York: Anchor Press/Doubleday, 1987.
———. *A Year to Live*. New York: Bell Tower, 1997.

Millman, Dan. *Way of the Peaceful Warrior*. Tiburon, CA: H. J. Kramer, Inc., 1980.

Moody, Raymond. *The Light Beyond*. New York: Bantam Books, 1988.

Moore, Thomas. *Care of the Soul*. New York: HarperPerennial, 1992.

Moss, Richard. *The Second Miracle: Intimacy, Spirituality, and Conscious Relationships*. Berkeley: Celestial Arts, 1995.

Moyers, Bill. *Healing and the Mind*. NY: Doubleday, 1993.

Murray, Michael, and Joseph Pizzorno. *Encyclopedia of Natural Medicine*. Revised 2nd edition. Rocklin, CA; Prima Publishing, 1998.

Myss, Caroline. *Anatomy of the Spirit*. New York: Harmony Books, 1996.

Ni, Maoshing, translator. *The Yellow Emperor's Classic of Medicine: The Essential Text of Chinese Health and Healing*. Boston: Shambala, 1995.

Ornish, Dean. *Love and Survival: The Scientific Basis for the Healing Power of Intimacy*. NY: HarperCollins, 1998.

Ornstein, Robert, and David Sobel. *Healthy Pleasures*. New York: Addison-Wesley, 1989.

Orr, Leonard, and Sondra Ray. *Rebirthing in the New Age*. Berkeley: Celestial Arts, 1977.

Pearson, Durk, and Sandy Shaw. *Life Extension: A Practical Scientific Approach*. NY: Warner Books, 1982.

Peck, M. Scott. *The Road Less Traveled*. New York: Simon & Schuster, 1978.

Pelletier, Kenneth. *Sound Mind, Sound Body: A New Model for Lifelong Health*. New York: Simon and Schuster, 1994.

Pert, Candace B. *Molecules of Emotion: Why You Feel the Way You Feel*. New York: Scribner, 1997.

Progoff, Ira. *At a Journal Workshop: Writing to Access the Power of the Unconscious and Evoke Creative Ability*. New York: Tarcher, 1992.

Reid, Clyde. *Celebrate the Temporary*. New York: Harper & Row, 1972.

Robbins, John. *Reclaiming Our Health: Exploding the Medical Myth and Embracing the Source of True Healing*. Tiburon, CA: Kramer, 1996.

Rossman, Martin L. *Healing Yourself*. New York: Pocket Books, 1987.

Scarf, Maggie. *Intimate Partners*. New York: Random House, 1987.

Schulz, Mona Lisa. *Awakening Intuition: Using Your Mind-Body Network for Insight and Healing*. New York: Harmony Books, 1998.

Siegel, Bernie. *Love, Medicine and Miracles*. New York: HarperCollins, 1986.

Van de Castle, Robert L. *Our Dreaming Mind*. New York: Ballantine Books, 1994.

Weil, Andrew. *Spontaneous Healing: How to Discover and Enhance Your Body's Natural Wisdom to Maintain and Heal Itself*. New York: Knopf, 1995.

Zi, Nancy. *The Art of Breathing: Thirty Simple Exercises for Improving Your Performance and Well-Being*. New York: Bantam Books, 1986.

Zukav, Gary. *The Seat of the Soul*. New York: Fireside, 1989.

PART TWO

Respiratory Disease

Alexander, Dale. *The Common Cold and Common Sense*. New York: Fireside Books, 1981.

Braly, James. *Dr. Braly's Food Allergy and Nutrition Revolution*. New Canaan, CT: Keats Publishing, 1992.

Firshein, Richard N. *Reversing Asthma*. New York: Warner Books, 1996.

Ivker, Robert S. *Sinus Survival: The Holistic Medical Treatment for Allergies, Asthma, Bronchitis, Colds, and Sinusitis*. NY: Tarcher/Putnam, 1995.

Null, Gary. *No More Allergies*. New York: Villard Books, 1992.

Rapp, Doris. *Allergies and Your Family*. Buffalo, NY: Practical Allergy, 1990.

Psychological Disease

Beck, Aaron T. *Cognitive Therapy of Depression*. New York: Guilford Press, 1989.

Bloomfield, Harold. *Healing Anxiety with Herbs*. New York: HarperCollins, 1998.

Burns, David D. *The Feeling Good Handbook: Using the New Mood Therapy in Everyday Life*. New York: Penguin Books, 1989.

Carlson, Richard, and Wayne Dyer. *You Can Be Happy No Matter What: Five Principles Your Therapist Never Told You*. San Rafael: New World Library, 1997.

Cousens, Gabriel. *Depression-Free for Life*. NY: HarperCollins, 2000.

Dowling, Colette, et al. *You Mean I Don't Have to Feel This Way? New Help for Depression, Anxiety, and Addiction*. New York: Bantam Books, 1993.

Greensberger, Dennis. *Mind over Mood: Change How You Feel by Changing the Way You Think*. New York: Guilford Press, 1995.

O'Connor, Richard. *Undoing Depression: What Therapy Doesn't Teach You and Medication Can't Give You*. Boston: Little Brown, 1997.

Patent, Arnold. *You Can Have It All*. Great Neck, NY: Money Mastery, 1984.

Musculoskeletal Disease

Bresler, David E. *Free Yourself from Pain*. Topanga, CA: Bresler Center, 1992.

Brownstein, Art. *Healing Back Pain Naturally*. Gig Harbor, WA: Harbor Press, 1999.

Colbin, Annemarie. *Food and Our Bones: The Natural Way to Prevent Osteoporosis*. New York: Plume, 1998.

Gaby, Alan R. *Preventing and Reversing Osteoporosis*. Rocklin, CA: Prima, 1994.

Luke, Barbara. *Good Bones: The Complete Guide to Building and Maintaining the Healthiest Bones*. Menlo Park, CA: Bull Publishing, 1998.

Mandell, Marshall. *Dr. Mandell's Lifetime Arthritis Relief System*. New York: Putnam/Berkeley, 1985.

Prudden, Bonnie. *Pain Erasure*. New York: M. Evans, 1980.

Sarno, John. *Mind over Back Pain*. New York: Berkeley Books, 1986.

Schatz, Mary Pullig. *Back Care Basics: A Doctor's Gentle Yoga Program for Back and Neck Pain*. Berkeley: Rodmell Press, 1992.

Swayzee, Nancy. *Breathworks for Your Back*. New York: Avon Books, 1998.

Theodasakis, Jason. *The Arthritis Cure*. New York: St. Martin's Press, 1997.

Systemic Conditions

Collinge, William. *Recovering from Chronic Fatigue Syndrome*. New York: Body Press/Perigree Books, 1993.

Crook, William. *The Yeast Connection*. New York: Vintage Books, 1996.

Freide, Karyn. *Hope and Help for Chronic Fatigue Syndrome*. New York: Fireside Books, 1990.

Goldberg, Burton, et al. *Chronic Fatigue, Fibromyalgia and Environmental Illness*. Tiburon, CA: Future Medicine Publishing, 1998.

Rosenbaum, Michael, and Murray Susser. *Solving the Puzzle of Chronic Fatigue Syndrome*. Tacoma: Life Sciences Press, 1992.

Teitelbaum, Jacob. *From Fatigued to Fantastic*. Annapolis: Deva Press, 1995.

Truss, C. Orian. *The Missing Diagnosis*. Birmingham: Missing Diagnosis, 1985.

Men's Conditions

Chaitow, Leon. *Prostate Troubles*. Wellingborough, England: Thorsons Publishers, 1988.

Green, James. *The Male Herbal*. Freedom, CA: The Crossing Press, 1991.

Gurian, Michael. *The Wonder of Boys*. New York: Tarcher/Putnam, 1996.

Ivker, Robert, and Edward Zorensky. *Thriving: The Complete Mind/Body Guide for Optimal Health and Fitness for Men*. New York: Crown, 1997.

Lazear, Jonathan. *Meditations for Men Who Do Too Much*. New York: Simon and Schuster, 1992.

Pittman, Frank. *Man Enough: Fathers, Sons, and the Search for Masculinity*. New York: Perigee Books, 1993.

Gastrointestinal Disorders

Braly, James. *Dr. Braly's Food Allergy and Nutrition Revolution*. New Canaan, CT: Keats Publishing, 1992.

Guillory, Gerard. *IBS: A Doctor's Plan for Chronic Digestive Troubles*. Point Roberts, WA: Hartley & Marks, Inc., 1991.

Hoffman, Ronald. *Seven Weeks to a Healthy Stomach*. New York: Pocket Books, 1990.

Perkin, Steven. *Gastrointestinal Health*. New York: Harper Perennial, 1992.

Scala, James. *Eating Right for a Bad Gut*. New York: Plume, 1992.

Kidney Stones

Golomb, Gail. *The Kidney Stone Handbook: A Patient's Guide to Hope, Cure and Prevention*. Roseville, CA: Foor Geez Press, 1999.

Rodman, John, et al. *No More Kidney Stones*. New York: John Wiley and Sons, 1996.

Cancer

Austin, Steve, and Cathy Hitchcock. *Breast Cancer: What You Should Know (But May Not Be Told) about Prevention, Diagnosis, and Treatment*. Rocklin, CA: Prima Publishing, 1994.

Diamond, John W., and W. Lee Cowden. *Definitive Guide to Cancer*. Tiburon, CA: Future Medicine Publishing, 1997.

Dreher, Henry. *The Complete Guide to Cancer Prevention*. New York: Harper and Row, 1988.

Lerner, Michael. *Choices in Healing: Integrating the Best of Conventional and Complementary Approaches to Cancer.* Cambridge: MIT Press, 1994.

Moss, Ralph. *Cancer Therapy: The Independent Consumer's Guide to Non-Toxic Treatment and Prevention.* Brooklyn: Equinox Press, 1992.

Simone, Charles B. *Cancer and Nutrition.* Garden City, NJ: Avery, 1992.

Walters, Richard. *Options: The Alternative Cancer Therapy Book.* Garden City, NJ: Avery, 1993.

Cardiovascular Disease

Bennett, Charles. *Controlling High Blood Pressure Without Drugs.* New York: Doubleday, 1984.

Charash, Bruce D. *Heart Myths.* New York: Viking Penguin, 1992.

Cranton, Elmer. *Bypassing Bypass.* Troutdale, VA: Medex Publisher, 1992.

Goldberg, Burton, et al. *Heart Disease, Stroke and High Blood Pressure.* Tiburon, CA: Future Medicine Publishing, 1998.

Kwiterovich, Peter. *The John Hopkins Complete Guide for Preventing and Reversing Heart Disease.* Rocklin, CA: Prima Publishing, 1993.

Ornish, Dean. *Dr. Dean Ornish's Program for Reversing Heart Disease.* New York: Ballantine Books, 1990.

Whitaker, Julian. *Reversing Heart Disease.* New York: Warner Books, 1985.

Neurological Disease

Ingram, Cass. *Who Needs Headaches?* Cedar Rapids, IA: Literary Visions Publishing, 1991.

Khalsa, Dharma Singh. *Brain Longevity.* New York: Warner Books, 1997.

Lombard, Jay. *The Brain Wellness Plan.* Kensington Books, 1997.

Mansfield, John. *Migraine and the Allergy Connection.* Rochester, VT: Healing Arts Press, 1990.

Milne, Robert, and Blake More. *Definitive Guide to Headaches.* Tiburon, CA: Future Medicine Publishing, 1997.

Philpott, William, and Dwight Kalita. *Brain Allergies: The Psychonutrient Connection.* New Canaan, CT: Keats Publishing, 1980.

Stromfeld, Jan, and Anita Weil. *Free Yourself from Headaches.* Berkeley: Frog, Ltd., 1995.

Warren, Tom. *Beating Alzheimer's.* Garden City, NJ: Avery, 1991.

Obesity

Bailey, Covert. *The New Fit or Fat.* Boston: Houghton Mifflin, 1991.

Eades, Michael R., and Mary Dan Eades. *Protein Power: The High Protein/Low-Carbohydrate Way to Lose Weight, Feel Fit, and Boost Your Health in Just Weeks.* New York: Bantam Books, 1998.

Heller, Rachel F., and Richard F. *The Carbohydrate Addict's Diet: The Lifelong Solution to Yo-Yo Dieting.* New York: Signet, 1993.

Ornish, Dean. *Eat More, Weigh Less: Dr. Dean Ornish's Life Choice Program for Losing Weight Safely While Eating Abundantly.* New York: HarperCollins, 1993.

Women's Conditions

Boston Women's Health Collective. *The New Our Bodies, Ourselves.* New York: Simon and Schuster, 1992.

DeMarco, Carolyn. *Take Charge of Your Body.* Winlaw, B.C., Canada: Well Women Press, 1994.

Lark, Susan. *The Premenstrual Syndrome Self-Help Book.* Berkeley: Celestial Arts, 1993.

———. *The Menopause Self-Help Book.* Berkeley: Celestial Arts, 1990.

Lee, John, and Virginia Hopkins. *What Your Doctor May Not Tell You about Menopause: The Breakthrough Book on Natural Progesterone.* NY: Warner Books, 1996.

Love, Susan. *Dr. Susan Love's Book of Hormones: Making Informed Choices about Menopause.* New York: Random House, 1997.

Northrup, Christiane. *Women's Bodies, Women's Wisdom.* Revised 2nd edition. New York: Bantam Books, 1998.

Perry, Susan, and Katherine O'Hanlan. *Natural Menopause: Guide to a Woman's Most Misunderstood Passage.* New York: Addison-Wesley, 1992.

Wolfe, Honora. *Menopause: A Second Spring.* Boulder, CO: Blue Poppy Press, 1992.

Vision Problems

Bates. W. H. *The Bates Method for Better Eyesight Without Glasses.* New York: Henry Holt, 1981.

Cheney, E. *The Eyes Have It: A Self-Help Manual for Better Vision.* York Beach, ME: Samuel Weiser, 1987.

Kaplan, Michael R. *Seeing Beyond 20/20: Improve the Quality of Your Vision and Your Life.* Hillsboro, OR: Beyond Words Publishing, 1987.

Liberman, Jacob. *Light, Medicine of the Future: How We Can Use It to Heal Ourselves NOW.* Santa Fe: Bear, 1991.

———. *Take off Your Glasses and See: How to Heal Your Eyesight and Expand Your Insight.* New York: Crown Publishers, 1995.

Food Allergies and Sensitivities

Braly, James. *Dr. Braly's Food Allergy and Nutrition Revolution.* New Canaan, CT: Keats Publishing, 1992.

Crook, William. *Detecting Your Hidden Allergies.* Jackson, TN: Professional Books/Future Health, 1988.

Mandell, Marshall, and L. Scanlon. *Dr. Mandell's Five-Day Allergy Relief System.* New York: Harper and Row, 1988.

Null, Gary. *No More Allergies.* New York: Villard Books, 1992.

Randolph, Theron, and Ralph Moss. *An Alternative Approach to Allergies.* New York: Harper Perennial, 1990.

Rapp, Doris. *Allergies and Your Family.* Buffalo, NY: Practical Allergy, 1990.

———. *Is this Your Child? Discovering and Treating Unrecognized Allergies.* New York: William Morrow, 1991.

Endocrinological Disease

Langer, Stephen D., with James F. Scheer. *Solved: The Riddle of Illness.* New Canaan, CT: Keats Publishing, 1984.

Philpott, William, and Dwight Kalita. *Victory over Diabetes.* New Canaan, CT: Keats Publishing, 1992.

Whitaker, Julian. *Reversing Diabetes.* New York: Warner Books, 1987.

Resource Guide

THE FOLLOWING ORGANIZATIONS offer additional information about various aspects of holistic medicine and provide referrals to practitioners.

GENERAL RESOURCE ORGANIZATIONS

American Holistic Medical Association (AHMA)
6728 Old McLean Village Drive
McLean, VA 22101-3906
(703) 556-9728/Fax (703) 556-8729

> The nation's oldest advocacy group devoted to promoting, teaching, and researching holistic medicine. Provides a list of referrals nationwide of holistic physicians (M.D.s and D.O.s).

American Board of Holistic Medicine (ABHM)
614 Daniels Drive, NE
E. Wenatchee, WA 98802–4036

> The AHMA's sister organization, ABHM is the first organization to certify physicians in holistic medicine and to create an acceptable standard of holistic medical practice.

American Preventive Medical Association
459 Walker Road
Great Falls, VA 22066
(703) 759-0662/Fax (703) 759-6711

> Advocacy organization that lobbies for medical freedom of choice. Provides information on current and pending legislation concerning health care issues.

Center for Science in the Public Interest
1875 Connecticut Avenue NW, Suite 300
Washington, DC 20009
(202) 332-9110/Fax (202) 265-4954

> Clearinghouse for researchers and consumers alike on issues related to health and nutrition.

World Research Foundation
15300 Ventura Blvd., Suite 405
Sherman Oaks, CA 91403
(818) 907-5483

> Fee-based information source on research devoted to alternative health care treatments and alternative approaches for treating specific disease conditions.

ACUPUNCTURE TRADITIONAL CHINESE MEDICINE (TCM)

American Association for Oriental Medicine
433 Front Street
Catasauqua, PA 18032
(610) 266-1433/Fax (610) 264-2768

> Professional association for non-M.D. acupuncturists. Offers publications and referral directory of members nationwide.

American Academy of Medical Acupuncture

58200 Wilshire Blvd., Suite 500

Los Angeles, CA 90036

(213) 937-5514

> Professional association of physician acupuncturists (M.D.s and D.O.s). Provides educational materials, postgraduate courses, and a membership directory of members nationwide.

National Commission for the Certification of Acupuncturists

1424 16th St. NW, Suite 601

Washington, DC 20036

(202) 232-1404

> Provides information about acupuncture and offers a test used by various states to determine competency of acupuncture practitioners.

National Acupuncture Detoxification Association

3115 Broadway, Suite 51

New York, NY 10027

(323) 993-3100

> Leading organization of its kind. Conducts research on and provides training in the use of acupuncture to treat addiction, including alcoholism.

Qigong Institute/East-West Academy of Healing Arts

450 Sutter, Suite 916

San Francisco, CA 94108

(415) 788-2227

> Provides education, training, and research about qigong in relation to health and healing.

AYURVEDIC MEDICINE

Ayurvedic Institute

P.O. Box 23445

Albuquerque, NM 87192

(505) 291-9698/Fax (505) 294-7572

> Provides training and information in and offers publications about Ayurvedic medicine. Also provides referrals.

American School of Ayurvedic Sciences

10025 NE 4th Street

Bellevue, WA 98004

(206) 454-8022

> Provides training in Ayurvedic Medicine to both professional health care practitioners and laypeople.

The College of Maharishi Ayur-Veda Health Center

P.O. Box 282

Fairfield, IA 52556

(515) 472-5866

> Offers Ayurvedic-related health education programs and physician referrals.

BEHAVIORAL MEDICINE/ MIND-BODY MEDICINE

National Institute for the Clinical Application of Behavioral Medicine

P.O. Box 523

Mansfield Center, CT 06250

(860) 456-1153/Fax (860) 423-4512

> Provides conferences and information for practitioners.

Association for Humanistic Psychology

45 Franklin Street, Suite 315

San Francisco, CA 94102

(415) 864-8850

> Provides publications about humanistic psychology and a list of referrals.

The Academy for Guided Imagery

P.O. Box 2070

Mill Valley, CA 94942

(800) 726-2070

Center for Mind-Body Medicine

5225 Connecticut Avenue NW, Suite 414

Washington, DC 20015

(202) 966-7338

> An educational program for health and mental health professionals, and laypeople interested in exploring their own capacities for self-knowledge and self-care. Provides educational and support groups for people with chronic illness, stress management groups, and training and programs in mind/body health care.

Mind/Body Medical Institute

New Deaconess Hospital

185 Pilgrim Road

Boston, MA 02215

(617) 632-9530

> Provides research, training, and conferences related to behavioral medicine, stress reduction, yoga, and meditation.

BODYWORK/MASSAGE THERAPIES

American Massage Therapy Association

820 Davis Street, Suite 100

Evanston, IL 60201

(847) 864-0123

> Provides comprehensive information on most areas of bodywork and massage, including an extensive review of the latest scientific research. Also publishes Massage Therapy Journal, available at most health food stores and many newsstands nationwide.

Associated Bodywork and Massage Professionals

P.O. Box 489

Evergreen, CO 80439

(303) 674-8478

> Provides information and referrals.

Alexander Technique

North American Society of Teachers of the Alexander Technique

P.O. Box 5536

Playa del Rey, CA 90296

(800) 473-0620

> Provides referrals, information, and training.

The Feldenkrais Method

Feldenkrais Guild

P.O. Box 489

Albany, OR 97321

(503) 926-0981

> Provides information, training, certification, and referrals.

Hellerwork

The Body of Knowledge/Hellerwork

406 Berry Street

Mt. Shasta, CA 96067

(916) 926-2500

> Provides information, training and certification, and referrals.

Polarity Therapy

American Polarity Therapy Association

4101 Lake Boone Trail, Suite 201

Raleigh, NC 27607

(303) 545-2080

> Provides information and referral directory.

Rolfing

International Rolf Institute

302 Pearl Street

Boulder, CO 80306

(303) 449-5903

> Provides information, training, and referral directory.

Reflexology

International Institute of Reflexology
P.O. Box 12462
St. Petersburg, FL 33733
(813) 343-4811
> Provides information, training, and referrals.

CHIROPRACTIC

American Chiropractic Association
1701 Clarendon Blvd.
Arlington, VA 22209
(703) 276-8800
> Professional association offering education and research into chiropractic; also offers publications.

International Chiropractors Association
1110 North Glebe Road, Suite 1000
Arlington, VA 22201
(800) 423-4690
(703) 528-5000
> Professional association offering education and research into chiropractic; also offers publications.

CHELATION THERAPY

American College of Advancement in Medicine (ACAM)
23121 Verdugo Drive, Suite 204
Laguna Hills, CA 92653
(800) 532-3688
> Offers education on chelation therapy for physicians, as well as a treatment protocol, with recommendations for dosage, rates of administration, and dietary supplementation. Provides a directory of practitioners.

American Board of Chelation Therapy
1407-B North Wells Street
Chicago, IL 60610
(800) 356-2228

> Provides certification for physicians in chelation therapy and a referral list of certified practitioners.

CRANIOSACRAL THERAPY

Cranial Academy
8606 Allisonville Road, Suite 130
Indianapolis, IN 46268
(317) 594-0411/Fax (317) 594-9299
> Provides information and a referral list of craniosacral therapists.

Upledger Institute
11211 Prosperity Farms Road
Palm Beach Gardens, FL 33410
(407) 622-4706
Fax (407) 622-4771
> Offers training, information, and referrals.

DIET AND NUTRITION

American College for Advancement in Medicine (see under chelation)
> Provides information about the use of nutritional supplements and a referral directory of physicians worldwide who have been trained in nutritional medicine.

American College of Nutrition
722 Robert E. Lee Drive
Wilmington, NC 28480
(919) 452-1222
> Information resource for nutrition research.

Center for Science in the Public Interest (see under general resource organizations)
> Provides a directory of organic mail order suppliers, hormone-free beef suppliers, and general information on diet and nutrition.

American Natural Hygiene Society
11816 Racetrack Road
Tampa, FL 33626
(813) 855-6607
> Provides information, publications, and referrals.

American Dietetic Association
216 West Jackson, Suite 800
Chicago, IL 60606
(312) 899-0040
> Provides information and certification.

International Association of Professional Natural Hygienists
Regency Health Resort and Spa
2000 South Ocean Drive
Hallandale, FL 33009
(305) 454-2220
> Professional organization of physicians who specialize in therapeutic fasting.

ENERGY MEDICINE

International Society for the Study of Subtle Energies and Energy Medicine (ISSSEEM)
356 Goldco Circle
Golden, CO 80401
(303) 278-2228/Fax (303) 279-3539
> Research organization; provides education and information, as well as publications.

Therapeutic Touch

Nurse Healers Professional Associates, Inc.
1211 Locust Street
Philadelphia, PA 19107
(215) 545-8079
> Provides information on training, conferences, and referrals of TT practitioners. Also publishes a newsletter.

Healing Touch

Colorado Center for Healing Touch, Inc.
198 Union Blvd., Suite 204
Lakewood, CO 80228
> Provides information and referrals.

Reiki

Reiki Alliance
P.O. Box 41
Cataldo, ID 83810
(208) 682-3535
> Provides information and referrals.

Energy Devices

Tools for Exploration
9755 Independence Avenue
Chatsworth, CA 91311
(888) 748-6657
> Provides nonmedical energy machines and other devices. Free catalog available by request.

ENVIRONMENTAL MEDICINE

American Academy of Environmental Medicine
10 E. Randolph
New Hope, PA 18938
(215) 862-4544
> Provides referral list of physicians practicing environmental medicine, as well as a newsletter and other information.

Human Ecology Action League (HEAL)
P.O. Box 49126
Atlanta, GA 30359
(404) 248-1898
> Provides referrals to support groups that assist people suffering from environmental illness.

Immuno Labs

1620 West Oakland Park Blvd., Suite 300

Fort Lauderdale, FL 33311

(800) 321-9197

> A lab specializing an allergy testing. Also provides referrals to environmental physicians worldwide.

HERBAL MEDICINE

American Botanical Council

P.O. Box 201660

Austin, TX 78720

(512) 331-8868

> A nonprofit research organization and education council that serves as a clearinghouse of information for professionals and laypeople alike.

Herb Research Foundation

1007 Pearl Street

Boulder, CO 80302

(303) 449-2265

> Provides research information and referrals to resources on botanical medicine worldwide. Publishes HerbalGram.

American Herbal Products Association

P.O. Box 2410

Austin, TX 78768

(512) 320-8555

> The trade association for herbal products manufacturers.

HOMEOPATHY

International Foundation for Homeopathy

2366 Eastlake Avenue East, Suite 301

Seattle, WA 98102

(206) 324-8230

> Provides training in homeopathy and offers referrals.

National Center for Homeopathy

801 North Fairfax, Suite 306

Alexandria, VA 22314

(703) 548-7790

> Offers training in homeopathy and provides referrals.

NATUROPATHIC MEDICINE

American Association of Naturopathic Physicians

2366 Eastlake Avenue East, Suite 322

Seattle, WA 98102

(206) 323-7610

> Provides information, publications, and a referral directory of naturopathic physicians; is in the forefront in licensing of naturopaths throughout the United States.

The Institute for Naturopathic Medicine

66½ North State Street

Concord, NH 03301

(603) 255-8844

> A nonprofit organization promoting research about naturopathy. Offers information to professional and laypeople, along with the general media.

OSTEOPATHIC MEDICINE

American Academy of Osteopathy

3500 DePauw Blvd, Suite 1080

Indianapolis, IN 46268

(317) 879-1881

> Affiliate organization representing D.O.s who provide osteopathic manipulative treatments and/or cranial osteopathy as part of their practice.

American Osteopathic Association

142 East Ontario Street

Chicago, IL 60611

(312) 280-5800

The national organization representing all D.O.s.

INTERNET RESOURCES

1 Healthy Universe (1HU)

www.1healthyuniverse.com

Founded by Larry Trivieri Jr.; an Internet gateway to the online world of holistic, alternative, complementary, and integrative medicine. Provides visitors with an online self-care clinic by Dr. C. Norman Shealy, wellness tests, healthy diet and recipe sections, and modules devoted to overall wellness, Dr. Robert Ivker's men's health clinic, interviews with leading practitioners and researchers, and an online bookstore. Also publishes a newsletter and provides links to over four hundred other Websites devoted to various aspects of holistic medicine.

Sinus Survival

Founded by Dr. Robert Ivker as a resource for information, education, and products related to the Sinus Survival Program—a holistic approach to treating and preventing respiratory disease (see chapter 6).

Clinical Pathways

http://atlas.uchsc.edu/article

Dr. Bob Anderson's holistic medicine database. 3,500 annotated abstracts of medical and scientific holistic research.

Index

About the Authors

Robert S. Ivker, D.O.

Dr. Robert S. Ivker has been a family physician since 1972. For the past 12 years he has been practicing holistic medicine, with an emphasis on the treatment of chronic disease and the creation of optimal health. In 1996 he was elected President of the American Holistic Medical Association. He is Assistant Clinical Professor in the Department of Family Medicine and a Clinical Instructor in the Department of Otolaryngology at the University of Colorado School of Medicine. Dr. Ivker is also the author of the bestselling book, *Sinus Survival: The Holistic Medical Treatment for Allergies, Asthma, Bronchitis, Colds, and Sinusitis*; and co-author of *Thriving: The Holistic Guide to Optimal Health for Men*. Dr. Ivker and his wife Harriet, a psychiatric social worker, have been married for 31 years. They have two daughters, Julie and Carin. The Ivkers live at the foot of the Rocky Mountains in Littleton, Colorado.

Robert A. Anderson, M.D.

Robert Anderson, M.D., graduated with honors from medical school in 1957 and has been a family doctor for more than 40 years. He became a charter fellow of the American Academy of Family Physicians in 1962 and was a diplomate of the American Board of Family Practice from 1973 to 1991. He is a past Clinical Assistant Professor of Family Medicine at the University of Washington and a past president of the American Holistic Medical Association, and he was the Founding Chief of Staff at Stevens Memorial Hospital in Edmonds, Washington. He has authored two books, *Stress Power!* (1978) and *Wellness Medicine* (1987). Dr. Anderson currently holds positions in several undergraduate and graduate institutions, where he teaches nutrition, stress management, wellness education, family medicine, and psychoneuro-immunology. Between 1997 and the present he has co-chaired four medical school courses for physicians, entitled "The Art and Science of Holistic Medicine in Treating Chronic Disease." Dr. Anderson serves as president of the new American Board of Holistic Medicine. He lives in Wenatchee, Washington.

Larry Trivieri, Jr.

Larry Trivieri, Jr. is a leading lay expert in the health and wellness field, and has been exploring holistic approaches to healing and human transformation for more than 25 years. He has written articles for a variety of magazines and newspapers, and been a guest on radio and television talk shows nationwide. He has served as senior writer for the critically acclaimed bestseller, *Alternative Medicine: The Definitive Guide,* and as senior contributing editor for *You Don't Have To Die: Unraveling the AIDS Myth.* In 1998, he founded the online resource *www.1healthy-universe.com,* one of the top Internet consumer sites devoted to all aspects of holistic and alternative forms of healing, and serves as its publisher and editor-in-chief. Mr. Trivieri is also an accomplished poet, lecturer, and workshop leader. He lives in Utica, New York.

For further information about Dr. Ivker's lectures, workshops, *Sinus Survival* Program, and to order *Sinus Survival* products, contact:

SINUS SURVIVAL
8552 East Creek Place
Englewood, CO 80112
303-771-0033   888-434-0033
fax: 303-221-5320
e-mail: drivker@sinussurvival.com
http://www.sinussurvival.com

Other books by Dr. Ivker:

Sinus Survival: The Holistic Medical Treatment for Allergies, Asthma, Bronchitis, Colds, and Sinusitis

Thriving: The Holistic Guide to Optimal Health for Men